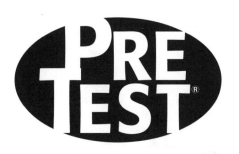

Pharmacology

PreTest® Self-Assessment

Notice

Medicine is an ever-changing science. As new research and clinical experience broaden our knowledge, changes in treatment and drug therapy are required. The authors and the publisher of this work have checked with sources believed to be reliable in their efforts to provide information that is complete and generally in accord with the standards accepted at the time of publication. However, in view of the possibility of human error or changes in medical sciences, neither the authors nor the publisher nor any other party who has been involved in the preparation or publication of this work warrants that the information contained herein is in every respect accurate or complete, and they disclaim all responsibility for any errors or omissions or for the results obtained from use of the information contained in this work. Readers are encouraged to confirm the information contained herein with other sources. For example and in particular, readers are advised to check the product information sheet included in the package of each drug they plan to administer to be certain that the information contained in this work is accurate and that changes have not been made in the recommended dose or in the contraindications for administration. This recommendation is of particular importance in connection with new or infrequently used drugs.

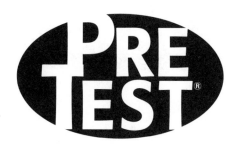

Pharmacology
PreTest® Self-Assessment and Review
Eleventh Edition

Marshal Shlafer, Ph.D.
Professor of Pharmacology
Director of Undergraduate Medical Pharmacology Education
Department of Pharmacology
University of Michigan Medical School
Ann Arbor, Michigan

McGraw-Hill
Medical Publishing Division

New York   Chicago   San Francisco   Lisbon   London   Madrid   Mexico City
Milan   New Delhi   San Juan   Seoul   Singapore   Sydney   Toronto

The McGraw·Hill Companies

Pharmacology: PreTest® Self-Assessment and Review, Eleventh Edition

Previous editions copyright © 2002, 1999, 1996, 1993, 1991, 1988, 1986, 1983, 1980, and 1976 by The McGraw-Hill Companies, Inc.

1 2 3 4 5 6 7 8 9 0 DOC/DOC 0 9 8 7 6 5 4

ISBN 0-07-143688-X

This book was set in Berkeley by North Market Street Graphics.
The editor was Catherine A. Johnson.
The production supervisor was Phil Galea.
Project management was provided by North Market Street Graphics.
The cover designer was Li Chen Chang/Pinpoint.
RR Donnelley was printer and binder.

This book is printed on acid-free paper.

Library of Congress Cataloging-in-Publication Data

Pharmacology: PreTest self-assessment and review.—11th ed. / [edited by] Marshal Shlafer.
    p. ; cm.
    Includes bibliographical references and index.
    ISBN 0-07-143688-X
    1. Pharmacology—Examinations, questions, etc. 2. Physicians—Licenses—United States—Examinations—Study guides. I. Shlafer, Marshal.
    [DNLM: 1. Pharmacology—Examination Questions. QV 18.2 P536 2004]
    RM301.13.P475 2004
    615'.1'076—dc22   2004052421

Student Reviewers

Stephen Clark
East Tennessee State University
Johnson City, Tennessee
Class of 2005

Alisa A. Meny
University of Medicine & Dentistry of New Jersey—
Robert Wood Johnson Medical School
Camden, New Jersey
Class of 2004

Sachin S. Parikh
University of Medicine & Dentistry of New Jersey—
Robert Wood Johnson Medical School
Camden, New Jersey
Class of 2004

Contents

Local Control Substances: Autacoids, Drugs for Inflammatory Processes

Gastrointestinal System and Nutrition (Vitamins)

Endocrine System

Anti-Infectives

Cancer Chemotherapy and Immunosuppressants

Toxicology

Preface

Welcome to this, the eleventh edition, of *Pharmacology: PreTest® Self-Assessment and Review*. We've made some significant changes to it, and hope that whether you're studying for a pharmacology course exam or Step 1 of the USMLE, you'll find it helpful.

Among the changes you'll find are:

- Nearly 300 new or extensively revised questions, many based on clinical vignettes, and nearly all pretested on hundreds of first- and second-year medical students

- A better blend of questions focusing on your basic science knowledge with those addressing clinical applications, and with information from other basic preclinical disciplines

- Clearer yet simpler explanations for why correct answers are correct and the others aren't

- More integration of question content between the various areas of pharmacology and therapeutics. This is a general "build upon the base" approach in which questions in later chapters encourage you to integrate new material with basic content presented earlier

- Placement of autonomic nervous system content "up front," right after the basic principles chapter, in recognition of autonomic aspects of drug action being so important in many more "specialized" areas of therapeutics

- Placement of renal and respiratory pharmacology into separate chapters to focus your review, but in such a way that you still maintain important integration with such pertinent topics as autonomics and cardiovascular

- Updates to all the text cross-references (in the answers) so you can easily find further explanations if you wish, and addition of cross-references to a third and commonly used medical pharmacology text

Introduction

Each *PreTest® Self-Assessment and Review* helps you assess and review your knowledge of a particular basic science—in this instance, pharmacology and therapeutics—in a way that addresses both your intensive and extensive knowledge of the subject, your expected knowledge of basic facts, and your ability to apply facts and concepts to some common (yet perhaps new, to you) clinical situations. Most of the questions you'll find here parallel the format and degree of difficulty of questions found in the United States Medical Licensing Examination (USMLE) Step 1.

Those who want to hone their skills before USMLE Step 2 or 3, or recertification, may find this to be a good beginning in their review process.

At the start of each chapter we provide a short list of key terms (mainly drug classes) to help orient you to the scope of the questions that follow. Each question is accompanied by an answer; explanations of a length, depth, and scope that we deem appropriate to understanding the answer; and cross-references to pages in one or more commonly used textbooks so you can get more information if you wish.

Study Tips

Each of you has a study and review method that has worked best for you. Go with what works best. It's gotten you into medical school and kept you there. But do prepare yourself to answer the questions in each chapter by reviewing the corresponding material from your notes and favorite (or, at least, assigned) text.

You should concentrate especially on prototype drugs. Then, mark your answer by each question, allowing yourself not more than one minute for each question. In this way you will be approximating the time limits imposed by the examination.

After you finish going through the questions in each section, spend as much time as you need verifying your answers and carefully reading the explanations provided. Pay special attention to the explanations for the questions you answered incorrectly—but read *every* explanation. I have designed the explanations to reinforce and supplement the information sought by the questions, and sometimes gently to encourage you to look at (usually earlier) parts of the book to see important connections.

Before you work on the questions or your studying overall, try organizing things in these ways, and aim to accomplish the following:

Be able to identify main drug classes, recognizing that sometimes we use more than one classification scheme, e.g., chemical, by main mechanism(s) of action, and by clinical use. And be able to cite a prototype drug for each. Conversely, give a prototype or otherwise representative drug, be able to work backward, and know the rest of the most relevant information.

For example, you can identify a group of drugs that are nonselective cyclooxygenase inhibitors, a main chemical class that includes acetylsalicylic acid (salicylates), that the prototype drug is aspirin, and that the main uses are for management of fever, inflammation, and mild pain.

Or, you could take a reverse approach by identifying propranolol as the prototype nonselective β-adrenergic blocker; identifying the main actions (due to blockade of β-adrenergic receptors, which implicitly means knowing what activating the β_1 and β_2 receptors does); and recognizing that propranolol has such uses as management of hypertension, certain types of angina pectoris, heart failure, tachycardia, and so on. You should be able to recognize the term catecholamine as applicable to a drug or drug group with structures and actions similar to epinephrine or norepinephrine.

Be able to recognize the most common and/or most important (e.g., serious or life-threatening) side effects or adverse responses for the main drugs or drug classes.

Often you know intuitively what these may be, since the most important side effects or adverse responses often are "extensions" of expected effects of the drug or class (e.g., most antihypertensive drugs can cause hypotension when blood levels are excessive), or where the drugs are eliminated (e.g., the common finding that many drugs cause hepatotoxicity or nephrotoxicity, because they are eliminated mainly by one of those organs). However, some drugs cause effects that are, for lack of a better phrase, unique or unexpected: ototoxicity from aminoglycoside antibiotics or loop diuretics; a lupus-like syndrome from hydralazine or isoniazid. Learn these "unique" responses.

Learn to recognize that intended effects or side effects that you simply should know give you a good idea of what relevant precautions or contraindications are, even if you haven't been taught about the latter, even if your learning focus hasn't been too clinical.

You should have learned that β-adrenergic blockers can reduce cardiac rate, or contractility, or electrical impulse conduction velocity (say, through the atrio-ventricular node), and sometimes these drugs are used for those effects. You should then realize that excessive doses may cause unwanted degrees of suppression of those cardiac parameters. And, although you may not have been taught explicitly, you should realize that the effects of these drugs warrant extra caution (or contraindicate altogether) the use of a β blocker in patients who already have bradycardia, reduced ventricular contractility, or with heart block. Making these associations or extrapolations is not rocket science that you must have been taught about explicitly. You should be able to use your basic knowledge of pharmacology and drug action, and of physiology and pathophysiology, to piece things together and get at the correct (or most logical) answer.

Depth and Scope of Questions and Answers

Students who have reviewed previous editions of *Pharmacology: PreTest* found the book to be extremely useful. However, some questions were cited as being "low-yield," "too basic," "too clinical," and the like.

Let me opine that, at this point in your medical education, you're probably not in the best position to make judgment calls on such matters. What students often cite as a low-yield question is actually basic but "must know" information, and just because you automatically know or recognize the answer doesn't mean that the information isn't important or that your ability to recognize it shouldn't be evaluated. Conversely, some students have called certain questions low yield simply because they haven't learned about the facts and concepts addressed in the question.

It is in some ways rewarding to answer an ostensibly complicated or detailed question correctly, but you don't want to find yourself so bogged down in knowing the details that you miss seeing the more important big picture. You have had an abundant amount of information about pharmacology presented to you, but that's only the foundation of a broad knowledge and experience base on which you'll build over the coming years. And your experiences from the course(s) you've taken may be quite different from those of students in other medical schools: after all, there is no one "standard" pharmacology curriculum for all medical schools, and points emphasized by a particular instructor that you've had can differ (sometimes markedly) in scope and orientation from those made by faculty elsewhere.

You may have had a stand-alone pharmacology course or two, perhaps with a focus on basic characteristics of drugs. That focus may have been on mechanisms of action or it may have been replete with issues of drug metabolism or structure. Or you may have had your pharmacology content integrated in some systems-based curriculum, which tends to teach and test on drug-related material in a very clinically oriented way. So for some of you it's tempting to view some questions as "too clinical." However, answering them is relatively simple if you think about the basic drug information you should have acquired, integrate it with what you should have learned in other courses (e.g., in a physiology or cell or molecular biology course), and do what you will soon have to do on the wards—make reasoned judgments based on applying your knowledge to a possibly new clinical picture.

So, what may be "too clinical" for some of you may be old hat for others. What may be a low-yield, no-brainer, or mere rat fact question to you might be assessing essential information overlooked by someone else who is studying just as hard, trying to achieve the same goal (passing Step 1, or a pharmy exam) as you.

Good luck.

Marshal Shlafer, Ph.D.
Professor, Department
    of Pharmacology
Director of Undergraduate Medical
    Pharmacology Education
University of Michigan Medical School
Ann Arbor, Michigan

Cross-References to Selected Pharmacology Texts

Explanations for the answers to the questions provided in this edition of *Pharmacology: PreTest* are cross-referenced to one or more basic pharmacology texts that are commonly used in medical schools throughout the country. We've used some shorthand to identify those texts as follows (see page 369 for complete, formal citations):

"Craig"—*Modern Pharmacology with Clinical Applications,* 6th edition, C. R. Craig and R. E. Stitzel, eds., 2004.

"Hardman"—*Goodman & Gilman's the Pharmacological Basis of Therapeutics,* 10th edition, J. G. Hardman and L.E. Limbird, eds., 2001.

"Katzung"—*Basic and Clinical Pharmacology,* 9th edition, B. G. Katzung, ed., 2004.

Please note the page cross-references apply to the latest available editions (at the time of this writing) of these texts, so if you have an earlier edition of any of these books you'll have to do a little looking to find the corresponding material.

Each of those texts excels in certain respects, yet each also has limitations—or, simply different emphases—compared with others. One may be more mechanistic or more detailed, another may be more clinical, one may paint a discussion about certain drugs or drug groups, or a particular medical condition, with broader brush strokes than another.

How pharmacology is presented and what "defines" the basics or core of the discipline vary tremendously from not only one text to another, but also from one medical school, or course, or instructor, to another. What you have learned from your lectures or from your assigned text inevitably reflects a bias on the part of the lecturers or the text book authors. And, just as your learning and testing experiences may vary, depending on where you are, so may the way you've prepared for a standardized exam that includes pharmacology (or other any preclinical) content. There is no standardized pharmacology curriculum, nor a standardized way to present it.

Thus, once you begin looking at my questions—and my answers to them—you may find that there is no explicit cross-reference to one of the above texts. You may find that the questions I ask, the way I ask them, or the answers I give, are different from what you have learned or how you learned it. They may be too clinical, or not mechanistic enough (or too mechanistic). They may address drugs you have not studied explicitly. Indeed, some questions may focus on drugs you haven't heard about at all (some drugs too new to make it into some of the older texts cited above are found below).

Don't worry. Study, read, review, and learn as you can from the questions and the explanations. Keep in mind that content in an ostensibly circumscribed area (or book chapter or lecture) can have significant ramifications on other areas. Appreciate the fact that in order to understand some concepts you have to integrate material from several disciplines or areas of pharmacology—and, of necessity, you may have to integrate material you have learned from such other basic biomedical disciplines as physiology, pathophysiology, biochemistry, molecular and cell biology, and many more.

Realize that regardless of the text or lecture material you have learned from, you may have to take whatever knowledge you have and apply it in new ways or in different situations.

List of Abbreviations and Acronyms

Note: We have omitted common symbols for chemical elements or their cationic or anionic forms (e.g., Ca, Cl), chemical formulae (e.g., NaCl), abbreviations of common biochemicals (ATP, ADP, DNA, etc.), units of measure (volume, weight, time), and Greek letters.

ACE—angiotensin-converting enzyme
ACh—acetylcholine
AChE—acetylcholinesterase
AChEI—acetylcholinesterase inhibitor
ACS—acute coronary syndrome
ACTH—adrenocorticotropic hormone
ADD—attention-deficit disorder
ADH—antidiuretic hormone [vasopressin (VP)]
ADHD—attention deficit hyperactivity disorder
AF (AFIB)—atrial fibrillation
AFL—atrial flutter
AIDS—acquired immunodeficiency syndrome
ALG—antilymphocyte globulin
ANS—autonomic nervous system
AUC—area under the (blood concentration vs. time) curve
AV—atrioventricular
B. fragilis—Bacteroides fragilis
BAL—British anti-Lewisite (dimercaprol)
BPH—benign prostatic hypertrophy
BPM—beats per minute
BUN—blood urea nitrogen
C_{av}—average (mean) plasma concentration
C_{max}—maximum plasma concentration
C_{min}—minimum plasma concentration
C_{ss}—steady-state plasma concentration
C. albicans—Candida albicans
C. botulinum—Clostridium botulinum
C. difficile—Clostridium difficile
C. neoformans—Cryptococcus neoformans
CAD—coronary artery disease
CCB—calcium channel blocker
CHD—coronary heart disease
CHF—congestive heart failure
CK—creatine kinase
Cl—clearance (of drug)
Cl^-—chloride
Cl_{total}—total body clearance

CNS—central nervous system
COMT—catechol-*O*-methyltransferase
COPD—chronic obstructive pulmonary disease
COX—cyclooxygenase(s); may be modified as COX-1 or COX-2
CRF—corticotropin-releasing factor
CSF—cerebrospinal fluid
CYP—cytochrome P450 (system or member of it)
D_2—dopamine D_2 receptor
DA—dopamine
DHT—dihydrotestosterone
DOPA (Dopa)—dihydroxyphenylalanine
DVT—deep venous thrombosis
E. coli—*Escherichia coli*
EDRF—endothelium-derived relaxing factor
EEG—electroencephalogram
EGF—epidermal growth factor
EKG—electrocardiogram
EPI—epinephrine
ER—endoplasmic reticulum
EtOH—ethanol
5-FU—5-fluorouracil
5-HT—5-hydroxytryptamine (serotonin)
FH_2—7,8-dihydrofolic acid
FH_4—5,6,7,8-tetrahydrofolic acid
FSH—follicle-stimulating hormone
FU—fluorouracil
G. lamblia—*Giardia lamblia*
G protein—guanine nucleotide-binding protein
GABA—γ-aminobutyric acid
G-CSF—granulocyte colony-stimulating factor
GERD—gastroesophageal reflux disease
GI—gastrointestinal
GM-CSF—granulocyte macrophage colony-stimulating factor
GnRH—gonadotropin-releasing hormone
GU—genitourinary
H. influenzae—*Haemophilus influenzae*
H. pylori—*Helicobacter pylori*
Hb—hemoglobin
hCG—human chorionic gonadotropin
HDL—high-density lipoprotein
HIV—human immunodeficiency virus
H^+,K^+,ATPase—hydrogen-potassium-adenosine triphosphatase; proton pump
hMG—human menopausal gonadotropin
HMG—CoA-β-hydroxy-β-methylglutaryl-coenzyme A
HRT—hormone replacement therapy

IgE, G (etc.)—immunoglobulin E, G
IL (-1, -2, etc.)—interleukin(s)-1, -2, etc.
IM—intramuscular(ly)
INH—isoniazid
IP_3—inositol-1,4,5-trisphosphate
IV—intravenous(ly)
k_e—elimination rate constant
K. pneumoniae—Klebsiella pneumoniae
L. pneumophilia—Legionella pneumophilia
L-dopa—levodopa
L-thyroxine (T_4)—levothyroxine
LDL—low-density lipoprotein
LHRH—luteinizing hormone-releasing hormone (hypothalamic)
LT—leukotriene
MAO—monoamine oxidase
MAO-A, -B—MAO type A, type B
MAOI—monoamine oxidase inhibitor
MDI—metered-dose inhaler
MI—myocardial infarction
mRNA—messenger ribonucleic acid
N_M receptors—nicotinic-skeletal muscle receptors (found at skeletal-somatic neuromuscular
    junction)
N_N receptors—nicotinic-neural receptors (found in parasympathetic ganglia and on cells of
    the adrenal medulla)
N. gonorrhoeae—Neisseria gonorrhoeae
NADH—nicotinamide adenine dinucleotide
NADPH—nicotinamide adenine dinucleotide phosphate
$Na^+,K^+,ATPase$—sodium-potassium-adenosine triphosphatase
NAPA—*N*-acetylprocainamide
NE—norepinephrine
NMDA—*N*-methyl-D-aspartate (glutamate channel)
NMS—neuroleptic malignant syndrome
NNRTI—nonnucleoside reverse transcriptase inhibitor
NPH—isophane (Neutral protamine Hagedorn) insulin
NPY—neuropeptide Y
NRTI—nucleotide reverse transcriptase inhibitor
NSAID—nonsteroidal anti-inflammatory drug (nonopioid analgesic/antipyretic)
P. aeruginosa—Pseudomonas aeruginosa
P. carinii—Pneumocystis carinii
P. vivax—Plasmodium vivax
PABA—*p*-aminobenzoic acid
PAM (2-PAM)—pralidoxime
PAS—*para*-aminosalicylic acid
PDGF—platelet-derived growth factor
PG—prostaglandin

PGE_1—prostaglandin E_1 (alprostadil)
PGE_2—prostaglandin E_2 (dinoprostone)
PGI_2—prostaglandin I_2 (prostacyclin)
PNS—parasympathetic nervous system
Po_2—partial pressure (tension) of oxygen
PPD—purified protein derivative of tuberculin
PTH—parathyroid hormone
PVC—premature ventricular contraction
RDA—recommended daily allowance
REM—rapid eye movement
6-MP—mercaptopurine
S. aureus—*Staphylococcus aureus*
S. haematobium—*Schistosoma haematobium*
SA—sinoatrial
SC—subcutaneous [administration route]
SH—sulfhydryl
SL—sublingual
SR—sarcoplasmic reticulum
SRS-A—slow-reacting substance of anaphylaxis
SSRI—selective serotonin reuptake inhibitor
SVT—supraventricular tachycardia
$t_{1/2}$—half-life (e.g., biologic or plasma half-life)
T_3—triiodothyronine
T_4—thyroxine
TB—tuberculosis
TG—triglyceride
TIA—transient ischemic attack
TNF—tumor necrosis factor
tPA—tissue plasminogen activator
TRH—thyroid/thyrotropin-releasing hormone
tRNA—transfer ribonucleic acid
TSH—thyroid-stimulating hormone
TXA_2—thromboxane A_2
UTI—urinary tract infection
V_d—volume of distribution (apparent)
VIP—vasoactive intestinal peptide
vitamin B_1—thiamine
vitamin B_2—riboflavin
vitamin B_6—pyridoxine
vitamin C—ascorbic acid
vitamin D—calcitriol [metabolite (active form: $1,25\text{-}(OH)_2D_3$)]
VLDL—very-low-density lipoprotein
VP—vasopressin [antidiuretic hormone (ADH)]
VT (VTACH)—ventricular tachycardia

General Principles

Biotransformation
Development of new drugs
Dosage regimens and pharmaco-
 kinetic profiles
Dose-response relationships
Drug names and nomenclature
Drug-receptor interactions

Factors affecting drug dosage
Molecular models of receptors and
 signal transduction mechanisms
Pharmacodynamics
Pharmacokinetics
Regulation by the Food and Drug
 Administration

Questions

DIRECTIONS: Each item contains a question or incomplete statement that is followed by several responses. Select the **one best** response to each question.

1. Azithromycin, an antibiotic, has an apparent volume of distribution (V_d) of approximately 30 L/kg. The correct interpretation of this information is that azithromycin is which of the following?

a. Effective only when given intravenously
b. Eliminated mainly by renal excretion, without prior metabolism
c. Extensively distributed to sites outside the vascular and interstitial spaces
d. Not extensively bound to plasma proteins
e. Unable to cross the blood-brain or placental barriers

2. Which of the following administration routes is most likely to subject a drug to a "first-pass" effect in the liver?

a. Inhalation
b. Intramuscular
c. Intravenous
d. Oral
e. Sublingual (SL)

3. Two drugs act on the same tissue or organ via activation of different receptors, resulting in effects that are qualitatively the opposite of one another. This represents which of the following types of antagonism?

a. Chemical
b. Competitive
c. Dispositional
d. Pharmacologic
e. Physiologic

Questions 4–7

A hypothetical aminoglycoside antibiotic was injected intravenously (5 mg/kg) into a 70-kg volunteer. The plasma concentrations of the drug were measured at various times after the end of the injection, as recorded in the table (on page 3) and shown in the figure below.

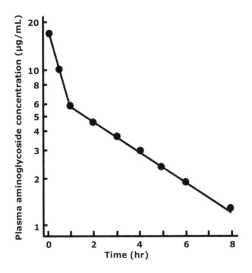

Time After Dosing Stopped (h)	Plasma Aminoglycoside Concentration (mcg/mL)
0.0	18.0
0.5	10.0
1.0	5.8
2.0	4.6
3.0	3.7
4.0	3.0
5.0	2.4
6.0	1.9
8.0	1.3

4. The elimination half-life ($t_{1/2}$) of the aminoglycoside in this patient was approximately:
a. 0.6 h
b. 1.2 h
c. 2.1 h
d. 3.1 h
e. 4.2 h

5. The elimination rate constant (k_e) of the aminoglycoside in this patient was approximately:
a. $0.15 \ h^{-1}$
b. $0.22 \ h^{-1}$
c. $0.33 \ h^{-1}$
d. $0.60 \ h^{-1}$
e. $1.13 \ h^{-1}$

6. The apparent volume of distribution (V_d) of the drug in this 70 kg patient was approximately:
a. 0.62 L
b. 19 L
c. 50 L
d. 110 L
e. 350 L

7. The total body clearance (Cl_{total}) of the drug in this patient was approximately:

a. 11 L/h
b. 23 L/h
c. 35 L/h
d. 47 L/h
e. 65 L/h

8. We are repeatedly administering a drug orally. Every dose is 50 mg; the interval between doses is 8 h, which is identical to the drug's plasma half-life. The bioavailability is 0.5. For as long as we conduct the experiment no interacting drugs are added or stopped, and there are no patient-related factors (excretion, metabolism) that might change the drug's pharmacokinetics.

Which of the following formulas results in the best *estimate* of how long it will take for the drug to reach steady-state serum concentrations (C_{SS})?

Abbreviations:
AUC = area under the concentration-time curve
Cl = clearance (mL/min)
D = dose (mg)
F = bioavailability (<1.0 for this drug given orally)
k_e = elimination rate constant
$t_{1/2}$ = half-life (h)
V_d = volume of distribution

a. $(0.693 \cdot V_d)/Cl$
b. $1/k_e$
c. $4.5 \cdot t_{1/2}$
d. $(t_{1/2}) \cdot (k_e)$
e. $D/(F \cdot t_{1/2})$

9. Which of the following pharmacokinetic values most reliably reflects the total amount of drug reaching the target tissue after oral administration?

a. Peak blood concentration
b. Time-to-peak blood concentration
c. Product of the V_d and the first-order rate constant
d. V_d
e. Area under the blood concentration-time curve (AUC)

10. Experiments show that 95% of an oral 80-mg dose of verapamil is absorbed in a 70-kg test subject. However, because of extensive biotransformation during its first pass through the portal circulation, the bioavailability was only 0.25 (25%). Assuming a liver blood flow of 1500 mL/min, which of the following is the hepatic clearance of verapamil in this situation?

a. 60 mL/min
b. 375 mL/min
c. 740 mL/min
d. 1110 mL/min
e. 1425 mL/min

11. Which of the following is calculated as the ratio of the area under the curve (AUC) obtained by oral administration vs. the AUC for intravenous administration of the same drug?

a. Absorption
b. Bioavailability
c. Clearance
d. Elimination rate constant
e. Extraction ratio
f. Volume of distribution

12. We administer an acidic drug (A) with a pK_a of 3.4 orally. Gut pH is 1.4, and plasma pH is 7.4. Assume the drug crosses membranes by simple passive diffusion (e.g., no transporters are involved). Which of the following observations would be true?

a. Only ionized forms of the drug, A−, will be absorbed from the gut into the plasma

b. The concentration ratio of *total* drug (A + HA⁻) would be 10,000:1 (gut > plasma)

c. The drug will be hydrolyzed by a reaction with HCl, and so cannot be absorbed

d. The drug will not be absorbed unless we raise gastric pH to equal pKa, as might be done with an antacid

e. The drug would be absorbed, and at equilibrium the plasma concentration of the nonionized moiety (HA) would be 10^4 times higher than the plasma concentration of A⁻

13. Identical doses of a drug are given orally (■) and intravenously (●), we sample blood at various times, measure blood concentrations of the drug, and plot the data. The data are shown below.

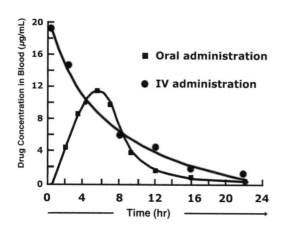

Further analysis of these data will allow us to determine which of the following?

a. Potency
b. Extent of plasma protein binding
c. Oral bioavailability
d. Therapeutic effectiveness
e. Elimination route(s)

14. Which of the following is a phase II biotransformation reaction?

a. Sulfoxide formation
b. Nitro reduction
c. Ester hydrolysis
d. Glucuronidation
e. Deamination

15. We start intravenous infusion of a drug using an infusion pump to ensure that the rate of drug delivery is constant over time. What one factor determines how long it will take for the drug to reach a steady-state concentration (C_{SS}) in the blood?

a. Apparent volume of distribution
b. Bioavailability
c. Clearance
d. Half-life
e. Infusion rate (mg of drug/min)

16. Yee et al. (Effect of grapefruit juice on blood cyclosporine concentration; Lancet 345:955–956, 1995) examined several pharmacokinetic variables related to oral cyclosporine administration with water, grapefruit juice, and orange juice:

	Grapefruit juice	Orange juice	Water	p^*
AUC (ng·h/mL)	7057 ± 2172	4871 ± 2045	4932 ± 1451	<0.0001
C_{max} (ng/mL)	1269 ± 381	972 ± 379	1080 ± 269	0.01
T_{max} (h)	2.86 ± 0.77	2.57 ± 0.85	2.36 ± 0.63	0.14

The numbers listed are arithmetic means ± one standard deviation of the mean. C_{max} is the peak blood concentration, and T_{max} is the time after administration at which peak serum concentrations of the drug are reached. p values are based on repeated-measures analysis of variance (ANOVA).

These data, and what you should have learned from your basic pharmacology studies, are consistent with the hypothesis that grapefruit juice does which of the following?

a. Activates an intestinal wall transporter for cyclosporine
b. Alters the route(s) of elimination for cyclosporine
c. Increases binding of cyclosporine to plasma proteins
d. Inhibits the first-pass metabolism of cyclosporine
e. Slows cyclosporine absorption

17. A 60-year-old man with aggressive rheumatoid arthritis will be started on an anti-inflammatory drug to suppress the joint inflammation. Published pharmacokinetic data for this drug include:

Bioavailability (*F*): 1.0 (100%)
Plasma half-life ($t_{1/2}$) = 0.5 h
Volume of distribution (V_d): 45 L

For this drug it is important to maintain an average steady state concentration 2.0 mcg/mL in order to ensure adequate and continued anti-inflammatory activity.

The drug will be given every 4 hours.

What dose will be needed to obtain an average steady-state drug concentration of 2.0 mcg/mL?

a. 5 mg
b. 100 mg
c. 325 mg
d. 500 mg
e. 625 mg

18. We take a blood sample from a patient (baseline) and then administer Drug A intravenously. We take additional blood samples periodically thereafter and measure drug concentration in each sample. We repeat the experiment, this time giving the same drug orally. If we then plot the logarithm of drug concentration vs. time, the *slope* of the resulting curve provides information about which of the following for Drug A?

a. Area under the curve (AUC)
b. Bioavailability
c. Elimination rate constant
d. Extraction ratio
e. Volume of distribution

Questions 19–21

For each description of a drug response below, choose the term with which it is most likely to be associated:

a. Supersensitivity
b. Tachyphylaxis
c. Tolerance
d. Hyposensitivity
e. Anaphylaxis

19. Immunologically mediated reaction to drug observed soon after administration

20. A rapid reduction in the effect of a given dose of a drug after only one or two doses

21. Hyperreactivity to a drug seen as a result of denervation

Questions 22–24

For each component of the time-action curve listed below, choose the lettered interval (shown on the diagram) representing the pharmacokinetic parameter:

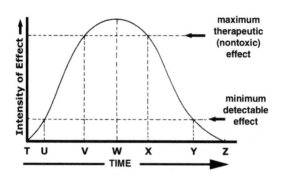

a. T to U
b. T to V
c. T to W
d. T to Z
e. U to V
f. U to W
g. U to X
h. U to Y
i. V to X
j. X to Y

22. Time to peak effect

23. Time to onset of action

24. Duration of action

Questions 25–27

For each numbered description below, select the lettered term that fits best. A letter may be used once, more than once, or not at all.

a. Filtration
b. Simple diffusion
c. Facilitated diffusion
d. Active transport
e. Endocytosis

25. Lipid-soluble drugs cross the membrane at a rate that is a function of their concentration gradient across the membrane and the lipid:water partition coefficient of the drug.

26. Bulk flow of water through membrane pores, resulting from osmotic differences across the membrane, transports drug molecules that fit through the membrane pores.

27. After binding to a proteinaceous membrane carrier, drugs are carried across the membrane (with the expenditure of cellular energy), where they are released.

Questions 28–30

Lipid-soluble xenobiotics are commonly biotransformed by oxidation in the microsomal mixed-function oxidase system. For each description below, choose the component with which it is most closely associated.

a. Nicotinamide adenine dinucleotide phosphate (NADPH)
b. Cytochrome *a*
c. Adenosine triphosphate (ATP)
d. NADPH-cytochrome P450 reductase
e. Monoamine oxidase (MAO)
f. Cyclooxygenase
g. Cytochrome P450

28. A group of iron (Fe)-containing isoenzymes that activate molecular oxygen to a form that is capable of interacting with organic substrates

29. The component that provides reducing equivalents for the enzyme system

30. A flavoprotein that accepts reducing equivalents and transfers them to the catalytic enzyme

Questions 31–32

A postoperative patient requires analgesia. We choose a drug that has the following pharmacokinetic properties:

Half-life: 12 h
Clearance: 0.08 L/min
Volume of distribution: 60 L

The patient has an indwelling venous catheter with a slow drip of 0.9% NaCl, and we will use this line to administer intermittent injections of the drug every 4 h.

The target blood level of the drug, following each injection, is 8 µg/mL.

31. With this administration plan, what dose should be injected every 4 h?
a.   0.960 mg (or 1 mg)
b.   6.4 mg (or 6 mg)
c.   25.6 mg (or 25 mg)
d.   150 mg
e.   550 mg

32. As we are calculating the dosage for intermittent injections, we realize we must control the patient's pain as soon as possible. Our target serum concentration, 8 µg/mL, is the same. However, we want to start with a loading dose for prompt effects. Which of the following would be the correct loading dose?
a.   0.48 mg (rounded to 0.5 mg)
b.   150 mg
c.   320 mg
d.   480 mg
e.   640 mg

33. We measure the heart rate of a healthy subject under the conditions noted below, allowing ample time for return to baseline conditions and full elimination of drugs between each . . .

1. at rest
2. during treadmill exercise sufficient to activate the sympathetic nervous system at a time when maximum heart rate is reached
3. after administration of acebutolol, a drug with affinity for β-adrenergic receptors
4. after giving acebutolol, followed by exercise at the same level used in condition 2

Acebutolol given at rest causes a slight but consistent increase of heart rate. Give a bigger dose at rest and heart rate rises a bit more.

When the patient exercises after receiving a low dose acebutolol, heart rate rises significantly less than it did in the absence of acebutolol. With exercise after the higher dose of acebutolol, the tachycardia is blunted even more.

The figure below summarizes the qualitative findings.

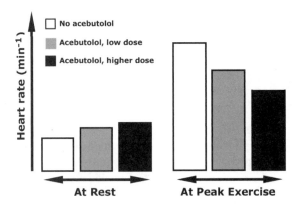

These findings suggest that, most likely, acebutolol:

a. Has higher affinity for adrenergic receptors than the endogenous agonists, epinephrine, and norepinephrine
b. Is a partial agonist for β-adrenergic receptors
c. Is activating spare receptors on myocardial cells
d. Is an irreversible or noncompetitive β-blocker
e. Is changing conformation of the adrenergic receptors

34. We are planning to infuse a drug intravenously at a constant amount per unit time (rate). It has a first-order elimination rate constant (k_{el}) of 0.35/h. No loading dose will be given. Approximately how long will it take for blood levels to reach steady state after the infusion begins?

a. 0.7 h
b. 1.2 h
c. 3.5 h
d. 9 h
e. 24 h

35. We want to calculate the apparent volume of distribution (V_d) for a hypothetical drug (Drug A) that has a half-life of 4 h. All (100%) of an absorbed dose of this drug undergoes Phase I oxidation, followed by conjugation (Phase II reaction).

We rapidly inject a known dose, and 30 min later begin taking serial blood samples (30 min apart) and quantifying drug concentration in each sample. What *one* other piece of information must we measure or otherwise determine to calculate V_d in the *easiest* possible way?

a. Area under the drug concentration-time curve (AUC)
b. Bioavailability
c. Clearance
d. Elimination rate constant (k_{el})
e. Maximum blood concentration immediately after the bolus injection (C_0)

36. We are working with a pharmacologically inert but easily measured substance, X. Its elimination shows linear kinetics (first-order plot of log drug concentration vs. time during elimination is a straight line). The plasma half-life is 30 min. Bolus IV doses well in excess of 100 mg must be given in order to saturate the enzymes responsible for metabolizing the drug, which will then lead to zero-order elimination kinetics.

We infuse a solution of X intravenously. The concentration of the solution is 2 μg/mL; the infusion rate is 1 mL/min and is kept constant at that. We continue the infusion for 24 h.

After allowing ample time for the drug to be eliminated completely, we repeat the administration. This time the concentration of the solution of X is 4 μg/mL, and we infuse it at a rate of 2 mL/min.

Which other variable will also be changed as a result of the stated changes of the stated infusion protocol?

a. Elimination rate constant
b. Half-life
c. Plasma concentration when C_{SS} is reached
d. Time to reach steady-state concentration (C_{SS})
e. Total body clearance
f. Volume of distribution

37. Which of the following is the general function or purpose served by *all* Phase I drug biotransformation reactions?

a. Add or unmask (expose) functional groups on a substrate, forming more polar molecules
b. Cleave azo, carbonyl, hydroxyl, nitro, or sulfate moieties from substrates
c. Convert substrates to metabolites that are less pharmacologically active or less toxic
d. Generate adequate levels of NADPH for use by other hepatocyte metabolic reactions
e. Prevent formation of epoxides or free radical forms of substrates

38. Dopamine, epinephrine (or norepinephrine), and histamine are important neurotransmitter agonists. When these ligands interact with their cellular receptors they elicit a response by:

a. Activating adenylyl cyclase, leading to increased intracellular cAMP levels
b. Activating phospholipase C
c. Inducing or inhibiting synthesis of ligand-specific intracellular proteins
d. Opening or closing ligand-gated ion channels
e. Regulating intracellular second messengers through G protein–coupled receptors

39. The FDA assigns the letters A, B, C, D, and X to drugs approved for human use. These classifications are about:

a. Amount of dosage reduction needed as serum creatinine clearances fall
b. Amount of dosage reduction needed in presence of liver dysfunction
c. Fetal risk when given to pregnant women
d. Relative margins of safety/therapeutic index
e. The number of unlabeled uses for a drug

General Principles

Answers

1. The correct answer is c. (*Craig, pp 28–29, 51–52. Hardman, p 20. Katzung, pp 34–38.*) For a 70-kg individual, *total* body water is about 40 L (≈0.6 L/kg); interstitial plus plasma water occupies about 12 L (≈0.17 L/kg).

Azithromycin, with a V_d of 30 L/kg, would be distributed in an apparent volume of about 2100 L in a typical 70-kg person.

Use simple logic to answer this question, but look at the answer to Question 6, if you wish. Even if you don't remember what total body water is (about 40 L or 0.6 L/kg), or the approximate value for interstitial plus plasma water (about 12 L or 0.17 L/kg), do the quick calculation. If you take the stated 30 L/kg and computed the total (and very hypothetical—apparent) volume for a 70-kg individual, you would arrive at 2100 L. That number not only reflects distribution into a hypothetical volume far in excess of vascular and interstitial volumes, but also far beyond what could ever be physically real. After all, 2100 L = 2100 kg; if we assumed the volume were pure water, you won't find human beings weighing that much!

Without more information, you cannot make definitive conclusions about the other properties listed as potential correct answers.

2. The answer is d. (*Craig, p 25; Hardman, pp 12, 23–24; Katzung, pp 42–43.*) The first-pass effect is commonly considered to involve the biotransformation of a drug during its first passage through the portal circulation of the liver. Drugs that are administered orally and rectally enter the hepatic portal circulation first and can be biotransformed there, extensively, before reaching the systemic circulation. Typically, and significantly, this can reduce oral bioavailability and systemic blood concentrations of the affected drug. Administration by the intravenous, intramuscular, and sublingual routes allows the drug to attain concentrations in the systemic circulation and to be distributed throughout the body before hepatic metabolism has had much of an impact on the administered dose "going in."

The lungs can subject some inhaled drugs to a significant "first-pass" effect, but such a situation is uncommon in the grander scheme of things.

3. The answer is e. (*Craig, pp 16–18; Hardman, pp 42, 54–55; Katzung, pp 14–17.*) *Physiologic,* or *functional, antagonism* occurs when two drugs produce opposite effects on the same physiologic function by interacting with different types of receptors. A practical example of this is the use of epinephrine as a bronchodilator to counteract the bronchoconstriction that occurs when the parasympathetic nervous system releases ACh or when we administer bethanechol or an acetylcholinesterase inhibitor to a patient with asthma. ACh constricts airway smooth muscle by acting as an agonist on muscarinic receptors. Epinephrine relaxes airway smooth-muscle cells and dilates the bronchi, through its agonist activity on β_2-adrenergic receptors.

Chemical antagonism occurs when two drugs combine with each other chemically and the activity of one or both is reduced or abolished. For example, dimercaprol chelates lead and reduces the toxicity of this heavy metal.

Competitive antagonism occurs when two compounds (drugs) compete for the same receptor site—both having affinity for the receptor, only one having efficacy. In most cases this is a reversible interaction—a surmountable ("overcomeable") one—and it is certainly the most common form of drug-drug antagonism when we think of often-used therapeutic agents. Thus, atropine (the prototype muscarinic receptor blocker) antagonizes the effects of ACh on the S-A node by competing for the same population of receptors. Propranolol does the same with respect to antagonizing the β-1-stimulatory effects of epinephrine, norepinephrine, and such other β-agonists on the heart.

Irreversible antagonism generally results from the binding of an antagonist to the same receptor site as the agonist by covalent interaction or by a very slowly dissociating noncovalent interaction. An example of this antagonism is the blockade produced by phenoxybenzamine on α-adrenergic receptors, resulting in a long-lasting reduction in the activity of norepinephrine.

Dispositional antagonism occurs when one drug alters the pharmacokinetics (absorption, distribution, biotransformation, or excretion) of a second drug so that less of the active compound reaches the target tissue. For example, phenytoin (anticonvulsant/antiepileptic drug) induces the hepatic metabolic inactivation of warfarin, reducing its anticoagulant activity.

4. The answer is d. (*Craig, pp 48–50; Hardman, pp 18–24; Katzung, pp 40–42.*) The figure provided with the question shows an elimination pattern with two distinct components—a two-compartment model. The upper (steep) portion of the line represents the α phase, which is the distribution of the drug from the tissues that receive high rates of blood flow [the central compartment (e.g., the brain, heart, kidney, and lungs)] to tissues with lower rates of blood flow [the peripheral compartment (e.g., skeletal muscle, adipose tissue, and bone)]. Once distribution to all tissue is complete, equilibrium occurs throughout the body. The elimination of the drug from the body (the β phase) is represented by the lower linear portion of the line; this part is used to determine the elimination half-life of the drug.

At 2 h after dosing, the plasma concentration was 4.6 mcg/mL; at 5 h, the concentration was 2.4 mcg/mL. Therefore, the plasma concentration of this aminoglycoside decreased to about one-half in approximately 3 h—its half-life. In addition, drug elimination usually occurs according to first-order kinetics [i.e., a linear relationship is obtained when the drug concentration is plotted on a log scale vs. time on a linear scale (semilog plot)].

5. The answer is b. (*Craig, pp 48–50; Hardman pp 20–22; Katzung, pp 40–42.*) The fractional change in drug concentration per unit of time for any first-order process is expressed by k_e. This elimination rate constant is related to the half-life ($t_{1/2}$) by the equation $k_e t_{1/2} = 0.693$. The units of k_e are time^{-1}, whereas the $t_{1/2}$ is expressed in units of time. Substitute the appropriate value for half-life estimated from the data from the graph or table accompanying the question (the β phase) into the preceding equation; rearrange to solve for k_e, and the answer is calculated:

$$k_e = \frac{0.693}{t_{1/2}} = \frac{0.693}{3.0\ h} = 0.23\ h^{-1}$$

$$k_e = 0.23\ h^{-1}$$

There are other mathematical approaches to arriving at the same answer. We show one here, but with the opinion that being able to recall this and actually do the calculations is beyond what you should reasonably be expected to do for a general pharmacology course or exam:

$$\log (A) = \log (A_0) - \left(\frac{k_e}{2.303}\right)(t)$$

where (A_0) is the initial drug concentration, (A) is the final drug concentration, t is the time interval between the two measurements of A, and k_e is the elimination rate constant. For example, by solving for k_e using the plasma concentration values at 2 and 5 h,

$$\log (2.4 \text{ mcg/mL}) = \log (4.6 \text{ mcg/mL}) - \left(\frac{k_e}{2.303}\right)(3 \text{ h})$$

k_e will equal 0.22 h^{-1}.

6. The answer is c. (*Craig, pp 51–52; Hardman, pp 20–22; Katzung, pp 34–35.*) The apparent V_d is defined as the volume of fluid into which a drug appears to distribute with a concentration equal to that of plasma, or the volume of fluid necessary to dissolve the drug and yield the same concentration as that found in plasma. By convention, the value of the plasma concentration at zero time is used. In this problem, a hypothetical plasma concentration of the drug at zero time (7 mcg/mL) can be estimated by extrapolating the linear portion of the elimination curve (the β phase) back to zero time. Therefore, the apparent V_d is calculated by

$$V_d = \frac{\text{Total amount of drug in the body}}{\text{Drug concentration in plasma at time zero}}$$

Since the total amount of drug in the body is the intravenous dose (complete, or 100%, bioavailability), 350 mg (i.e., 5 mg/kg × 70 kg), and the estimated plasma concentration at zero time is 7 mcg/mL, substitution of these numbers in the equation (and keeping our units straight) yields the apparent V_d:

$$V_d = \frac{350 \text{ mg}}{0.007 \text{ mg/mL}} = 50,000 \text{ mL} = 50 \text{ L}$$

. . . or, if you wish to normalize V_d to body weight, about 0.7 L/kg.

7. The answer is a. (*Craig, pp 50–51; Hardman, pp 18–20; Katzung, pp 34–38.*) Clearance by an organ is defined as the apparent volume of a biologic fluid from which a drug is removed by elimination processes per unit of time. The total body clearance (Cl_{total}) is defined as the sum of clearances of all the organs and tissues that eliminate a drug. Cl_{total} is influenced by the apparent V_d and k_e. The more rapidly a drug is cleared, the greater is the value of Cl_{total}. Therefore, for the new aminoglycoside in this patient,

$$Cl_{total} = V_d k_e = (50 \text{ L}) (0.22 \text{ h}^{-1}) = 11 \text{ L/h}$$

8. The answer is c. (*Craig, pp 49–51; Hardman, pp 23–24; Katzung, pp 44–46.*) This question, with its many variables and equations, was written intentionally to see whether you would take a needlessly complicated approach to a very straightforward concept. If you give doses of a drug repeatedly (and this works best when the dosing interval is identical to the drug's half-life) and hold every other pertinent variable constant (dose, route, elimination status, etc.), you simply multiply the half-life by 4 or 5 (hence, our use of 4.5) to arrive at the approximate time until C_{ss}—the time at which "drug in = drug out"—is reached.

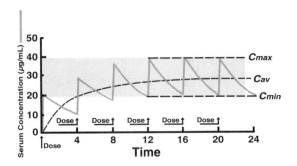

You can see it here, with repeated administration of a drug at intervals equal to the drug's half-life; note that the *average serum concentration* (C_{av}) does not appear to "flatten-out," or reach a plateau, until at least 4 doses have been given.

Note: the equation $(0.693 \cdot V_d)/Cl$ (answer a), is the equation for calculating the half-life.

9. The answer is e. (*Craig, pp 49–50; Hardman, pp 18–20; Katzung, pp 41–42.*) The fraction of a drug dose absorbed after oral administration is affected by a wide variety of factors that can strongly influence the peak blood levels and the time-to-peak blood concentration. The V_d and the total body clearance ($V_d \infty$ first-order k_e) also are important in determining the amount of drug that reaches the target tissue. Only the area under the blood concentration-time curve, however, reflects absorption, distribution, metabolism, and excretion factors; it is the most reliable and popular method of evaluating bioavailability.

10. The answer is d. *(Craig, pp 49–50; Hardman, pp 18–20; Katzung, pp 41–42.)* *Bioavailability* is defined as the fraction or percentage of a drug that becomes available to the systemic circulation following administration by any route. This takes into consideration that not all of an orally administered drug is absorbed and that a drug can be removed from the plasma and biotransformed by the liver during its initial passage through the portal circulation. A bioavailability of 25% indicates that only 20 mg of the 80-mg dose (i.e., 80 mg × 0.25 = 20 mg) reached the systemic circulation. Organ clearance can be determined by knowing the blood flow through the organ (Q) and the extraction ratio (ER) for the drug by the organ, according to the equation:

$$Cl_{organ} = Q \cdot ER$$

The extraction ratio is dependent on the amounts of drug entering the organ (arterial side; C_A) and leaving it on the venous side (C_V).

$$ER = \left(\frac{C_A \cdot C_V}{C_A} \right)$$

In this problem, the amount of verapamil entering the liver per unit time was 76 mg (80 mg × 0.95) and the amount leaving was 20 mg. Therefore,

$$ER = \frac{76 \text{ mg} - 20 \text{ mg}}{76 \text{ mg}} = 0.74$$

$$Cl_{liver} = (1500 \text{ mL/min}) (0.74) = 1110 \text{ mL/min}$$

11. The answer is b. *(Craig, pp 50–51; Hardman, pp 23–24; Katzung, pp 41–42.)* Among other things, knowing the AUC of a drug given intravenously (which, by definition, is associated with a bioavailability of 1.0, or 100%) is a prerequisite for knowing the bioavailability of the same drug given by any other route; bioavailability is calculated as the ratio of AUC for any non-IV route and the AUC_{IV}.

12. The answer is e. (*Craig, pp 20–22; Hardman, p 4; Katzung, pp 7–8.*) Recall the two Henderson-Hasselbach equations, which apply to how local pH affects the ionization of molecules in an aqueous environment. And, recall, that all other things being equal, that we assume membranes are permeable only to nonionized (and lipid-soluble) forms of a drug:

For acidic drugs: $pH = pK_a + \log [A^-]/[AH]$

For basic drugs: $pH = pK_a = \log [B]/[BH^+]$

Our drug was an acid with $pK_a = 3.4$. In the stomach (pH 7.4) the ratio of nonionized to ionized molecules will be 1:0.01. The nonionized molecules will diffuse across the membrane. Once in the plasma, pH 7.4, the ratio of HA:A$^-$ will become 1:10,000. And the concentration ratio of total drug across the membrane will be 10:000:1, but with the larger amount being in the plasma, not the gut.

You might also want to look at the figure, below, to get a "big picture" of how changing pH changes the ionization of acidic and basic drugs.

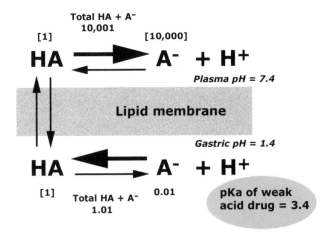

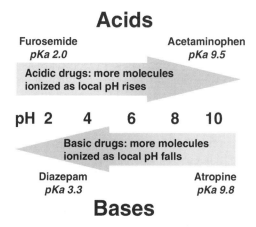

Acids

Furosemide
pKa 2.0

Acetaminophen
pKa 9.5

Acidic drugs: more molecules
ionized as local pH rises

pH 2   4   6   8   10

Basic drugs: more molecules
ionized as local pH falls

Diazepam
pKa 3.3

Atropine
pKa 9.8

Bases

13. The answer is c. (*Craig, pp 50–51; Hardman, pp 23–24; Katzung, p 41.*) We are making this data comparison to determine the drug's bioavailability. We define the bioavailability of a drug given intravenously as 1.0 (100%), since with IV administration we avoid all the applicable barriers to drug absorption. But, of course, it's important to know how much total drug, over a period of time, gets into the bloodstream with other administration routes that we might want to use clinically. Drugs given by routes other than IV must be absorbed (and be exposed to all the barriers that limit or slow or otherwise affect absorption); and because they might not be absorbed from their administration site, or might be susceptible to such processes as hepatic first-pass metabolism, they usually have a bioavailability < 1.0.

The calculation of bioavailability is based on the ratio of the area under the concentration-time curve (AUC) for the administration route being considered (oral, IM, etc.) and the AUC obtained with IV administration:

$$\frac{AUC_{\text{other route}}}{AUC_{IV}}$$

Measurement of blood levels of a drug at a single time point will not give us the information we need to determine bioavailability.

Note that with oral absorption there is a delay until there is some detectable drug in the blood; that reflects both the time needed for absorption of the drug and, in most cases, the sensitivity of the assay to measure the drug. With IV administration blood levels rise instantaneously. Note, too, that as blood levels of the drug rise toward the peak with oral administration, rates of drug entry into the blood exceed rates of elimination (whether by metabolism, excretion, or both, depending on what the drug is). Likewise, once blood concentrations start to fall the amount of drug entering the system becomes less than the amount being eliminated, per unit time. That is, "amount in < amount out."

Finally—and although you can't tell precisely from the graph—the half-lives for the drug, measured under different experimental conditions, are identical: in general (and it depends on the drug and its blood level), the drug will be eliminated at the same rate (based on usual kinetic influences, such as first-order kinetics) regardless of administration route.

None of the other choices in the question (i.e., potency, effectiveness, or plasma protein binding) can be evaluated using this type of comparison.

14. The answer is d. (*Craig, pp 37–38; Hardman, pp 12–14; Katzung, pp 52–56.*) Biotransformation reactions involving the oxidation, reduction, or hydrolysis of a drug are classified as Phase I (or nonsynthetic) reactions; these reactions may result in either the activation or inactivation of a pharmacologic agent. There are many types of these reactions; oxidations are the most numerous. Phase II (occasionally called synthetic) reactions, which almost always result in the formation of an inactive product, involve *conjugation* of the drug (or its derivative) with an amino acid, carbohydrate, acetate, sulfate—or glucuronic acid as noted in the question. The conjugated form(s) of the drug or its derivatives may be more easily excreted than the parent compound.

15. The answer is d. (*Craig, pp 48–49; Hardman, pp 26–27; Katzung, pp 39; 44–46.*) With intravenous infusions of a drug, only the drug's half-life determines how long it will take for blood levels to reach a steady state (on average, neither rising nor falling thereafter) so long as the infusion rate is not changed. By definition, when steady state is reached, the amount of drug entering the blood per unit time is equal to the rate at which drug is being eliminated, whether by excretion, metabolism, or a combination of both (depending on the drug).

The apparent volume of distribution has no impact on time to C_{ss}. Bioavailability does not, either, because with intravenous drug administration the bioavailability is 1.0 (100%). Clearance, a parameter that relates elimination rate of a drug to the drug's concentration [Cl = rate of elimination (mg/h)/drug concentration (mg/mL)]. Because clearance considers a rate of drug elimination, it affects the C_{ss}, but it is not a determinant of it. The infusion rate clearly affects the blood concentration reached at steady state, but it does not affect the time needed to reach C_{ss}. For example, if we had a drug with a half-life of 4 h, infused it at a rate of x mg/min, and then repeated the experiment with the same drug at an infusion rate of $2x$ mg/min, blood concentrations at steady state would clearly be different. However, it would still take the same amount of time (roughly 4 to 5 half-lives), to reach steady state.

16. The answer is d. (*Craig, p 36; Hardman, pp 16–17; Katzung, p 62.*) Grapefruit juice (but not most other citrus juices) contains compounds that can inhibit the metabolism of several drugs, one of which is cyclosporine. The effect is especially important for first-pass hepatic metabolism of oral drugs that are susceptible to the first-pass effect. (Other drugs include verapamil, some of the statin-type cholesterol-lowering medications, and most of the second generation antihistamines, including fexofenadine.) The result is increased bioavailability of an orally administered dose and increased AUC. Peak and total (integrated over time) plasma levels of the interactant typically are increased, and one potential (if not likely) outcome is excessive (toxic) effects.

The "grapefruit juice effect" does not alter the main route(s) of drug absorption or elimination, nor affect plasma protein binding capacity, because those are properties related to the drug, not how or how well or quickly, it enters the circulation. Note that these data are consistent with the hypothesis that grapefruit juice does not statistically significantly slow entry of cyclosporine entry into the blood; it is mainly an effect on "how much," not on "how fast."

17. The answer is d. (*Craig, pp 52–53; Hardman, pp 26–27; Katzung, pp 45–46.*) Here is how you solve the problem. Note: It's easy to be misled by inconsistent use of units of measurement (mcg vs. mg, mL vs. L), so be sure you convert units as necessary.

First calculate the drug's elimination rate constant:

$$k_e = 0.693/t_{1/2} \quad \text{or}$$

$$k_e = 0.693/0.5 \text{ h} = 1.386/\text{h}$$

Then calculate the clearance:

$$Cl = k_e \cdot V_d \quad \text{or}$$

$$Cl = 1.386/\text{h} \cdot 45 \text{ L, which equals } 62.37 \text{ L/h, or } 62,370 \text{ mL/h}$$

Recall that $C_{ave} = (F/Cl) \cdot (\text{Dose}/\tau)$, where τ represents the dosing interval (given as 4 h).

Rearrange to solve for the dose.

$$\text{Dose} = (C_{ave} \cdot Cl \cdot \tau)/F, \text{ or}$$

$$\text{Dose} = [(2 \text{ mcg/mL}) \cdot (62,370 \text{ mL/h}) \cdot 4 \text{ h}]/1.0$$

Thus, Dose = 499,000 mcg, or 499 mg (close enough to 500 mg).

18. The correct answer is c. (*Craig, pp 49–50; Hardman, pp 20–21; Katzung, pp 34–47.*) Regardless of which administration route has been used, if we plot the log of blood concentration of a drug vs. time (and assuming first-order kinetics, which applies to the elimination of most drugs), we get a straight line. It is described by the equation

$$\ln C = \ln C_0 - Kt$$

The slope of this line, κ, is the *elimination rate constant*.

An arguably more useful (and familiar) measure of the rate at which a drug is eliminated is the half-life ($t_{1/2}$). It is equal to $0.693/\kappa$, and is defined as the time it takes for the concentration of a drug in the blood to fall to precisely one half of what it is now (or at any specified time).

The *area under the curve* (AUC) is the integration of a time vs. concentration plot for a drug. It is a linear—not a logarithmic or semilog—plot. One use for plots of AUC is to estimate one's "total exposure" to a drug, usually from "time zero" (instantaneously upon administration) until blood concentrations of drug are no longer reliably detectable or further measurements are impractical. The AUC can be used to estimate total body clearance of a drug, without the need to know the drug's volume of distribution or its half-life, since

$$\text{Clearance} = \frac{\text{Dose}}{\text{AUC}}$$

Determining AUC also enables us to calculate a drug's *bioavailabity*. Bioavailability (F) is a measure of the fraction of an administered dose that is absorbed systemically and is detectable in the plasma. Note that when a drug is given intravenously, bioavailability is, by definition, 1.0 (100%), since there are no barriers that might prevent the absorption of drug from the administration site. So by administering a drug intravenously, and also giving it by another route, we can calculate bioavailability. For example, assume the other route we use is oral (PO).

$$\text{Bioavailability} = \left(\frac{\text{Dose}_{\text{IV}}}{\text{Dose}_{\text{PO}}} \right) \times \left(\frac{\text{AUC}_{\text{PO}}}{\text{AUC}_{\text{IV}}} \right)$$

If we do our bioavailability determinations by giving the same dose of the drug, the dosage units in the above equation cancel out, and so

$$\text{Bioavailability} = \frac{\text{AUC}_{\text{PO}}}{\text{AUC}_{\text{IV}}}$$

The *extraction ratio* (E) is a measure of a drug's removal from the blood as it passes through an organ (e.g., the liver) that can metabolize (or otherwise extract) it, e.g., from the arterial to the venous side of that organ.

The rate of drug entry to an organ is the product of blood flow (Q) and the arterial concentration of the drug (C_A). The rate at which the drug leaves is flow × the venous concentration (C_V). If flow into and out of an organ are identical (as it often is), then the extraction ratio can be expressed as

$$E = \frac{(C_A - C_V)}{C_A}$$

We can also use the extraction ratio to calculate the organ clearance of a drug—i.e., the volume per unit time from which an organ removes a drug

$$\text{Organ clearance} = \text{Blood flow} \times \text{Extraction ratio}$$

The *volume of distribution* (V_d) relates the amount of drug in the body to its concentration in the blood (or plasma). It is typically calculated as the administered dose divided by the concentration of drug in the blood

$$V_d = \frac{D}{C}$$

To simplify things, we typically give the drug intravenously (so we know how much drug enters the system) and measure the concentration immediately thereafter (or use a plot of the log of drug concentration vs. time) to extrapolate drug concentration at "time zero" (the y-axis intercept).

19–21. The answers are 24-e, 25-b, 26-a. *(Hardman, pp 56–57; Katzung, p 31.)*
Anaphylaxis refers to an acute hypersensitivity reaction that appears to be mediated primarily by immunoglobulin E (IgE). Specific antigens can interact with these antibodies and cause sensitized mast cells to release vasoactive substances, such as histamine. Anaphylaxis to penicillin is one of the best-known examples; the drug of choice to relieve the symptoms is epinephrine.

Decreased sensitivity to a drug, or tolerance, is seen with some drugs such as opiates and usually requires repeated administration of the drug. *Tachyphylaxis,* in contrast, is tolerance that develops rapidly, often after a single injection of a drug. In some cases, this may be due to what is termed as the *downregulation of a drug receptor,* in which the number of receptors becomes decreased.

A person who responds to an unusually low dose of a drug is often said to be *hyperreactive* to that drug. Supersensitivity refers to increased responses to low doses only after denervation of an organ. At least three mechanisms are responsible for supersensitivity: (1) increased receptors, (2) reduction in tonic neuronal activity, and (3) decreased neurotransmitter uptake mechanisms.

22–24. The answers are 22-c, 23-a, 24-h. *(Craig, pp 48–49; Hardman, pp 25–26; Katzung, pp 41–46.)*
Time-action curves relate the changes in intensity of the action of a drug dose and the times that these changes occur. There are three distinct phases that characterize the time-action pattern of most drugs: (1) The time to onset of action is from the moment of administration (T on the figure that accompanies the question) to the time when the first drug effect is detected (U). (2) The time to reach the peak effect is from administration (T) until the maximum effect has occurred (W), whether this is above or

below the level that produces some toxic effect. (3) The duration of action is described as the time from the appearance of a drug effect (U) until the effect disappears (Y). For some drugs, a fourth phase occurs (interval Y to Z), in which residual effects of the drug may be present. These are usually undetectable, but may be uncovered by readministration of the same drug dose (observed as an increase in potency) or by administration of another drug (leading to some drug-drug interaction).

25–27. The answers are 25-b, 26-a, 27-d. *(Craig, pp 20–24; Hardman, pp 3–5; Katzung, pp 5–7)*
The absorption, distribution, and elimination of drugs require that they cross various cellular membranes. The descriptions that are given in the question define the various transport mechanisms. The most common method by which ionic compounds of low molecular weight (100 to 200) enter cells is via membrane channels. The degree to which such filtration occurs varies from cell type to cell type because their pore sizes differ.

Simple diffusion is another mechanism by which substances cross membranes without the active participation of components in the membranes. Generally, lipid-soluble substances employ this method to enter cells. Both simple diffusion and filtration are dominant factors in most drug absorption, distribution, and elimination.

Pinocytosis is responsible for the transport of large molecules such as proteins and colloids. Some cell types (e.g., endothelial cells) employ this transport mechanism extensively, but its importance in drug action is uncertain, at best. In the grander scheme of things, it is not particularly important.

Membrane carriers are proteinaceous components of the cell membrane that are capable of combining with a drug at one surface of the membrane. The carrier-solute complex moves across the membrane, the solute is released, and the carrier then returns to the original surface where it can combine with another molecule of solute. There are two primary types of carrier-mediated transport: (1) active transport and (2) facilitated diffusion. During active transport, (1) the drug crosses the membrane against a concentration gradient, (2) the transport mechanism becomes saturated at high drug concentrations and thus shows a transport maximum, and (3) the process is selective for certain structural configurations of the drug. Active transport is responsible for the movement of a number of organic acids and bases across membranes of renal tubules, choroid plexuses, and hepatic cells. With facilitated diffusion, the transport process is selective and saturable, but the drug is not transferred against a concentration gradient and does not require the expenditure of cellular energy. Glucose transport into erythrocytes is a good example of this process. In both situations, if two compounds are transported by the same mechanism, one will competitively inhibit the transport of the other, and the transport process can be inhibited noncompetitively by substances that interfere with cellular metabolism.

28–30.   The answers are 28-g, 29-a, 30-d. *(Craig, pp 34–37; Hardman, pp 12–14; Katzung, pp 52–53.)*
There are four major components to the mixed-function oxidase system: (1) cytochrome P450, (2) NADPH, or reduced nicotinamide adenine dinucleotide phosphate, (3) NADPH-cytochrome P450 reductase, and (4) molecular oxygen. The figure below shows the catalytic cycle for the reactions dependent on cytochrome P450.

Cytochrome P450 catalyzes a diverse number of oxidative reactions involved in drug biotransformation; it undergoes reduction and oxidation during its catalytic cycle. A prosthetic group composed of Fe and protoporphyrin IX (forming heme) binds molecular oxygen and converts it to an activated form for interaction with the drug substrate. Similar to hemoglobin, cytochrome P450 is inhibited by carbon monoxide. This interaction results in an absorbance spectrum peak at 450 nm, hence the name P450.

NADPH gives up hydrogen atoms to the flavoprotein NADPH-cytochrome P450 reductase and becomes $NADP^+$. The reduced flavoprotein transfers these reducing equivalents to cytochrome P450. The reducing equivalents are used to activate molecular oxygen for incorporation into the

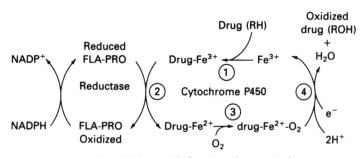

(From DiPalma and DiGregorio, with permission.)

substrate, as described above. Thus, NADPH provides the reducing equivalents, whereas NADPH-cytochrome P450 reductase passes them on to the catalytic enzyme cytochrome P450.

Monoamine oxidase (MAO) is a flavoprotein enzyme that is found on the outer membrane of mitochondria. It oxidatively deaminates short-chain monoamines only, and it is not part of the drug-metabolizing microsomal system. ATP is involved in the transfer of reducing equivalents through the mitochondrial respiratory chain, not the microsomal system.

31. The answer is d. (*Hardman, pp 18–29; Katzung, pp 44–50.*) The dose to give equals the product of the target blood concentration and the drug's clearance.

$$D = C_{desired} \times Cl$$

To simplify things, let's get the units of volume the same for both clearance and concentration. The clearance of 0.08 L/min = 80 mL/min.
Therefore

$$D = 8 \text{ mcg/mL} \times 80 \text{ mL/min}$$
$$= 640 \text{ mcg/min}$$

The stated dosing interval is 4 h, so

$$640 \text{ mcg/min} \times 60 \text{ min/h} \times 4 \text{ h} = 153,500 \text{ mcg}$$

which (rounded) is 150 mg.

32. The answer is d. (*Hardman 10e, pp 25–29*) Here the loading dose equals the product of the target blood concentration and the volume of distribution

$$D = C_{desired} \times V_d$$

Again, we convert units to make things consistent. The volume of distribution, 60 L, is, of course 60,000 mL

$$D = 8 \text{ mcg/mL} \times 60,000 \text{ mL}$$
$$= 480,000 \text{ mcg}$$
$$= 480 \text{ mg}$$

33. The answer is b. *(Craige, pp 113–114; Hardman, pp 39–43; Katzung, pp 16–17.)* Partial agonists have both the ability to bind to receptors (affinity), and the ability to evoke a response by activating those receptors (efficacy), albeit weakly, under basal conditions. Thus, when acebutolol is administered at rest (a condition under which endogenous catecholamine levels are low), heart rate rises slightly due to β-1 receptor activation via weak agonist activity. However, the occupation of adrenergic receptors by this weak agonist reduces the number of receptors available to bind and respond to stronger agonists (epinephrine, norepinephrine). As a result, the magnitude of the response to stronger agonists in the presence of the partial agonist is lower than in the absence of it (all other things being equal).

34. The answer is d. *(Hardman, pp 24–29; Katzung, pp 40–47.)* With first-order elimination of a drug, we get a straight line if we plot the log of drug concentration in the blood vs. time. The slope of the line is the elimination rate constant (k_{el}). The drug's half-life—a value we will need to use momentarily—is related to k_{el} as follows: $t_{1/2} * (k_{el}) = 0.693$. So, for the drug noted in the question, $t_{1/2} = 0.693/0.35$, or approximately 2 h. It takes approximately 4 to 5 half-lives to reach a steady-state blood concentration. Do the simple math and you will see that the time for this drug is approximately 9 h.

35. The answer is e. *(Craig, pp 48–52; Hardman, pp 24–29; Katzung, pp 40–47.)* You should recall that $V_d = \text{dose}/C_0$. We know what the dose is. What we must calculate is the initial drug concentration (C_0)—the peak drug concentration that is reached "instantaneously" after giving the IV bolus dose. Unfortunately, we've waited 30 min before taking our first blood sample, but that is not a problem: plot the log of drug concentration vs. time and extrapolate to where the line intercepts the log-concentration axis (t_0). This gives us C_0.

Plug the extrapolated C_0 into the equation and you have your answer.

Note that bioavailability is not a factor in this instance, because with IV administration bioavailability is 1.0 (100%). Knowing or calculating the elimination rate constant won't help either, because it is inextricably linked to the half-life, which we already know $(k_{el} = 0.693/t_{1/2})$. Calculating the AUC (concentration vs. time integral) with a bolus injection will give us no information more useful than what we already have. Clearance (generally referring to renal clearance) is irrelevant in this situation: we've stated that the drug is completely metabolized to other products; thus, there is no Drug A to measure in the urine.

36. The answer is c. *(Craig, pp 48–52; Hardman, pp 24–29; Katzung, pp 34–43.)* Only the drug concentration at steady state will change (it will be greater with this altered protocol). Do not be misled by the numbers. The time to reach C_{SS} with a constant drug infusion is a function of half-life (or the elimination rate constant, which is related to it: $k_{el} = 0.693/t_{1/2}$), and that will not change under the conditions stated. Likewise, with the vast majority of drugs eliminated by first-order kinetics, there will be no change of total body clearance or of volume of distribution. (Note: We described Substance X as being pharmacologically inert simply so you didn't conjure up confounding but largely irrelevant issues, such as an active drug that is able to cause residual or long-lasting effects on its elimination or elimination rate, e.g., a drug that caused long-lasting induction of hepatic drug-metabolizing enzymes.)

37. The answer is a. *(Craig, p 34; Hardman, pp 12–13; Katzung, pp 52–56.)* The general outcome of Phase I reaction is the formation of one or more metabolites that are more polar than the substrate; this is accomplished (whether through oxidation, hydroxylation, deamination, etc.) either by adding or exposing a particular functional group on the substrate. This increased polarity of the product(s) either facilitates excretion directly or prepares the product for subsequent conjugation reactions (glucuronidation, glutathione conjugation, glycine conjugation, etc.) by a Phase II reaction.

Recall that it is the lipophilicity of drugs that enables them to pass through biological membranes (e.g., to be absorbed to cause effects), yet this very same physicochemical property hinders their elimination from the body—were it not for Phase I metabolic reactions.

It is true that most Phase I reactions lead to less active or less toxic products, but not all do. Prodrugs, for example, are pharmacologically inactive substances that are given with the expectation (knowledge) that they will be metabolized (by a Phase I reaction) to the active species that ultimately causes effects.

38. The answer is e. *(Craig, pp 11–12, 98–100; Hardman, pp 34–36; Katzung, pp 16–27.)* The key concept is that these very important agonists, and many others, "transduce" their signals and eventually change a characteristic of cell function (cause a response) through G proteins—a family of guanine nucleotide-binding proteins. These ligands bind to the extracellular face of the transmembrane protein. The various G proteins (e.g., Gi, Gq, Gs) bind to intracellular portions of the receptor. They then couple the initial ligand interaction to the eventual response through a series of effector enzymes or enzyme systems that are G protein-regulated.

For example, adenylyl cyclase can be activated, catalyzing the formation of cAMP that then activates one or several kinases that phosphorylate specific intracellular proteins. But the actual steps that occur after ligand binding depend on what the ligand is, what specific G protein is involved, and which kinases are activated and what proteins they phosphorylate. And what happens (i.e., what the response is) depends on all of the above and, of course, which cell type is being affected.

For example, activation of adenylyl cyclase and increased cAMP levels may occur in one system, but the opposite may occur in another. Some signal transduction pathways involve phospholipase C, others do not. A calcium channel may be affected in one system and a potassium channel (or no ion channel) in others.

By way of review, recall that there are three other main mechanisms or pathways for signal transduction about which we have reasonable knowledge.

One mechanism or pathway uses a receptor protein that spans the cell membrane, but G proteins are not involved. On the inner membrane face it possesses enzymatic activity that is regulated by the presence or absence of ligand bound to the extracellular face of the protein. The tyrosine kinase pathway is an example, and the overall pathway is responsible for the activity of various growth factors, including insulin.

Another is used by very lipid-soluble ligands that cross cell membranes easily and act on some intracellular receptor (e.g., glucocorticosteroids), which act in the nucleus and, through interaction with heat-shock protein (hsp90), eventually alters changes in transcription of specific genes.

The third involves transmembrane ion channels, the "open" or "closed" states of which are controlled by ligand binding to the channel. This process applies to some of the important neurotransmitters, especially those in the brain (GABA, the main inhibitory neurotransmitter) and such amino acids as glycine, which exert "excitatory" actions. The nicotinic receptor for ACh fits in this category too.

39. The answer is c. (*Craig, p 382; Hardman, pp 53–54; Katzung, pp 68–70, 996–998.*) These are pregnancy classifications. Drugs in pregnancy Category A have been evaluated in controlled clinical studies in all trimesters, and they are deemed safe enough to pose only a remote risk of fetal harm. With categories B, C, and D, there is increasing evidence, whether from animal or human studies (or both), of increasing risks. Drugs in Category D have demonstrable risk, but may be used when, for example, the purpose is to manage a life-threatening condition and no safer alternatives are available. Notice of such must be included in the package insert's Warning section. Classification X also means proven fetal harm, but the risks of administering to a pregnant woman far exceed the potential benefits. This warning is put in the Contraindications section of the package insert.

Autonomic Nervous System

Adrenergic agonists
Adrenergic antagonists
Cholinergic agonists
Cholinergic antagonists

Ganglionic antagonists
Monoamine oxidase inhibitors
Skeletal muscle relaxants
Skeletal neuromuscular blockers

Questions

DIRECTIONS: Each item contains a question or incomplete statement that is followed by possible responses. Select the **one best** response to each question.

Questions 40–45

The diagram on the next page shows the main elements of the efferent pathways in the autonomic (parasympathetic and sympathetic; PNS, SNS, respectively) and somatic nervous systems.

Some of the questions that follow have you respond by selecting the letter representing one of the nerves, above. Those nerves are

a. Preganglionic parasympathetic
b. Postganglionic parasympathetic
c. Preganglionic sympathetic
d. Postganglionic sympathetic to structures other than sweat glands
e. "Preganglionic" (functionally equivalence) sympathetic to adrenal medulla
f. Preganglionic sympathetic, sweat gland innervation
g. Postganglionic sympathetic to sweat glands
h. Motor nerve, somatic nervous system

Schematic of Efferent Pathways in the Peripheral Nervous Systems

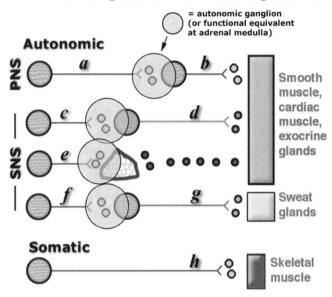

= autonomic ganglion (or functional equivalent at adrenal medulla)

Autonomic

PNS

a

b

Smooth muscle, cardiac muscle, exocrine glands

c

d

e

f

g

Sweat glands

Somatic

h

Skeletal muscle

40. Which nerve in the schematic is adrenergic—synthesizing and releasing norepinephrine (NE) as its neurotransmitter?

a. a
b. b
c. c
d. d
e. e
f. f
g. g
h. h

41. Pancuronium or tubocurarine blocks activation of certain structures by a neurotransmitter. Which nerve innervates those structures?

a. a
b. b
c. c
d. d
e. e
f. f
g. g
h. h

42. *Reuptake* (into the nerve) is the main physiologic process for terminating the postsynaptic activity of a peripheral nervous system neurotransmitter. For which nerve does this process apply?

a. a
b. b
c. c
d. d
e. e
f. f
g. g
h. h

43. Of all the nerves shown on the previous page, which of the following is unique about *nerve g*?

a. Cocaine blocks release of its neurotransmitter
b. Is adrenergic
c. Is cholinergic, but anatomically and functionally part of the SNS
d. Its neurotransmitter acts on nicotinic receptors
e. Uses epinephrine as its neurotransmitter

44. On which receptor type does the neurotransmitter released from *nerve g* act?

a. α_1 adrenergic
b. α_2 adrenergic
c. Muscarinic
d. Nicotinic
e. β_1 adrenergic
f. β_2 adrenergic

45. On which receptor type does the neurotransmitter released from *nerve d* act? Remember: you can select only one answer.

a. α_1 adrenergic
b. α_2 adrenergic
c. Muscarinic
d. Nicotinic
e. β_1 adrenergic
f. β_2 adrenergic
g. It depends

46. Of the several types of adrenergic receptors found throughout the body, which is responsible for the cardiac stimulation that is observed following an intravenous injection of epinephrine?

a. α_1
b. α_2
c. β_1
d. β_2
e. β_3

47. Echothiophate, which is used mainly for its ophthalmic actions, inhibits:

a. Tyrosine hydroxylase
b. Acetylcholinesterase (AChE)
c. Catechol-O-methyltransferase (COMT)
d. Monoamine oxidase (MAO)
e. DOPA decarboxylase

48. We want to prescribe scopolamine, as a transdermal drug delivery system (skin patch), for a patient who will be leaving for an expensive cruise. Which finding would rule-out prescribing the drug, because it is likely to pose adverse effects or be truly contraindicated?

a. Angle-closure (narrow-angle) glaucoma
b. Bradycardia
c. History of diarrhea from shellfish
d. Resting blood pressure of 112/70
e. Hypothyroidism, mild
f. Parkinson's disease (early onset, not currently treated)

49. Which β-adrenergic blocker also competitively blocks α-adrenergic receptors?

a. Labetalol
b. Metoprolol
c. Nadolol
d. Pindolol
e. Timolol

50. A male patient who has been "surfing the Web" in search of an aphrodisiac or some other agent to enhance "sexual prowess and performance" discovers yohimbine. He consumes the drug in excess and develops symptoms of toxicity that require your intervention. You consult your preferred drug reference and learn that yohimbine is a selective α_2-adrenergic antagonist. Which would you expect as a response to this drug?

a. Bradycardia
b. Bronchoconstriction
c. Excessive secretions by exocrine glands (salivary, lacrimal, etc.)
d. Hypertension
e. Reduced cardiac output from reduced left ventricular contractility

51. Which is a reversible cholinesterase inhibitor that is indicated for the treatment of Alzheimer's disease?

a. Tacrine
b. Edrophonium
c. Neostigmine
d. Pyridostigmine
e. Ambenonium

52. Hypotension, bradycardia, respiratory depression, and muscle weakness, all unresponsive to atropine and neostigmine, would most likely be due to:

a. Scopolamine
b. Isofluorophate
c. Tubocurarine
d. Nicotine
e. Pilocarpine

53. Ritodrine hydrochloride is used in the treatment of:

a. Parkinson's disease
b. Bronchial asthma
c. Depression
d. Hypertension
e. Premature labor

54. A patient receives bethanechol after abdominal surgery. Her heart rate falls slightly and she experiences some wheezing. These cardiac and pulmonary responses represent or reflect:

a. Expected side effects
b. Idiosyncrasy
c. Parasympathetic ganglionic activation
d. Reflex (baroreceptor) suppression of cardiac rate
e. Undiagnosed asthma

55. A predictably dangerous side effect of nadolol that constitutes a contraindication to its clinical use in susceptible patients is the induction of:

a. Hypertension
b. Cardiac arrhythmia
c. Asthmatic attacks
d. Respiratory depression
e. Hypersensitivity

56. All the following drugs are used topically in the treatment of chronic wide-angle glaucoma. Which one reduces intraocular pressure by decreasing the formation of the aqueous humor?

a. Timolol
b. Echothiophate
c. Pilocarpine
d. Isofluorphate
e. Physostigmine

57. We give an "effective dose" of atropine to a person who is poisoned with an AChE inhibitor. Which structure will continue to be overactivated by the excess ACh after this drug is given?

a. Airway smooth muscle
b. S-A node of the heart
c. Salivary and lacrimal glands
d. Skeletal muscle
e. Vascular smooth muscle

58. Guanadrel is an antihypertensive drug: it reduces arteriolar constriction and in doing so lowers blood pressure, by reducing the amount of norepinephrine in peripheral adrenergic nerves. Lowered blood pressure is not accompanied by reflex tachycardia, and bradycardia is the more common outcome. The main ocular effect of guanadrel is miosis. The widespread abolition of sympathetic influences throughout the body often causes diarrhea and urinary frequency.

   Based on this description, guanadrel is most similar to:

a. Acetylcholine
b. Atropine
c. Epinephrine
d. Isoproterenol
e. Norepinephrine
f. Propranolol
g. Reserpine

59. Which is a muscarinic receptor–blocking drug that is administered by inhalation to cause bronchodilation for patients with emphysema [chronic obstructive pulmonary disease (COPD)]?

a. Albuterol
b. Diphenhydramine
c. Ipratropium
d. Pancuronium
e. Pilocarpine

60. Which of the following is the acetylcholinesterase inhibitor that is used in the diagnosis of myasthenia gravis?

a. Edrophonium
b. Ambenonium
c. Malathion
d. Physostigmine
e. Pralidoxime
f. Pyridostigmine

61. It is common to include small amounts of epinephrine in solutions of local anesthetics that will be administered by infiltration (injection around sensory nerve endings), as when a skin laceration needs suturing. Which of the following is a main reason for including the epinephrine?

a. To antagonize the otherwise intense and common vasodilator effects of the anesthetic
b. To counteract cardiac depression caused by the anesthetic
c. To prevent anaphylaxis in patients who are allergic to the anesthetic
d. To reduce the risk of toxicity caused by systemic absorption of the anesthetic
e. To shorten the duration of anesthetic action

62. Which of the following is the drug of choice for treating anaphylaxis?

a. Epinephrine
b. Norepinephrine
c. Isoproterenol
d. Diphenhydramine
e. Atropine

63. Which of the following applies to both phentolamine and prazosin?

a. Are competitive antagonists at α_1-adrenergic receptors
b. Profoundly inhibit gastric acid secretion
c. Cause a high incidence of bronchoconstriction in asthmatics
d. Cause bradycardia
e. Are used chronically for the treatment of primary hypotension

64. Left ventricular contractile force improves when dobutamine is given to a 60-year-old man with low cardiac output due to reductions of both heart rate and stroke volume. What is the main mechanism by which dobutamine is causing this effect?

a. α-adrenergic agonist
b. α-adrenergic antagonist
c. β_1-adrenergic agonist
d. β_1-adrenergic antagonist
e. Mixed α and β agonist
f. Mixed α and β antagonist

65. We observe a rise of arterial *pulse pressure* during slow IV infusion of a drug to a normal subject. The agent that will do this is which of the following?

a. Albuterol
b. Amphetamine
c. Epinephrine
d. Metoprolol
e. Phenylephrine

66. What accounts for the *main* physiologic process by which the actions of norepinephrine, released from an adrenergic nerve, are terminated?

a. Metabolism by enzyme(s) located near the postsynaptic receptor(s) and/or in the synaptic cleft
b. Reuptake into the nerve ending
c. Metabolism by catechol-O-methyltransferase (COMT)
d. Degradation by mitochondrial monoamine oxidase (MAO)
e. Conversion to a "false neurotransmitter" in the nerve ending

67. In which condition is administration of a β blocker (nonselective or otherwise) generally acceptable, appropriate, and safe?

a. Angina, vasospastic ("variant"; Prinzmetal's)
b. Asthma
c. Bradycardia
d. Diabetes mellitus, insulin-dependent and poorly controlled
e. Heart block (second degree or greater)
f. Hyperthyroidism, symptomatic and acute
g. Severe congestive heart failure

68. A patient presents in the Emergency Department in great distress and with the following signs and symptoms:

bizarre behavior, delirium
facial flushing
clear lungs, no wheezing, rales, etc.
high heart rate
absence of bowel sounds
distended abdomen, full bladder
hot, dry skin
absence of lacrimal, salivary secretions
very high fever
dilated pupils that do not respond to light

Identify the drug class that was responsible.

a. AChE inhibitors
b. α-adrenergic blockers
c. Antimuscarinics
d. β-adrenergic blockers
e. Parasympathomimetics (muscarinic agonists)
f. Peripherally acting (neuronal) catecholamine depletors

69. Acebutolol and pindolol are classified as β blockers with *intrinsic sympathomimetic activity*. This means that they:

a. Are partial agonists (mixed agonist/antagonists)
b. Cause norepinephrine and epinephrine release
c. Induce catecholamine synthesis
d. Potentiate the actions of norepinephrine on α-adrenergic receptors
e. Would exert no effects if, somehow, we could completely deplete all the catecholamines in the body

70. A 10-year-old boy displays hyperactivity and is unable to focus on his schoolwork because of an inability to focus on the activity. Which of the following drugs might prove effective for relieving the boy's main symptoms?

a. Methylphenidate
b. Terbutaline
c. Dobutamine
d. Pancuronium
e. Prazosin
f. Scopalamine

71. We administer hexamethonium to a subject. He is in the supine position. Which of the following responses would you expect in response to this drug?

a. Bradycardia
b. Increased GI tract motility, possible spontaneous defecation
c. Increased salivary secretions
d. Miosis
e. Vasodilation

72. Which class of drug can mask one of the major symptoms of hypoglycemia in a person with diabetes mellitus?

a. α-adrenergic agonist
b. α-adrenergic antagonist
c. β-adrenergic agonist
d. β-adrenergic antagonist
e. Cholinergic agonist
f. Cholinergic antagonist

73. A patient with chronic open-angle glaucoma is treated with a topical ophthalmic β blocker. Which of the following is the most likely mechanism by which this drug lowers intraocular pressure?

a. Decreasing aqueous humor synthesis/secretion
b. Contracting the iris dilator muscles
c. Dilating the uveoscleral veins
d. Directly opening the trabecular meshwork
e. Contracting the circular pupillary constrictor muscle

Questions 74–75

For each numbered item, select the letter representing the drug that was given to the subject.

a. Baclofen
b. Doxazosin
c. Mivacurium
d. Phentolamine
e. Propantheline
f. Scopolamine
g. Timolol

74. A 65-year-old man complains of losing his vision. Retinal examination reveals optic nerve cupping. Peripheral vision loss is observed on visual field tests, and his intraocular pressure is increased. Following treatment with the drug, he has improved visual acuity and decreased intraocular pressure.

75. A 30-year-old woman is being prepared for anesthesia before exploratory surgery for a mass in her neck. In addition to using an inhalation anesthetic, we give a drug that causes complete paralysis of the skeletal muscles.

76. To facilitate or ease learning about the autonomic nervous system (or most other things), it's sometimes helpful to identify a generally applicable "rule" and then learn the one or two main exceptions to it. So: sympathetic innervation of which structure is the exception to the general rule that "all postganglionic sympathetic nerves are adrenergic?"

a. Arterioles in the skin
b. Arterioles in the viscera
c. Radial muscle in the iris of the eye
d. Sinoatrial node of the heart
e. Sweat glands

77. A patient with a history of asthma experiences significant bronchoconstriction and urticaria, and histamine is a main mediator in these responses. Which of the following drugs may pose extra risks for this patient—not because it has any bronchoconstrictor effects in its own right, but because it quite effectively releases histamine from mast cells?

a. Atropine
b. Isoproterenol
c. Neostigmine
d. Pancuronium
e. Propranolol
f. *d*-tubocurarine

78. A patient receives a single injection of succinylcholine to facilitate an endoscopic procedure. The dose is correct for the vast majority of patients, and normally effects of this drug abate spontaneously over a couple of minutes. This gentleman remains apneic for an extraordinarily long time. A genetically based aberrant cholinesterase is eventually determined to be the cause. What would we administer if we were concerned about this unusually lengthy drug response?

a. Atropine
b. Bethanechol
c. Neostigmine
d. Nothing
e. Physostigmine
f. Tubocurarine

79. We administer an "effective" dose of a drug and observe the following responses

Stimulates the heart
Dilates some blood vessels but constricts none
Dilates the bronchi
Raises blood glucose levels
Neither dilates nor constricts the pupil of the eye

Which of the following drug caused these responses?

a. Atropine
b. Epinephrine
c. Isoproterenol
d. Norepinephrine
e. Phenylephrine

80. "First-generation" (older) histamine H_1 blockers such as diphenhydramine, phenothiazine antipsychotic drugs (e.g., chlorpromazine), and tricyclic antidepressants (e.g., imipramine) have pharmacologic actions, side effects, toxicities, and contraindications that are very similar to those of which of the following?

a. Atropine
b. Bethanechol
c. Isoproterenol
d. Neostigmine
e. Propranolol

81. Physostigmine is the antidote for poisoning with antimuscarinic drugs (e.g., atropine). Another AChE inhibitor, neostigmine, is not suitable. That is because neostigmine cannot overcome the adverse effects of the antimuscarinic drug in or on which of the following?

a. Central nervous system (e.g., the brain)
b. Exocrine glands
c. Heart
d. Skeletal muscle
e. Smooth muscle

Questions 82–84

For each patient, select the mechanism of action that is most likely associated with the named drug.

a. α-adrenergic activation (agonist)
b. β-adrenergic blockade
c. Calcium channel blockade
d. Histamine (H_1) receptor blockade
e. MAO inhibition
f. Muscarinic receptor blockade
g. Serotonin receptor blockade

82. A 26-year-old woman has a runny nose and itchy eyes from a bout with the common cold. Diphenhydramine provides symptomatic relief.

83. A 36-year-old man with essential hypertension has a resting blood pressure of 140/94 mmHg. We give metoprolol, and over a period of about two months his blood pressure falls to 130/86.

84. During the past year, a 38-year-old woman has become progressively depressed and now refuses to leave her house. Physical examination and blood chemistries are negative. She is given phenelzine, which diminishes her depression and enables her to leave her house.

85. You are volunteering in a hospital in a very poor part of the world. Their drug selection is limited. A patient presents with acute cardiac failure, for which your preferred drug is dobutamine, given intravenously. However, there is none available. Which other drug, or combination of drugs, would be a suitable alternative? (All these drugs are available in parenteral formulations.)

a. Dopamine (at a very high dose)
b. Ephedrine
c. Ephedrine plus propranolol
d. Norepinephrine plus phentolamine
e. Phenylephrine plus atropine

86. A patient presents with food poisoning that is attributed to botulism (*Botulinus* toxin poisoning). Which would be a correct characteristic, finding, or mechanism associated with this toxin?

a. Complete failure of all cholinergic neurotransmission
b. Favorable response to administration of pralidoxime
c. Impairment of parasympathetic, but not sympathetic, nervous system activation
d. Massive overstimulation of all structures having muscarinic cholinergic receptors
e. Selective paralysis of skeletal muscle

87. In general, structures that are affected by sympathetic activation respond to both sympathetic neural activation and to the hormonal component, epinephrine released from the adrenal medulla. Which structure/function is unique in that it responds to epinephrine, but not norepinephrine, and has no direct neural control?

a. Airway (tracheal, bronchiolar) smooth muscle: relaxation
b. Atrioventricular node: increased automaticity and conduction velocity
c. Coronary arteries: constriction
d. Iris of the eye: dilation (mydriasis)
e. Renal juxtaglomerular apparatus: renin release

Questions 88–94

The figure below shows some of the main elements of norepinephrine (NE) synthesis, release, actions, and other steps in adrenergic neurotransmission. Use it to refresh your memory so you can answer the next 7 items. Note that the effector (target) cell will have either an α-adrenergic receptor or a β-adrenergic receptor, not both, depending what the effector cell is.

Adrenergic Neuroeffector Junction

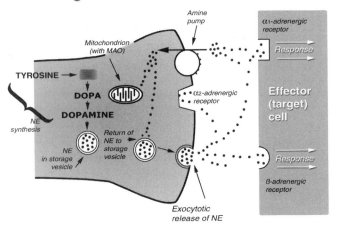

88. Which of the following is the main role of intraneuronal (mitochondrial) monoamine oxidase (MAO)?

a. To convert (metabolize) dopamine to NE
b. To facilitate exocytotic NE release
c. To metabolically degrade NE that is free in the nerve terminal
d. To provide metabolic energy for nonexocytotic (direct) release of NE in response to certain catecholamine-releasing drugs
e. To synthesize ATP that is required for postsynaptic effector (target) cell response to activation by NE

89. Which of the following prevents the entry of norepinephrine into neurotransmitter "storage vesicles" in adrenergic nerve endings?
a. Pargyline
b. Prazosin
c. Propranolol
d. Reserpine
e. Tyramine

90. We administer reserpine on a daily basis, at usual effective doses, for a time sufficient for the drug to exert its maximal and expected effects. Which would occur?
a. Accumulation of NE leading to excessive release and responses
b. Depletion of intraneuronal NE stores
c. Direct, nonexocytotic NE release
d. Inhibited NE synthesis
e. Subsensitivity of pre- and post-synaptic alpha-adrenergic receptors

91. We administer cocaine. In terms of how it affects processes sketched in the diagram above, which of the following would be the main action or effect?
a. Activation of α_2-adrenergic receptors leading to increased NE release
b. Blockade of NE reuptake by the amine pump
c. Dependent on what the postsynaptic effector cell is (i.e., muscle or gland, and type thereof)
d. Direct activation of postsynaptic adrenergic receptors, leading to a sympathomimetic response
e. Inhibition of MAO, leading to increased intraneuronal NE levels
f. Prevention of NE exocytosis

92. We administer a drug that is a selective agonist at the presynaptic alpha-receptors (α_2). The response is which of the following?
a. Activation of NE exocytosis
b. Activation of the amine pump, stimulation of NE reuptake
c. Dependent on what the postsynaptic effector cell is (i.e., muscle or gland, and type thereof)
d. Inhibition of NE release
e. Stimulation of intraneuronal MAO

93. Which would selectively block the postsynaptic α-adrenergic (α_1) receptors, but have no effect on presynaptic α-adrenergic receptors (α_2) or postsynaptic β-adrenergic receptors found on structures regulated by the sympathetic nervous system?

a. Ephedrine
b. Labetalol
c. Phentolamine
d. Phenylephrine
e. Prazosin

94. If we introduced amphetamine into the above system, which would occur?

a. Activation of MAO
b. Blockade of the amine pump
c. Displacement, release of neuronal NE
d. Enhanced NE synthesis
e. Neuronal stabilization via activation of α_2 receptors

95. The figure below shows several responses measured in a subject (healthy; receiving no other drugs) at rest and after receiving a dose of an unknown drug. Note: The blood pressures shown can be considered mean blood pressure; the fall caused by the unknown was mainly due to a fall of diastolic pressure.

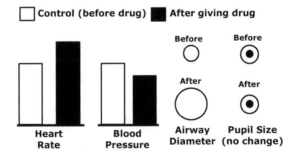

Which one of the following drug most likely caused the observed responses?
a. Atropine
b. Isoproterenol
c. Neostigmine
d. Phenylephrine
e. Propranolol

Questions 96–97

The following scenario applies to both questions. Note: the correct answers are based on solid pharmacologic principles; altered drug responses are not due to idiosyncrasy or any other unusual causes.

You have treated dozens of patients with acute hypotension from various causes, including overdoses of drugs that can cause hypotension. Your usual approach to restoring blood pressure, and one that has worked well every time, is to inject x mg of phenylephrine intravenously. Today a patient with severe drug-induced hypotension presents. He has been taking this drug for many months. You give the phenylephrine at the same dose and by the same route as you always have.

96. Phenylephrine causes no change of blood pressure. Which of the following drugs did the patient take and overdose on?
a. Atenolol
b. Bethanechol
c. Prazosin
d. Propranolol
e. Reserpine

97. Phenylephrine causes a vasopressor response that is far greater than you've ever encountered before using x mg of phenylephrine; systolic pressure rises dramatically, if not dangerously. Which of the following drugs did the patient take and overdose on?
a. Atenolol
b. Bethanechol
c. Prazosin
d. Propranolol
e. Reserpine

98. What property of edrophonium makes it the preferred agent for making the differential diagnosis between a myasthenic and a cholinergic crisis?

a. Crosses blood-brain barrier easily, directly activates respiration in medulla
b. Effects limited to skeletal muscle
c. Fast onset, very short duration
d. Has antimuscarinic (atropine-like) effects that eliminate parasympathetic side effects
e. Margin of safety (therapeutic index) so high that serious/fatal responses cannot occur

99. A patient received a single dose of succinylcholine for preoperative intubation. Skeletal muscle paralysis during a 3-h surgery is maintained by a long-acting nondepolarizing type (i.e., curare-like) neuromuscular blocker. Surgery is over and the plan is to reverse the skeletal muscle paralysis.

What adjunct is administered first to block unwanted effects of the reversing agent on smooth muscles and glands, and then what drug is used to actually reverse the skeletal muscle paralysis?

a. Atropine to control smooth muscle, cardiac, and gland responses, then neostigmine to reverse skeletal muscle paralysis
b. Belladonna alkaloids to block smooth muscle, cardiac, and gland responses, then pralidoxime to restore skeletal muscle function
c. β-blocker first to control cardiac responses, physostigmine for reversal
d. Epinephrine first to control smooth muscle and glands, acetylcholine to reactivate skeletal muscle
e. Physostigmine to control smooth muscles and glands, succinylcholine again for reversal

Autonomic Nervous System

Answers

40. The answer is d. (*Craig, pp 83–87; Hardman, pp 115–118, pp 129–135; Katzung, pp 75–76.*) Postganglionic sympathetic nerves to all structures innervated by the SNS, with the exception of those innervating sweat glands (see question 43), are adrenergic.

41. The answer is h. (*Craig, pp 338–340, 342–344; Hardman, pp 144–145, 196–200; Katzung, pp 75–76.*) Pancuronium and tubocurarine (as well as metocurine and several related drugs) are skeletal neuromuscular blockers. They specifically and competitively block activation of nicotinic receptors on skeletal muscle by ACh.

42. The answer is d. (*Craig, pp 89–92; Hardman, pp 134–135; Katzung, pp 75–76.*) The actions of norepinephrine are terminated as a result of neuronal reuptake, and only postganglionic sympathetic nerves to structures other than sweat glands (*d*) use NE as the neurotransmitter. All the other nerves shown in the diagram are cholinergic; the actions of the ACh they release are terminated promptly by hydrolysis (via acetylcholinesterase).

43. The answer is c. (*Craig, pp 83–84; Hardman, pp 116 overleaf, 120; Katzung, pp 75–76, 84–86.*) The postganglionic sympathetic fibers innervating sweat glands are cholinergic. That is the exception to the rule "all postganglionic sympathetic fibers are adrenergic."

44. The answer is c. (*Craig, pp 84, 92–93, 121–123; Hardman, pp 116 overleaf, 120; Katzung, pp 75–76, 87–86.*) The nerve is cholinergic, so the neurotransmitter it acts on, postsynaptically, must be either nicotinic or muscarinic. Nicotinic receptors are found on cell bodies of all postganglionic nerves (in both SNS and PNS), on the adrenal medulla, and on skeletal muscle (somatic nervous system). Cholinergic receptors at all other sites are muscarinic, "defined" by the fact that those receptors are competitively blocked by atropine.

45. The answer is g. (*Craig, p 93; Hardman, pp 116 overleaf, 129–140; Katzung, pp 76, 84–86.*) The neurotransmitter released from nerve d, the postganglionic sympathetic fibers (to structures other than sweat glands), is norepinephrine. NE can activate α-adrenergic receptors (both α_1 and α_2), and β_1 receptors (not β_2). Of course, different structures have different subtypes of adrenergic receptors; e.g., β_1s are found in the heart, while αs are found on such structures as arterioles and the iris dilator muscle. So, the only correct response to the question "which receptors are activated" really depends on which structure is being innervated.

46. The answer is c. (*Craig, p 93; Hardman, pp 119–120, 220–225; Katzung, p 129–130.*) Both the contractile and rhythmic effects of epinephrine on the heart are mediated through activation of β_1-adrenergic receptors. These receptor sites mediate an epinephrine-induced increased firing rate of the SA node (spontaneous, or Phase 4, depolarization), increased conduction velocity through the AV node and the His-Purkinje system, and increased contractility and conduction velocity of atrial and ventricular muscle. Epinephrine activation of α adrenoceptors does not affect cardiac function in any physiologically or therapeutically important way—except for the crucial role of α adrenoceptors as mediators of coronary artery vasoconstriction (clearly a vascular smooth muscle, not cardiac muscle, phenomenon). The β_2-adrenergic receptors play virtually no direct role in cardiac stimulation. They are more important in the relaxation of tracheobronchial smooth muscle, dilation of arterioles that serve skeletal muscles, increased secretion of insulin by the pancreas, and to a lesser degree relaxation of the detrusor of the urinary bladder. (Lipolysis in fat cells and melatonin secretion by the pineal gland appear to involve stimulation of β_3-adrenergic receptors. However, we do not have any clinically useful drugs that selectively activate or block the β_3 receptors, and so you might want to question how much you learn about the β_3s.)

47. The answer is b. (*Craig, p 130; Hardman, pp 176–189; Katzung, pp 101–104.*) Echothiophate iodide is a long-acting ("irreversible," which basically means "very long acting" in terms of the duration of clinical effects) acetylcholinesterase inhibitor. It is used topically on the eye for the treatment of various types of glaucoma. Maximum reduction of intraocular pressure occurs within 24 h, and the effect may persist for several days. The drug is water-soluble, which affords a practical advantage over the lipid-soluble isofluorphate (another cholinesterase inhibitor used to treat glaucoma). (Had we listed a drug with a generic name ending in the suffix "-stigmine," you no doubt would have answered correctly and immediately. However, echothiophate is one of those cholinesterase inhibitors that is not a stigmine. If you're unfamiliar with the drug—this one or any one as you work your way through the questions—by all means look it up!)

48. The answer is a. *(Craig, pp 138–139; Hardman, pp 163–167; Katzung, p 118.)* With any antimuscarinic drug—and scopolamine certainly is one—narrow-angle glaucoma (which accounts for only about 10% of all glaucomas) is the biggest concern. The drug might provoke significant rises of intraocular pressure as it further reduces aqueous humor drainage, causing not only pain but vision problems that might be severe or permanent. Bradycardia is not a concern; if anything, the scopolamine would increase heart rate a bit. Should the patient eat some bad shellfish, the diarrhea might be reduced or prevented altogether by the scopolamine. A resting blood pressure of 112/70 (or thereabouts) is not at all uncommon (wish mine were that, without drugs) or worrisome, and not likely to be changed at all by the drug. Hypothyroidism typically is associated with slight bradycardia; again, no envisaged problem with scopolamine. And if our patient had mild Parkinson's disease, we might actually, eventually, see a little improvement with this drug. Recall, one strategy to manage parkinsonism—basically a central imbalance between dopamine and ACh, is to block the muscarinic receptors (with such drugs as benztropine or trihexyphenidyl; see CNS chapter).

49. The answer is a. *(Craig, pp 113, 116–117; Hardman, p 255; Katzung, p 142.)* Labetalol is a competitive antagonist at both α- and β-adrenergic (both β_1 and β_2) receptors. This might help you remember that labetalol blocks both main types of adrenergic receptors: take the first two letters of the generic name and reverse them—*la* becomes *al,* as in *a*lpha—and then add the next four letters—beta. La(pha) + beta. (This trick will not help you remember the name of another important α/β blocker, carvedilol. Note, too, that the generic names of all the drugs listed end in *-olol.* Can you think of a major drug's generic name that ends in -olol and is *not* a β blocker? There isn't any. Might this help your learning?)

Labetalol's α-blocking actions are weak compared with actions at the β receptors. This relative difference is somewhat serum concentration-dependent: at relatively low serum levels, as might be achieved with typical oral doses, it is about three times more potent as a β blocker than as an α blocker (do not commit this to memory!). With higher serum concentrations, such as those often achieved with parenteral (e.g., IV) dosing, the intensity of β blockade increases considerably with little increase in α-blocking efficacy (another ultimately important point, but not priority knowledge now!). One of labetalol's main uses is for managing essential hypertension (all the orally administered β blockers are indicated for essential hypertension, and most are indicated for chronic-stable angina). Given parenterally (IV), it is often a first-choice agent for managing urgent hypertensive crises when more efficacious (and potentially more dangerous) IV drugs aren't indicated or cannot be given safely.

Metoprolol (and atenolol and acebutolol, not listed) have a preferential effect on β_1 receptors ("cardioselectivity") vs. β_2, and have no α-blocking actions. Nadolol and timolol are nonselective β blockers. (One property to remember for nadolol is its relatively long half-life; for timolol you might want to recall that a topical ophthalmic dosage form is often used for chronic open-angle glaucoma.) Pindolol has the property of ISA—intrinsic sympathomimetic activity.

50. The answer is d. (*Craig, p 94; Hardman, pp 137, 146, 242, 249; Katzung, pp 81, 84, 146, 189.*) Whether you memorize that yohimbine is a selective α_2 antagonist is up to you, but you should know what the main effects of an α_2 antagonist are. That, of course, depends on knowing what α_2 receptors—at least in the peripheral autonomic nervous system—do. Recall that the preponderance of physiologically important α_2 receptors are located on adrenergic nerve terminals or adrenergic nerve "endings." When stimulated by a suitable agonist, the response is a turning-off of further norepinephrine release. Because norepinephrine is the neurotransmitter released from adrenergic nerves and it is an excellent α agonist, the presynaptic α_2 receptors upon which norepinephrine acts serve as the main physiologic mechanism for regulating neurotransmitter release.

So, when we activate those receptors with yohimbine, we enhance overall activity of the sympathetic nervous system by interfering with norepinephrine's ability to turn-off its own release. Of the responses listed, only hypertension (owing to the vasoconstrictor effects of norepinephrine on postsynaptic α-adrenergic receptors) occurs as a result of yohimbine (or of norepinephrine excess).

51. The answer is a. (*Craig, pp 128, 130, 371; Hardman, pp 186–189, 561; Katzung, pp 105, 1010–1011.*) Patients with Alzheimer's disease present with progressive impairment of memory and cognitive functions such as a lack of attention, disturbed language function, and an inability to complete common tasks. Although the exact defect in the central nervous system (CNS) has not been elucidated, evidence suggests that a reduction in cholinergic nerve function is largely responsible for the symptoms.

Tacrine has been found to be somewhat effective in patients with mild-to-moderate symptoms of this disease for improvement of cognitive functions. The drug is primarily a reversible cholinesterase inhibitor that increases the concentration of functional ACh in the brain. However, the pharmacology of tacrine is complex; the drug also acts as a muscarinic receptor modulator in that it has partial agonistic activity, as well as weak antagonistic activity on muscarinic receptors in the CNS. In addition, tacrine appears to enhance the release of ACh from cholinergic nerves, and it may alter the concentrations of other neurotransmitters such as dopamine and NE.

Of all of the reversible cholinesterase inhibitors, only tacrine and physostigmine cross the blood-brain barrier in sufficient amounts to make these compounds useful for disorders involving the CNS. Physostigmine has been tried as a therapy for Alzheimer's disease; however, it is more commonly used to antagonize the effects of toxic concentrations of drugs with antimuscarinic properties, including atropine, antihistamines, phenothiazines, and tricyclic antidepressants. Neostigmine, pyridostigmine, and ambenonium are used mainly in the treatment of myasthenia gravis; edrophonium is useful for the diagnosis of this disease.

52. The answer is d. (*Craig, pp 85, 92, 142–144; Hardman, pp 208–211; Katzung, pp 97, 106.*) Nicotine is a drug that initially stimulates and then blocks nicotinic muscular (NM) (skeletal muscle) and nicotinic neural (NN) (parasympathetic ganglia) cholinergic receptors. Blockade of the sympathetic division of the autonomic nervous system (ANS) results in arteriolar vasodilation, bradycardia, and hypotension. Blockade at the neuromuscular junction leads to muscle weakness and respiratory depression caused by interference with the function of the diaphragm and intercostal muscles. Atropine, a muscarinic receptor blocker, would be an effective antagonist, as would neostigmine, a cholinesterase inhibitor. Pilocarpine and isofluorphate are cholinomimetics and can be antagonized by atropine; the effects of tubocurarine can be inhibited by neostigmine. Diazoxide, a vasodilator, would cause tachycardia, rather than bradycardia.

53. The answer is e. *(Craig, p 720; Hardman, pp 231, 860; Katzung, pp 135, 138.)* Ritodrine hydrochloride is a selective β_2-adrenergic agonist that relaxes uterine smooth muscle. It also has the other effects attributable to β-adrenergic receptor stimulants, such as bronchodilation, cardiac stimulation, enhanced renin secretion, and hyperglycemia.

54. The answer is a. *(Craig, pp 93, 123–126; Hardman, pp 157–161; Katzung, pp 98–100.)* These are expected side effects from bethanechol, which is a muscarinic agonist (parasympathomimetic drug). They occur even though the effects of the drug—the ones for which the drug is given—are "predominately" on the bladder musculature. These effects are common, not at all an idiosyncratic reaction. Bethanechol has no sympathetic (or parasympathetic) ganglionic blocking actions. If the patient had undiagnosed asthma (and the presence of asthma would contraindicate use of the drug), the pulmonary response would be much more significant than "some wheezing." Potentially fatal bronchospasm could occur, because the airway smooth muscles of asthmatic individuals are exquisitely (hyper)sensitive to muscarinic agonists, with even small doses of those drugs capable of causing a lethal outcome.

55. The answer is c. *(Craig, pp 115–117; Hardman, pp 250–253, 257–258, 1834–1836; Katzung, pp 148–154, 157.)* The chief danger of therapy with β-adrenergic blocking agents, such as nadolol and propranolol, is associated with the blockade itself. β-adrenergic blockade results in an increase in airway resistance that can be fatal in asthmatic patients. Hypersensitivity reactions such as rash, fever, and purpura are rare and necessitate discontinuation of therapy.

56. The answer is a. *(Craig, p 115; Hardman, pp 254, 260, 1834–1836; Katzung, pp 156.)* When applied topically to the eye, both the direct-acting cholinomimetic agents (e.g., pilocarpine) and those cholinomimetic drugs that act by inhibition of AChE (e.g., echothiophate, isofluorphate, and physostigmine) cause miosis by contracting the sphincter muscle of the iris and reducing ocular pressure by contracting the ciliary muscle. In patients with glaucoma, this latter effect permits greater drainage of the aqueous humor through the trabecular meshwork in the canal of Schlemm and a reduction in resistance to outflow of the aqueous humor. Certain β-adrenergic blocking agents (e.g., timolol and levobunolol) applied to the eye are also very useful in treating chronic wide-angle glaucoma. These drugs appear to act by decreasing the secretion (or formation) of the aqueous humor by antagonizing the effect of circulating catecholamines on β-adrenergic receptors in the ciliary epithelium.

57. The answer is d. *(Craig, pp 126–129, 131, 134–137; Hardman, pp 162–165, 184–185; Katzung, pp 102–103, 116–117.)* In "cholinesterase poisoning" we are dealing with overstimulation (from accumulated ACh) of both peripheral muscarinic and nicotinic receptors. Recall that atropine is a specific muscarinic receptor blocker, and the muscarinic receptors are the ones found on such structures as smooth muscle, cardiac nodal tissue, and exocrine glands. In contrast, the cholinergic receptor on skeletal muscle is nicotinic, so skeletal muscle isn't affected by atropine. If one receives a lethal dose of a cholinesterase inhibitor, he or she may be a little more comfortable (less defecation, urination, respiratory tract gurgling and constriction, and all that), but they are still likely to die from skeletal muscle (nicotinic) overstimulation and then fatigue and paralysis (of which paralysis of the diaphragm and intercostals muscles are the most lethal consequences).

58. The answer is g. *(Craig, pp 94, 234–235; Hardman, pp 143–145, 881–882; Katzung, pp 90, 167–170.)* You have learned about a very similar drug, reserpine, but probably haven't heard about guanadrel in particular. It is basically very much like reserpine, a prototypic slow-acting catecholamine depletor. By chemically "wiping out" the sympathetic nervous system parasympathetic influences (e.g., miosis, diarrhea, urination) predominate; arterioles dilate and blood pressure falls (because there's little/no norepinephrine to be released, because it's been depleted from the nerve endings), and heart rate does not increase reflexly because it can't (again, no norepinephrine to be released to stimulate the heart).

59. The answer is c. *(Craig, pp 138, 461, 464; Hardman, pp 168–169; Katzung, pp 115, 327–328.)* Ipratropium, a quaternary antimuscarinic drug, is FDA-approved for use as an inhaled bronchodilator for COPD. (It is used, but not FDA-approved for, some cases of asthma.) Albuterol certainly is an inhaled bronchodilator for asthma or COPD, but it works, of course, as a β_2-adrenergic agonist. Diphenhydramine has bronchodilator activity (by blocking both histamine H_1 and muscarinic receptors), but it is not given by inhalation; moreover, for ambulatory patients with asthma the mucus-thickening effects of muscarinic receptor blockade can do more harm than good. Pancuronium is a curare-like skeletal neuromuscular blocker (nicotinic/skeletal muscle competitive antagonist of ACh). Pilocarpine is a muscarinic agonist, used mainly for causing miosis in patients with angle-closure glaucoma. It will cause bronchoconstriction— an effect that may be harmful for patients with COPD and certainly would be harmful for asthmatics. A wide variety of clinical conditions are treated with antimuscarinic drugs. Dicyclomine hydrochloride and methscopolamine bromide are used to reduce GI motility, although side effects—dryness of the mouth, loss of visual accommodation, and difficulty in urination—may limit their acceptance by patients. Cyclopentolate hydrochloride is used in ophthalmology for its mydriatic and cycloplegic properties during refraction of the eye. Trihexyphenidyl hydrochloride is one of the important antimuscarinic compounds used in the treatment of parkinsonism. For bronchodilation in patients with bronchial asthma and other bronchospastic diseases, ipratropium bromide is used by inhalation. Systemic adverse reactions are low because the actions are largely confined to the mouth and airways.

60. The answer is a. *(Craig, pp 126–130, 347; Hardma, pp 176, 186–188; Katzung, pp 101–104.)* Although all of the listed compounds inhibit the activity of the cholinesterases, only edrophonium chloride is used in the diagnosis of myasthenia gravis. The drug has a more rapid onset of action (1 to 3 min following intravenous administration) and a shorter duration of action (approximately 5 to 10 min) than pyridostigmine bromide. It is more water-soluble than physostigmine salicylate and, therefore, produces no clinically significant adverse effects on the CNS.

Pyridostigmine bromide is used in the treatment of this muscle weakness disease. Physostigmine salicylate is indicated topically for the treatment of glaucomas and is also a valuable drug for treating toxicity of anticholinergic drugs such as atropine. Malathion is an anticholinesterase that is used topically for the treatment of head lice and is never used internally.

61. The answer is d. (*Craig, pp 334–335; Hardman, pp 240, 377–378; Katzung, p 137.*) There are several reasons for and outcomes of adding a vasoconstrictor (usually epinephrine) to some local anesthetics, including those given by infiltration. The vasoconstrictor confines the local anesthetic to the desired site of action (site of administration) by reducing local blood flow and the rate of anesthetic entry into the bloodstream. It is the bloodstream (or, more precisely, it is the presence of anesthetic in the systemic distribution system) that delivers the drug to sites where signs and symptoms of toxicity occur. Slow down anesthetic absorption rates and the drug will enter the circulation slowly enough that it can be metabolized (inactivated) fast enough to prevent accumulation to toxic levels. That is, we reduce the risk of systemic toxicity with added vasoconstrictor.

Another outcome of including a vasoconstrictor is to prolong (and certainly not shorten) the duration of local anesthetic effect. That occurs also because reduced local blood flow keeps the anesthetic in the vicinity of sensory nerves longer (since the anesthetic is not being removed as quickly by blood flow).

More on this issue will be presented in the CNS questions. But for now: Local anesthetics (except cocaine) *can* cause vasodilation, but unless the dosages are quite high (toxic), the vasodilation is not intense; hypotension is uncommon with usual dosages. Likewise, cardiac depression can occur, but again that is a manifestation of overdose. We don't routinely include epinephrine in a local anesthetic to combat or prevent these problems, and the amount of epinephrine found in these preparations is far too low to do anything meaningful to remedy these adverse responses should they occur. Likewise, the amounts of vasoconstrictor are far too low to prevent (or treat) anesthetic-induced anaphylaxis—a reaction that requires only a few molecules of antigen to occur.

So what the vasoconstrictor does is essentially cause a pharmacologic tourniquet, reducing regional blood flow that otherwise would quickly "wash away" the anesthetic. This essentially confines the anesthetic to the desired site longer than otherwise, and decreases the potential systemic reactions. Some local anesthetics cause vasodilation, which allows more compound to escape the tissue and enter the blood. Procaine is an ester-type local anesthetic with a short duration of action due to rather rapid biotransformation in the plasma by cholinesterases. The duration of action of the drug during infiltration anesthesia is greatly increased by the addition of epinephrine, which reduces the vasodilation caused by procaine.

62. The answer is a. (*Craig, p 104; Hardman, pp 71, 240; Katzung, p 138.*) Epinephrine is the drug of choice to relieve the symptoms of an acute, systemic, immediate hypersensitivity reaction to an allergen (anaphylactic shock). Subcutaneous administration of a 1:1000 solution of epinephrine rapidly relieves itching and urticaria, and this may save the life of the patient when laryngeal edema and bronchospasm threaten suffocation and severe hypotension, and cardiac arrhythmias become life-endangering. Norepinephrine, isoproterenol, and atropine are ineffective therapies. Angioedema is responsive to antihistamines (e.g., diphenhydramine), but epinephrine is necessary in the event of a severe reaction.

63. The answer is a. (*Craig, pp 111–113; Hardman, pp 242–248; Katzung, pp 142–146.*) Both phentolamine and prazosin competitively block the postsynaptic (α_1) adrenergic receptors. Phentolamine, but not prazosin, also blocks α_2 (presynaptic) receptors.

[There are some other minor properties of phentolamine: it directly (via a nonadrenergic mechanism) relaxes arterioles, but that is not the main mechanism of its antihypertensive effects, and has some ability to block effects of serotonin and increase gastric acid and pepsin secretion in the stomach, neither of which provides a clinical use for the drug.]

Phentolamine, a parenteral drug, is used for acute hypertension, whether drug-induced or due to such pathologic processes as pheochromocytoma. The drug triggers significant reflex tachycardia, which poses major clinical problems. For that reason, and others, phenylephrine is being used less and less. When adrenergic blockade is indicated for rapid control of hypertension due to causes other than overdoses with a pure α agonist (e.g., phenylephrine), the combined α/β blocker labetalol is almost always used instead.

Prazosin, as you certainly know, is a selective α_1-adrenergic receptor blocker that, at therapeutic doses, has little activity at α_2-adrenergic receptors. and clinically insignificant direct vasodilating activity. This oral drug is usually selected as a second-line agent for managing essential hypertension or as an adjunct to managing pheochromocytoma long-term. Since prazosin has no appreciable α_2-blocking effects, it does not interfere with the ability of norepinephrine to suppress its own neuronal release. This is one of the reasons why reflex tachycardia is more severe and common with phentolamine than with prazosin.

64. The answer is e. *(Craig, p 105; Hardman, pp 228–229, 238–239; Katzung, pp 133, 136, 208–209.)* Dobutamine raises LV developed pressure by acting as a β_1-selective agonist, and that is the mechanism by which it causes its positive inotropic effect (and, to a lesser degree, positive chronotropy).

To be precise, the drug is a racemic mixture: the (+) isomer, which is a potent β_1 agonist that also has some α_1 antagonist effects; the (–) isomer is an efficacious and potent α_1 agonist. So, there are probably several ways that we might classify the drug.

Nonetheless, when the drug is used for acute heart failure the intent of its use—and, indeed the main mechanism by which it does what we want—is to activate β_1 receptors. The positive inotropic and chronotropic effects raise myocardial oxygen demand, which may be problematic for patients with ischemic heart disease. On occasion, the drug may cause significant increase of blood pressure, mainly through α-mediated vasoconstriction. That is a dose-dependent phenomenon; the cardiac stimulant effects persist after the dose is dropped. Dobutamine is used clinically as a β_1-selective agonist. It is useful in CHF because of its ability to increase cardiac output while causing a decrease in ventricular filling pressure. It may not benefit patients with ischemic heart disease because it tends to increase heart rate and myocardial oxygen demand.

65. The answer is c. *(Craig, pp 100–102; Hardman, pp 221–222, 228; Katzung, pp 129–131.)* Recall that pulse pressure is the difference between systolic and diastolic pressures. Epinephrine's β_1 activity increases left ventricular pressure development, which leads to an increase in peak systolic arterial pressure. Its peripheral vasoconstricting effect (in some vascular beds), mediated by α-agonist activity, increases systolic pressure further. However, the drug also causes dilation in some other peripheral vascular beds (e.g., large arterioles in the extremities). This occurs via β_2 activation and tends to lower diastolic pressure (under the conditions we described). So, pulse pressure is increased by the epinephrine.

66. The answer is b. (*Craig, pp 90–92; Hardman, pp 134–135; Katzung, pp 81–83.*) Norepinephrine (and other monoamine neurotransmitters such as dopamine) is removed from its receptors by an "amine pump" located in the neuronal membrane. Recall that this process can be blocked by (among other drugs) cocaine and tricyclic antidepressants. (You might ask "what about 'stimulation' of presynaptic α_2 receptors?" Well, that answer might work, but it wasn't one of the choices here. Moreover, presynaptic α_2 receptor activation only inhibits release of additional NE; it does not stop the effects of NE that has already been released.)

Catechol-O-methyltransferase (COMT), and to a greater degree monoamine oxidase (MAO), are enzymes responsible for metabolic degradation of norepinephrine. However, they are not important in terminating the actions of released norepinephrine to the extent that they account for the physiologic "turning-off" of norepinephrine's actions.

67. The answer is f. (*Craig, pp 113–117; Hardman, pp 249–253, 257–261; Katzung, pp 154–156.*) The tachycardia associated with symptomatic, untreated hyperthyroidism reflects to a great degree thyroid hormone-related hyperreactivity of β-adrenergic receptors to catecholamines. The untoward and potentially dangerous cardiac response can be managed, symptomatically, with a β blocker. Of the conditions listed, this is the only indication for propranolol or virtually any other β blocker; and the only one that is not likely to worsen some aspect of the current clinical presentation.

Recall from your studies of cardiovascular pharmacology that β blockers (particularly such ones as carvedilol, which also has α-blocking activity) now play important roles in managing congestive heart failure, so long as the degree of failure is not "severe" (i.e., so long as cardiac output/ejection fraction, or heart rate, are not so low that reducing them further could be life-threatening).

Recall, too, that even very small doses of a β blocker (even a topical β blocker that might be used for glaucoma, and even the so-called selective β_1 blockers such as atenolol or metoprolol) can prove lethal for some asthmatics.

β-blockers may pose significant problems for patients with severe, poorly controlled diabetes mellitus. They can, for example, prevent tachycardia that is one signal to the patient that blood glucose levels are too low, and they can delay the recovery of blood glucose levels following an episode of hypoglycemia. However, for many patients with mild and well-controlled diabetes (especially type 2), in such conditions as mild-to-moderate heart failure (and others), judicious use of a β blocker may provide more benefit than harm. Bradycardia or heart (A-V nodal) block can be worsened by any β blocker. Administration of any β blocker to a patient with second or third degree (complete) heart block can have devastating consequences.

68. The answer is c. *(Craig, p 138; Hardman, pp 167–168; Katzung, pp 116–117.)* These are among the classic signs and symptoms of atropine (antimuscarinic) poisoning. Although you may have not learned this this way, put a Lewis Carroll/Alice in Wonderland spin on what the main findings are. Maybe that will help your memory. The antimuscarinic drug-poisoning syndrome has the patient

red as a beet (characteristic facial flushing; a so-called "atropine flush");

dry as a bone (no exocrine gland secretions, no fecal or urinary output because bowel and bladder motility are inhibited);

hot as a furnace (profound fever; a CNS "problem" compounded by a lack of body heat loss normally afforded by sweating);

blind as a bat (paralysis of accommodation and dilated pupils do not respond to even very bright light);

mad as a hatter (CNS problems, including delirium).

You may never see true atropine poisoning. As you know, that prototype antimuscarinic is not used clinically that much, except in some particular specialties. However, you should realize that many common groups of drugs (see Question 80), some of which are available over-the-counter, exert strong antimuscarinic effects; the signs and symptoms of "atropine poisoning" are an important component of their overdose syndromes.

69. The answer is a. *(Craig, pp 113–114; Hardman, pp 253–256; Katzung, p 150, 153–154.)* The β blockers with intrinsic sympathomimetic activity (ISA) are partial agonists. At usual doses, and in the presence of low (e.g., resting) sympathetic tone, they act as weak agonists for β-adrenergic receptors. Under these conditions, then, they may actually but slightly increase such β-mediated responses as heart rate. However, while these drugs are occupying the β-adrenergic receptors, they simultaneously block (antagonize) the effects of more efficacious ("stronger") β agonists, e.g., epinephrine and norepinephrine. Thus, although they weakly increase resting heart rate, when catecholamine levels are high (as with stress, or exercise), such β-mediated responses as acceleration of heart rate are less intense than they would be had these drugs with ISA not been present. See Question 33 (in the General Principles section) for more information, because it was based on the effects of a β blocker with ISA/partial agonist activity.

70. The answer is a. *(Craig, pp 94, 106, 349–351; Hardman, pp 237, 241; Katzung, p 134, 139.)* Methylphenidate is similar to amphetamine and acts as a CNS stimulant, with more pronounced effects on mental than on motor activities. It is used to treat narcolepsy and attention-deficit hyperactivity disorders.

71. The answer is e. *(Craig, pp 141–142, 145–146; Hardman, pp 145, 196, 207–208, 210–211; Katzung, pp 118–120.)* Answering this question requires knowledge of two things: how hexamethonium is classified (what it does) and which branch of the autonomic nervous system, parasympathetic or sympathetic, exerts "predominant resting tone" over various structures and their functions. (If you have not specifically learned or read about hexamethonium, perhaps you know about largely similar ones, trimethaphan or mecamylamine. It's OK to consider them equivalent for the purpose of answering this question.)

Hexamethonium is an autonomic ganglionic blocking drug. So by blocking neurotransmission across all autonomic ganglia (and activation of the adrenal medulla), we essentially denervate distal structures. Now we observe how things change.

For the structures and functions listed (and several others that weren't), it is the parasympathetic nervous system that exerts the predominant resting tone. Only control of vascular smooth muscle tone (and, therefore, of blood pressure) is primarily regulated by the sympathetic nervous system.

Block the ganglia and vasodilation will occur as predominant SNS influences are removed. As far as the other structures go—all of which are mainly influenced by the PNS at rest—we would observe a rise of heart rate, decreases of bladder and gut tone (e.g. reduced tone of the bladder detrusor and longitudinal muscles of the gut), mydriasis, and reduced salivary secretions (xerostomia). Sweat gland secretions, which also have predominant sympathetic control, would decrease too.

72. The answer is d. *(Craig, p 116; Hardman, pp 257–258; Katzung, p 153.)* β-adrenergic antagonists should be used with caution in diabetic patients who are prone to hypoglycemia because β-adrenergic antagonists may mask the tachycardia that is one of several symptoms the diabetic can "use" to sense dangerous falls of blood glucose. The β blockers also inhibit hepatic glycogenolysis, and the mobilization of glucose, in response to hypoglycemia that is stimulated by catecholamines. There's also evidence that β blockers slow the recovery of blood glucose levels from hypoglycemic levels once the problem is detected and attempts to correct it are started.

73. The answer is a. (*Craig, pp 113–115; Hardman, pp 260, 1834–1837; Katzung, pp 151–152.*) The secretion of aqueous humor occurs in response to activating β-adrenergic receptors located on ciliary epithelia. β-adrenergic antagonists decrease secretory activity and lower intraocular pressure. Muscarinic agents induce contraction in the circular pupillary constrictor muscles. Ciliary muscle contraction facilitates opening of the trabecular meshwork, leading to better outflow of aqueous humor. α-adrenergic agonists cause contraction of the radially oriented pupillary dilator muscles.

74. The answer is g. (*Craig, pp 113–114; Hardman, pp 262–254; Katzung, p 152.*) Timolol is a nonselective (propranolol-like) β_1/β_2-adrenergic receptor antagonist. For ophthalmologic use it is given to lower intraocular pressure in patients with chronic open-angle glaucoma (presumably by decreasing production of aqueous humor).

75. The answer is c. (*Craig, pp 341–344; Hardman, pp 196–206; Katzung, pp 429–434.*) Mivacurium is a nondepolarizing neuromuscular blocking agent (same class as tubocurarine, atracurium, pancuronium, and several others). It and the related drugs are competitive antagonists of ACh at the nicotinic receptors at the myoneural junction of skeletal muscle. At therapeutic doses, these drugs can induce complete paralysis of skeletal muscles, unlike the weaker, centrally acting skeletal muscle relaxants (e.g., baclofen, diazepam, cyclobenzaprine), which reduce skeletal muscle spasm but do not completely block contractions. The primary therapeutic use of atracurium and other curariform drugs is as an adjunct in surgical anesthesia to relax the skeletal musculature and facilitate surgical manipulation.

76. The answer is e. (*Craig 11e, pp 84, 93; Hardman 10e, pp 116 overleaf, 118–119.*) By way of (essential) review of a point made earlier: sympathetic innervation of sweat glands involves postganglionic sympathetic nerves that are cholinergic, not adrenergic. We know that the neurotransmitter is ACh, and more specifically that they are muscarinic, because sweat gland activation can be competitively blocked by atropine or other drugs with antimuscarinic activity. We know that this innervation is part of the sympathetic nervous system because (1) sweating occurs as part of the sympathetic "fight or flight" response to stress; and (2) anatomically, the preganglionic cell bodies and the ganglia in the efferent pathway located at sites consistent with the rest of the sympathetic nerves [i.e., thoracic and lumbar origins, paravertebral ganglia].

77. The answer is f. (*Craig, p 343; Hardman, p 203; Katzung, p 438–439.*) Tubocurarine, arguably the prototypic nondepolarizing skeletal neuromuscular blocker (competitive antagonist of the effects of ACh on skeletal muscle nicotinic receptors), differs from most of the other nondepolarizing neuromuscular blockers (including pancuronium) because it quite effectively triggers histamine release. It is a "direct" effect on mast cells, not one involving activation of antibodies on the mast cells. This effect is not clinically significant for patients who do not have asthma, but for many who do, the bronchoconstriction can be problematic (even though the patient is intubated while they are receiving the blocker). In the absence of (released) histamine, curare and the other neuromuscular blockers would have no effect on airway smooth muscle activity.

Atropine causes bronchodilation by blocking muscarinic receptors on airway smooth muscle cells. Isoproterenol, the β_1/β_2 agonist, is a bronchodilator. Propranolol triggers airway smooth muscle contraction in asthmatics, but that is due to blockade of epinephrine's agonist (bronchodilator) actions on β_2 receptors. Histamine is not involved in the responses to any of these drugs.

78. The answer is d. (*Craig, p 342; Hardman, pp 203, 205; Katzung, p 433.*) While this may seem like a trick question, the point is that even with markedly deficient cholinesterase activity, the succinylcholine eventually will be metabolized and its effects will disappear. All that needs to be done is to maintain adequate mechanical ventilatory support.

Succinylcholine exerts its effects by activating nicotinic receptors on skeletal muscle (powerfully but normally briefly, owing to prompt metabolism) and depolarizing the myocytes. Atropine will not work. It blocks only muscarinic receptors. Bethanechol is a muscarinic agonist. Although it may have some nicotinic activating actions at extraordinarily high doses, that effect would add to, not resolve, the effects of the succinylcholine. Some texts note that under some conditions succinylcholine can cause what is termed Phase II block: a type of neuromuscular blockade that is curare-like (i.e., nondepolarizing).

Because nondepolarizing blockade can be (and is, clinically) reversed with acetylcholinesterase inhibitors (mainly neostigmine; physostigmine would work but is not used because of its CNS effects), the implication is that we could administer a cholinesterase inhibitor here and reverse the paralysis. However, this so-called Phase II block is a manifestation of excessive (toxic) doses of succinylcholine and is not likely to apply here. Regardless, the approach is to give nothing and to ventilate the patient as long as needed, as noted above.

79. The answer is c. (*Craig, pp 93, 102; Hardman, pp 118–119, 221–222, 228; Katzung, pp 128–131.*) Piece things together. Some tip-offs to help arrive at the correct answer: no effect on the size of the pupil, so rule out any drug that has effects on the "parasympathetic" side, whether as an agonist or antagonist (here, atropine), and rule out any drug with α effects. (As noted above, no β receptors control the size of the pupil of the eye.)

Does isoproterenol fit all the other criteria/properties? Yes. And none of the other choices have *all* the stated properties, only some of them.

80. The answer is a. (*Craig, p 138; Hardman, pp 164–167, 452–455, 487–490, 657; Katzung, pp 109–115.*) These drugs all possess antimuscarinic (atropine-like) actions that often are sufficiently strong to cause all the side effects and adverse responses associated with atropine itself. Likewise, it is prudent to assume they share all the contraindications and precautions associated with atropine and that managing severe overdoses of those drugs or drug groups will resemble (and need to be treated) in quite the same way as those of the prototype antimuscarinic. That would include the potential need to administer physostigmine, the acetyl-cholinesterase inhibitor that plays an important role in managing atropine poisoning.

Note that of all the drugs with atropine-like actions, diphenhydramine (and, to a somewhat lesser extent the other first generation antihistamines) are available over-the-counter. Although you may do your best to avoid pre-scribing drugs with atropine-like actions for patients who should not receive them, atropine-like problems can arise in patients who self-prescribe these nonprescription medications.

Clearly, the effects of bethanechol (muscarinic agonist) and neostigmine (acetylcholinesterase inhibitor) are the opposite of those you'd expect to see with atropine (muscarinic receptor blocker). You might argue that isoproterenol (β_1 and β_2 agonist) causes some effects (e.g., tachycardia) that you would expect with atropine. True. However, despite any similarities in appearance, the mechanism is quite different, the spectrum of all effects caused by the drug is different, and certainly most contraindications and toxic manifestations are very different. Propranolol (prototype nonselective β blocker) is radically different from atropine in nearly every important way.

81. The answer is a. *(Craig, pp 126–131; Hardman, pp 168, 175, 183, 188; Katzung, pp 101–104.)* Physostigmine is basically the only clinically useful AChE inhibitor that gets into the brain, a major target of atropine/antimuscarinic poisoning. That is because it lacks the quaternary (charged at virtually all pH values likely to be found in the a living person, outside of the stomach) structure that nearly all the other common alternatives possess, and lacking that structure it can cross the blood-brain barrier.

Alternatives such as neostigmine, pyridostigmine, and others will combat peripheral effects of atropine poisoning, just as physostigmine will. Unfortunately, some of the CNS manifestations (e.g., severe fever, leading to seizures) contribute greatly to the morbidity and mortality associated with high does of antimuscarinics, and the quaternary agents simply will not combat them in the CNS.

By the way, basically the only clinical use for physostigmine is for managing atropine/antimuscarinic poisoning. You won't encounter too many patients overdosed on atropine itself, but you'll see many poisoned with older antihistamines (e.g., diphenhydramine), older (tricyclic or tetracyclic) antidepressants (e.g., imipramine), some of the centrally acting antimuscarinics that are used for parkinsonism (e.g., benztropine and trihexyphenidyl); scopolamine (used for motion sickness), and most of the phenothiazine antipsychotics (e.g., chlorpromazine). Owing to the often strong antimuscarinic side effects of these drugs, treating overdoses of any of them probably will involve managing what amounts to "atropine poisoning"—and many other problems too.

(You may not know this, and perhaps it will have some meaning or help jog your memory: the trade name for physostigmine is Antilirium. Recall that one of the hallmark CNS signs of atropine/antimuscarinic poisoning is delirium. Hence, anti-lirium.)

82. The answer is f. (*Craig, pp 138t, 453–455; Hardman, pp 652–653; Katzung, pp 109, 266.*) You may have chosen e (histamine H_1 receptor blocker) to answer this question. You are correct in identifying diphenhydramine as a member of that class of drugs. However, histamine plays a minor role in the symptoms of rhinovirus infections. The drying up of nasal secretions afforded by diphenhydramine in this instance is due to the drug's rather intense muscarinic receptor-blocking actions.

83. The answer is b. (*Craig, pp 114–115, 227, 232–233; Hardman, pp 652–653; Katzung, pp 148–150, 153, 171.*) Metoprolol preferentially blocks β_1-adrenergic receptors. It lowers blood pressure primarily by decreasing peak left ventricular systolic pressure development, but also inhibits renin release. Both effects involve β_1 blockade. All other β blockers except those that have α-blocking activity (labetalol, carvedilol) lower blood pressure by this β_1-related action, even those with β_2-blocking activity (e.g., propranolol, many others).

84. The answer is e. (*Craig, pp 94t, 391–393; Hardman, pp 452, 462, 472; Katzung, pp 483 ,492, 494.*) Most MAOIs are nonselective for MAO-A and -B. MAOIs mainly act on tissues regulated by or that synthesize sympathomimetic amines and serotonin. MAO-B is more or less selectively inhibited by such drugs as selegiline, which is indicated for management of Parkinson's disease.

85. The answer is d. (*Craig, pp 101–102, 112t; Hardman, p 228; Katzung, pp 136–137, 212–213.*) Dobutamine behaves, for all practical purposes, as a selective β_1 agonist. Norepinephrine is a β_1 agonist that also activates α-adrenergic receptors effectively. However, when it is administered with phentolamine (prototype α blocker) its spectrum of activity is, qualitatively, identical to that of dobutamine.

High doses of dopamine cause positive inotropic and chronotropic effects, but also release neuronal norepinephrine and probably activate α-adrenergic receptors directly (causing unwanted vasoconstriction). These vasoconstrictor effects would negate vasodilator effects due to stimulation of dopamine D_1 receptors found in some arterioles, and of D_2 receptors found on some ganglia, and in the cardiovascular control center of the CNS.

Ephedrine weakly activates all adrenergic receptors and also leads to norepinephrine release. Overall, its effects are quite similar to those produced by norepinephrine itself. Regardless, if one administers ephedrine with propranolol, the prototypic nonselective (β_1 and β_2) beta blocker, ephedrine's remaining actions amount to selective α-adrenergic activation (i.e., phenylephrine-like)—not at all like dobutamine.

Phenylephrine (α agonist) plus atropine (muscarinic antagonist) causes effects that in no way resemble those of dobutamine or the norepinephrine-phentolamine combination.

86. The answer is a. (*Craig, pp 67t, 94t, 340–341; Hardman, pp 143–144; Katzung, p 90.*) Botulinus (botulinum) toxin prevents release of acetylcholine (from storage vesicles) by virtually all cholinergic nerves. Thus, there is no activation of any cholinergic receptors, whether nicotinic or muscarinic. Noteworthy findings, then, include an inability to activate all postganglionic neurons (sympathetic and parasympathetic), no physiologic release of epinephrine from the adrenal medulla, and flaccid skeletal muscle paralysis due to failure of ACh release from motor nerves. The cause of death is ventilatory failure because the intercostals muscles and diaphragm are nonfunctional.

Pralidoxime is a cholinesterase reactivator, an antidote for poisonings with "irreversible" cholinesterase inhibitors such as soman, sarin ("nerve gases"), and many organophosphorus insecticides. Because no ACh is being released in botulinus poisoning, "reactivation" of the enzyme that normally metabolizes the neurotransmitter is irrelevant (and ineffective).

87. The answer is a. (*Craig, pp 93, 103; Hardman, pp 118–119; Katzung, p 130.*) With only one major exception (sweat glands), the neurotransmitter released by postganglionic sympathetic nerves (adrenergic nerves) to activate their targets is norepinephrine (NE). Of course, NE is a "good" agonist for only α- and β_1-adrenergic receptors. In contrast, epinephrine (from the adrenal medulla) is a good agonist for both classes of adrenergic receptors and their main subtypes, including β_2. Of the responses listed in the question, only airway smooth-muscle relaxation is a process that involves (depends on) activation of β_2-adrenergic receptors. There is no innervation of these muscles, and so no NE to be released. Even if NE were injected, its lack of β_2 agonist activity would render it ineffective as a bronchodilator.

88. The answer is c. (*Craig, pp 89–92; Hardman, pp 132–135, 144–145; Katzung, pp 81–82, 90.*) While mitochondria in virtually all cells in which they are found are important for oxidative phosphorylation and ATP synthesis, we asked about the MAO that is rich in adrenergic neurons. There MAO will degrade NE that is free (i.e., not safely stored away) in the storage vesicles. If that intravesicular uptake is inhibited, NE stores will be depleted.

89. The answer is d. (*Craig 11e, pp 89–92; Hardman 10e, pp 132–135, 144–145; Katzung 9e, pp 81–82, 90.*) Reserpine blocks intraneuronal storage of NE, thereby exposing the free NE to degradation by MAO. Pargyline is a MAO inhibitor. Prazosin and propranolol are adrenergic receptor blockers (α_1 and β, respectively) and have no direct effect on NE storage. Tyramine is an indirect-acting sympathomimetic that releases neuronal NE via a process that does not involve exocytosis.

90. The answer is b. (*Craig, pp 89–92, 94; Hardman, pp 132–135, 144–145; Katzung, pp 81–90.*) Reserpine blocks NE entry into the storage vesicles, rendering the neurotransmitter vulnerable to inactivation by MAO. Ultimately, neuronal NE stores are depleted. Because physiologic activation of postsynaptic structures depends on NE release, and in reserpine-treated individuals the amount of NE available for release is diminished, it appears as if the overall activity of the sympathetic nervous system has been "ratcheted down"—and normally opposing parasympathetic influences become unmasked and predominate.

We should note that concomitant with NE depletion and reduced physiologic stimulation of adrenergic receptors (due to diminished NE release), the postsynaptic adrenergic receptors become supersensitive (not subsensitive) because of what amounts to chemical denervation. Those receptors will have heightened responses (in terms of intensity) to a given dose of an exogenous α or β agonist.

91. The answer is b. (*Craig, pp 89–92, 94, 407; Hardman, pp 132–135, 144–145; Katzung, pp 81, 90.*) Cocaine and tricyclic antidepressants are classic examples of drugs that inhibit NE reuptake by the amine pump, which is the main process by which released NE re-enters the neuron. In the presence of cocaine or a tricyclic, released NE lingers and accumulates in the synapse (neuroeffector junction), and so pertinent adrenergic responses appear heightened or more intense, and prolonged. Provided an adrenergic nerve is present (as it is in the diagram), the effects of cocaine or a tricyclic antidepressant are not affected by or dependent on whether the effector (target) is smooth muscle, cardiac muscle, or an exocrine gland of any sort.

There is no direct functional link between the amine pump and such processes as NE release (exocytotically or otherwise) or activation of presynaptic (α_2) adrenergic receptors.

92. The answer is d. *(Craig, pp 235–237; Hardman, pp 132–135, 144–145; Katzung, pp 81–90, 125, 134, 165–167.)* The adrenergic neuronal α_2 receptor, when activated by a suitable agonist, signals the neuron to stop further NE release. Norepinephrine itself is one such agonist; its activation of the presynaptic α_2 receptor [which occurs concomitant with activation of postsynaptic (α_1 or β_1) adrenergic receptors] provides the physiologic "feedback" signal that halts further NE release. That is, released NE regulates the release of more NE from the very neuron from which the neurotransmitter came.

Although activation of both the presynaptic α_2 receptors and NE reuptake by the amine pump occur simultaneously, there is no direct functional linkage between the two. That is, activating (or blocking) the α_2 receptor will not directly affect NE reuptake, nor will drugs that affect the amine pump necessarily have any effect on the α_2 receptors and the function they serve.

93. The answer is e. *(Craig, pp 111–113, 231; Hardman, pp 144–145, 246–247; Katzung, p 172.)* Prazosin selectively blocks α_1 adrenergic receptors and, unlike many other α-blockers (phentolamine, phenoxybenzamine) has virtually no presynaptic effects. None of the other drugs fit the bill: epinephrine, strong agonist for all adrenergic receptors; labetalol, (α/β blocker, nonselective); and phenylephrine is a strong agonist for all (α-adrenergic receptors).

94. The answer is c. *(Craig, pp 105–106, 349–351; Hardman, pp 133, 203–204; Katzung, pp 81–90.)* Amphetamines can be classified as indirect-acting sympathomimetics. They are taken into the adrenergic nerve ending by the amine pump and then displace NE from its storage vesicles and cause the neurotransmitter to be released into the synaptic space where all the expected effects of NE ultimately occur.

95. The answer is b. *(Craig, p 93; Katzung, pp 86, 129–131.)* To me, the tip-off that helps get to the correct answer is to focus (no pun intended) on the fact that the unknown drug did not change the size of the pupil of the eye. (See Question 95 also.) Of all the main autonomic receptors, adrenergic and cholinergic, only the β receptors play no role in regulating the size of the pupil. That narrows things down to isoproterenol or propranolol. Propranolol might lower BP (particularly in a hypertensive patient), but it would not raise heart rate or dilate the bronchi. Only isoproterenol fits the bill.

And the other answers? Atropine might raise heart rate, it is not likely to lower BP, it will dilate the airways, but it would also cause mydriasis. Neostigmine would slow heart rate, maybe lower BP (probably not), and constrict the airways and pupils. Phenylephrine would raise BP, and if the BP rise is sufficiently high and quick, reflexly lower heart rate. It would do nothing to airway diameter, but would cause mydriasis.

96. The answer is c. *(Craig, pp 105, 111–113; Katzung, pp 122–124, 130–131, 142–145.)* Phenylephrine raises blood pressure by activating α-adrenergic receptors on vascular smooth-muscle cells. Prazosin competitively blocks those receptors, and when present at sufficiently high doses (as might occur with an acute, severe overdose) may eliminate the vasopressor response to even higher than usual doses of phenylephrine. β blockers (atenolol, propranolol) have no α-blocking activity and so won't reduce the vasopressor response to phenylephrine. Nor will bethanechol, which causes vasodilation by activating muscarinic receptors for ACh. And reserpine? See the answer to question 111.

97. The answer is e. *(Craig, pp 94, 97; Hardman, pp 123, 132t, 204, 791–792; Katzung, p 89.)* Reserpine treatment of sufficient duration depletes neuronal norepinephrine. This accounts for the lowered blood pressure with therapeutic doses or frank hypotension with overdoses. One consequence of this, long-term, is development of adrenergic receptor supersensitivity because the receptors just aren't being activated as they should. And a consequence of that, in turn, will be heightened (and sometimes extreme) responses to a given dose of adrenergic agonists that can activate adrenergic receptors (α or β) directly, including the phenylephrine you administered. (That is, the dose-response curve for direct-acting adrenergic agonists is "shifted to the left" after long-term reserpine treatment.)

98. The answer is c. (*Craig, pp 126–130, 347; Hardman, pp 186–187; Katzung, pp 101–104.*) Edrophonium's actions occur quickly (so the diagnosis can be made quickly), and they are short-lived (so adverse effects, should they occur, will resolve spontaneously and quickly). Edrophonium does not cross the blood-brain barrier or directly activate ventilation centrally. Its effects are not at all limited to skeletal muscle: the drug inhibits metabolism and causes a synaptic build-up, of ACh wherever it is released by postganglionic cholinergic nerves and somatic motor nerves. Thus, and especially in patients who were experiencing a cholinergic crisis, all the effects typically associated with parasympathetic activation will occur, along with sweating (since innervation of sweat glands by the sympathetic nervous system involves ACh release by the postganglionic nerves). The drug has no intrinsic antimuscarinic activity to block or reduce these muscarinic responses. Regardless of what the drug's margin of safety may be (and we don't know or need to know), when it is given to a patient experiencing a cholinergic crisis one potential (and not at all rare) outcome is ventilatory arrest: intercostal muscles and the diaphragm, which are already overstimulated and "fatigued" with excess AChE inhibitor doses, are likely to cease functioning altogether—albeit briefly—when additional cholinesterase inhibitor is introduced through edrophonium administration.

99. The answer is a. (*Craig, p 137; Hardman, pp 150–153, 158; Katzung, p 440–441.*) Skeletal muscle paralysis from curare-like drugs involves competitive blockade of skeletal muscle nicotinic receptors. We reverse that by administering an ACh esterase inhibitor (e.g., neostigmine). Of course, the increased peripheral ACh levels will not only overcome skeletal muscle blockade, but also exert expected muscarinic-activating effects of various smooth muscles (e.g., the airways), the heart, and exocrine glands. We prevent those unwanted "parasympathomimetic" effects by giving atropine (antimuscarinic) right before giving the cholinesterase inhibitor. None of the other approaches are rational or used for "reversal."

Central Nervous System

Antidepressants and other mood-stabilizing drugs
Antiepileptics
Antiparkinson's
Antipsychotics
Anxiolytics
Central nervous system stimulants and anorexigenic agents
Ethanol and related alcohols
General anesthetics
Intravenous anesthetics and anesthesia adjuncts
Opioid analgesics and antagonists
Psychotomimetics
Sedatives, hypnotics

Questions

DIRECTIONS: Each item contains a question or incomplete statement that is followed by possible responses. Select the **one best** response to each question.

100. A person who was physically dependent on and an abuser of heroin is now maintained on methadone. He succumbs to temptation and buys an opioid on the street. He takes it and rapidly goes into withdrawal. Which of the following drugs did he take?

a. Meperidine
b. Heroin
c. Pentazocine
d. Codeine
e. Propoxyphene

101. A major problem that must be faced when administering anticonvulsants with many other medications (including other antiepileptic drugs) involves drug interactions due to altered metabolism. Which of the following drugs is likely to cause excessive or toxic effects from certain other drugs by inhibiting their metabolism?

a. Carbamazepine
b. Ethosuximide
c. Phenobarbital
d. Phenytoin
e. Valproic acid

102. Which of the following local anesthetics is useful for topical (surface) administration only?

a. Procaine
b. Bupivacaine
c. Etidocaine
d. Benzocaine
e. Lidocaine

103. A woman develops akathisia, a Parkinson-like syndrome, galactorrhea, and amenorrhea, during drug therapy. These responses reflect which of the following?

a. Blockade of muscarinic receptors
b. Blockade of α-adrenergic receptors
c. Blockade of dopamine receptors
d. Supersensitivity of dopamine receptors
e. Stimulation of nicotinic receptors

104. Diphenhydramine is prescribed as an adjunct to other drugs being used to manage a patient with Parkinson's disease. What is the main and most likely purpose of adding this drug?

a. To counteract sedation that is likely to be caused by the other medications
b. To help correct further the dopamine-ACh imbalance that accounts for parkinsonian signs and symptoms
c. To manage cutaneous allergic responses that are so common with "typical" antiparkinson drugs
d. To prevent the development of manic/hypomanic responses to other antiparkinson drugs
e. To reverse tardive dyskinesias if the parkinsonism was induced by an antipsychotic drug

105. Inhibitors of serotonin (5-HT) uptake, such as paroxetine, can cause clinically significant drug interactions with which of the following?

a. Diazepam
b. Digoxin
c. Halothane
d. Phenobarbital
e. Tranylcypromine

106. Which of the following antidepressants selectively inhibits neuronal serotonin (5-HT) reuptake and has minimal effect on the reuptake of norepinephrine or dopamine?

a. Bupropion
b. Fluoxetine
c. Imipramine
d. Maprotiline
e. Venlafaxine

107. A patient on the trauma-burn unit receives a drug to ease dressing changes. They experience good, prompt analgesia, but despite the absence of pain sensation their heart rate and blood pressure rise much as if the sympathetic nervous system were activated by painful responses. As the effects of the drug develop their skeletal muscle tone progressively increases. They appear awake at times because their eyes periodically open. As drug effects wear off they hallucinate and behave in a very agitated fashion. Which drug was given?

a. Fentanyl
b. Ketamine
c. Midazolam
d. Succinylcholine
e. Thiopental

108. A patient who has been treated with levodopa is switched to a regimen with a proprietary product that contains both levodopa and carbidopa. What is the main role of carbidopa in this approach?

a. Block ACh release in the CNS, thereby facilitating levodopa's ability to restore a dopamine-ACh balance
b. Help activate dietary vitamin B_6, a deficiency of which occurs during levodopa therapy
c. Increase permeability of the blood-brain barrier to levodopa, giving levodopa better access to the CNS
d. Inhibit metabolic conversion of levodopa to dopamine in the gut
e. Reduce levodopa-induced hypotension by blocking vascular dopamine receptors

109. Which of the following is a competitive benzodiazepine receptor antagonist?

a. Chlordiazepoxide
b. Flumazenil
c. Ketamine
d. Midazolam
e. Triazolam

110. There should be little argument that nowadays the only medically justified long-term use of phenobarbital is for managing which of the following conditions?

a. Alcohol withdrawal signs/symptoms
b. Anxiety management
c. Certain epilepsies
d. Endogenous depression (adjunct to SSRIs)
e. Sleep disorders such as insomnia

111. A patient develops status epilepticus. Which of the following is the best *first* IV drug to give?

a. Carbamazepine
b. Lorazepam
c. Phenobarbital
d. Phenytoin
e. Valproic acid

112. One reason for the declining use of tricyclic antidepressants is the prevalence of side effects or adverse responses, even with therapeutic serum levels. One of those "very common" side effects is due to which of the following?

a. Anticholinergic effects
b. Arrhythmias
c. Hepatotoxicity
d. Nephrotoxicity
e. Seizures

113. A patient is started on oral therapy with a drug, and dosages are increased incrementally by x mg in an attempt to control symptoms. Up to a point, each dosage increase of x mg leads to an approximately proportional increase in serum concentrations. We are now at a therapeutic serum level.

The next dosage increase of x mg raises the serum concentration by an amount that is far greater than what occurred with prior increases. The patient suddenly experiences signs and symptoms of toxicity (overdose).

The drug is stopped. Serial blood samples are taken to track the drug's elimination. Until serum concentrations fall below the therapeutic range, the data reveal zero-order elimination kinetics.

This description of unusual pharmacokinetics is typical of which of the following?

a. Chlorpromazine
b. Diazepam
c. Morphine
d. Phenobarbital
e. Phenytoin

114. Which of the following drugs is a selective inhibitor of monoamine oxidase type B (MAO-B) and is useful in treating some cases of parkinsonism?

a. Bromocriptine
b. Carbidopa
c. Phenelzine
d. Selegiline
e. Tranylcypromine

115. A patient with severe, acute trauma pain requires analgesia. The physician orders morphine. Which of the following coexisting conditions would pose the greatest risk from morphine's use in this case?

a. Acute pulmonary edema
b. Closed head injury
c. Compound fractures of both femurs
d. Hypertension
e. Opioid abuse, recent history of
f. Recent myocardial infarction

116. Meperidine is similar to morphine in many ways. However, with very high blood levels or with true overdoses, meperidine—but not morphine—can be expected to cause which of the following?

a. Constipation
b. Heightened response to pain
c. Intense biliary tract spasm
d. Miosis
e. Psychosis-like state, possibly seizures
f. Respiratory depression

117. Which of the following drugs specifically enhances the activity of brain dopamine by inhibiting the metabolic inactivation of dopamine?

a. Benztropine
b. Selegiline
c. Trihexyphenidyl
d. Bromocriptine
e. Chlorpromazine

118. Which of the following is a dopamine receptor *agonist* that is useful in the therapy of Parkinson's disease?

a. Selegiline
b. Bromocriptine
c. Apomorphine
d. Amantidine
e. Belladonna

119. Chlorpromazine is prescribed for a patient with schizophrenia. Which other signs/symptoms that the patient may also have might be beneficially affected by the drug?

a. Epilepsy
b. Hypotension
c. Nausea and vomiting
d. Urinary retention, as from prostatic hypertrophy
e. Xerostomia (dry mouth)

120. Morphine may be characterized best by which statement?
a. Is classified as a mixed agonist-antagonist drug
b. Used medically to inhibit withdrawal symptoms in persons who are dependent on heroin
c. High doses, it causes death by respiratory depression
d. Is a pure opioid antagonist at the μ, κ, and δ receptors
e. Has an addiction potential equal to that of codeine

121. Given the concern about cocaine abuse, and deaths from it, which of the following statements correctly characterizes this drug?
a. Produces bradycardia and vasodilation
b. Its central effects are effectively antagonized by naloxone
c. Is metabolized by the hepatic mixed-function oxidases
d. Blocks nerve conduction effectively
e. Blocks both α- and $β_1$-adrenergic receptors

122. Which of the following is a selective dopamine receptor (D_2) agonist?
a. Fluphenazine
b. Bromocriptine
c. Promethazine
d. Haloperidol
e. Chlorpromazine

123. In comparing side effects profiles of chlorpromazine and haloperidol, we find that haloperidol tends to cause or is associated with which of the following?
a. A higher incidence of extrapyramidal reactions
b. Intense atropine-like side effects
c. More frequent and lethal blood dyscrasias
d. More frequent orthostatic hypotension
e. Very slow onset of psychomotor symptom control

124. A 33-year-old woman patient treated with haloperidol for a history of schizophrenia is seen in the emergency department (ED) because of complaints of fever, stiffness, and tremor. Her temperature is 104°F, and her serum creatine kinase (CK) level is elevated. What has occurred?
a. Overdose
b. Allergy
c. Neuroleptic malignant syndrome (NMS)
d. Tardive dyskinesia
e. Parkinsonism

125. Phencyclidine (PCP) may best be characterized by which of the following statements?

a. It has opioid activity
b. Its mechanism of action is related to its anticholinergic properties
c. It can cause significant hallucinogenic activity
d. It causes significant withdrawal symptoms
e. Treatment of overdose is with an opiate

126. In comparing neuroleptics, which of the following is most likely associated with skeletal muscle rigidity, tremor at rest, flat facies, uncontrollable restlessness, and spastic torticollis?

a. Clozapine
b. Haloperidol
c. Olanzapine
d. Sertindole
e. Ziprasidone

127. In comparing neuroleptics, which of the following is most likely to cause constipation, urinary retention, blurred vision, and dry mouth?

a. Chlorpromazine
b. Clozapine
c. Haloperidol
d. Olanzapine
e. Sertindole

128. A patient exhibiting multiple facial tics, aggressive outbursts of behavior, and spontaneous repetitive foul language. This syndrome is managed appropriately with which of the following drugs?

a. Clozapine
b. Haloperidol
c. Levodopa
d. Thioridazine
e. Trazodone

129. After a few weeks on a drug, a patient reports profound thirst and the production of copious volumes of clear (dilute) urine each day. This is a fairly common, and unique, side effect of which of the following?

a. Diazepam
b. Fluoxetine
c. Haloperidol
d. Lithium
e. Phenytoin

130. You have a patient with severe postoperative pain who is not getting adequate analgesia from usually effective doses of morphine. The physician orders an immediate switch to a high dose of pentazocine. Which of the following is the most likely outcome?

a. Abrupt, added respiratory depression
b. Acute development of physical dependence
c. Coma
d. Seizures
e. Worsening of pain

131. A patient is on long-term methadone therapy. Which of the following is a characteristic of this drug?

a. Useful for maintenance therapy in opioid- (e.g., heroin-) dependent individuals, but lacks clinically useful analgesic effects
b. It has greater oral bioavailability than morphine, especially when oral administration is started
c. Causes pentazocine-like activation of κ receptors and blockade of μ receptors
d. When abruptly stopped after long-term administration, causes a withdrawal syndrome that is more intense, but briefer, than that associated with morphine or heroin withdrawal
e. Remarkably devoid of such typical opioid analgesic side effects as constipation and respiratory depression

132. We prescribe fluoxetine for a 40-year-old man with repetitive obsessive behavior that prevents him from carrying out simple tasks. This drug is classified as which of the following?

a. MAO inhibitor (MAOI)
b. Tricyclic nonselective amine reuptake inhibitor
c. Heterocyclic nonselective amine reuptake inhibitor
d. Selective serotonin reuptake inhibitor
e. α_2-adrenergic receptor inhibitor
f. Muscarinic receptor inhibitor

133. A 25-year-old man with difficulty sleeping and poor appetite associated with weight loss is placed on amitriptyline. This drug is classified as which of the following?

a. MAO inhibitor
b. Tricyclic nonselective amine reuptake inhibitor
c. Heterocyclic nonselective amine reuptake inhibitor
d. Selective serotonin reuptake inhibitor
e. α_2-adrenergic receptor antagonist

134. Clozapine is prescribed for a patient with a psychiatric disorder. Which of the following is the most serious side effect or adverse response for which we must monitor?

a. Agranulocytosis
b. Extrapyramidal side effects (parkinsonian)
c. Hypoglycemia
d. Hypotension, severe
e. Ventilatory depression or arrest

135. Which of the following drugs is effective in minimizing emotional bluntness and social withdrawal seen in schizophrenia?

a. Chlorpromazine
b. Fluphenazine
c. Haloperidol
d. Olanzapine
e. Thiothixene

136. A 26-year-old woman with reactive depression complains of missing her period and having milk discharge from her breasts (galactorrhea). Pregnancy tests are negative. Which of the following is most likely to have caused these findings?

a. Amoxapine
b. Clomipramine
c. Fluoxetine
d. Sertraline
e. Tranylcypromine

137. A 12-year-old boy has been treated with methylphenidate for the last three years. His younger sister finds the bottle of pills and consumes enough to cause significant toxicity. Which of the following findings would you expect?

a. Hypertension, tachycardia, seizures
b. Hypotension, bronchospasm
c. Drowsiness, obtunded reflexes, diarrhea
d. Miosis, bradycardia, profuse salivation, sweating
e. Hypothermia, skeletal muscle weakness or paralysis, pupils that are not responsive to light

138. When a local anesthetic is administered, which function or sensation is first to disappear as the drug's effects build and the last to reappear as the drug's effects wear off?

a. Autonomic efferent function
b. Motor nerve activity
c. Pain
d. Pressure (deep or heavy pressure)
e. Temperature

Questions 139–140

A 55-year-old woman undergoes surgery. She receives several drugs for preanesthesia care, intubation, and intraoperative skeletal muscle paralysis; and a mixture of inhaled anesthetics to complete the balanced anesthesia. Toward the end of the procedure she develops hyperthermia, hypertension, hyperkalemia, tachycardia, muscle rigidity, and metabolic acidosis.

139. Which of the following drugs is most likely to have participated in this reaction?

a. Fentanyl
b. Halothane
c. Ketamine
d. Midazolam
e. Propofol

140. In managing the reaction noted in Question 139, what should be administered specifically in an attempt to correct the abnormal skeletal muscle activity that is mainly responsible for all the other secondary signs and symptoms we described?

a. Baclofen
b. Diazepam
c. Cyclobenzaprine
d. Dantrolene
e. Halothane

141. Two inhaled general anesthetics, A and B, have the following MAC values:

A. MAC = 2%
B. MAC = 100%

Based on this information alone, which of the following statements is true?

a. Drug A has a longer duration of action than Drug B
b. Drug A is more soluble in the blood than Drug B
c. Drug B causes greater analgesia and skeletal muscle relaxation than Drug A
d. The concentration of drug in inspired air that is needed to cause adequate surgical anesthesia is higher for Drug B than for Drug A
e. The time to onset of adequate general anesthesia is 50 times longer for Drug B than for Drug A

142. A 30-year-old alcohol abuser decides to abstain from alcohol. Liver function tests are, fortunately, normal. Shortly after abstaining he becomes agitated, anxious, has visual hallucinations, is generally totally disoriented, and suffers bouts of insomnia. Which of the following agents would be indicated for managing these signs and symptoms?

a. Amitriptyline
b. Carbamazepine
c. Dextroamphetamine
d. Diazepam
e. Disulfiram
f. Valproic acid

143. Although a patient was instructed not to use alcohol because of a medication he is taking, he ignored advice and decided to have a cocktail. Within minutes he develops flushing, a throbbing headache, nausea, and vomiting. Which of the following medications was he taking?

a. Naltrexone
b. Diazepam
c. Disulfiram
d. Phenobarbital
e. Tranylcypromine

144. An SSRI antidepressant (e.g., fluoxetine) will be prescribed for an adult patient. You should advise him or her that two most likely side effects or adverse responses that may eventually occur at therapeutic blood levels are which of the following?

a. Intense dizziness upon standing (orthostatic hypotension) and palpitations (reflex cardiac stimulation)
b. Migraine headache and involuntary skeletal muscle twitching
c. Polyuria (diabetes insipidus-like condition) and insatiable thirst
d. Seizures and bradycardia
e. Sexual dysfunction and weight gain

Questions 145–147

Each group of questions below consists of lettered options followed by a set of numbered items. For each numbered item, select the one lettered option with which it is most closely associated. Each lettered option may be used once, more than once, or not at all.

For each patient, select the drug of choice.

a. Alprazolam
b. Diazepam
c. Ethosuximide
d. Midazolam
e. Oxazepam
f. Phenytoin

145. A 14-year-old girl is brought to the ED by her mother, who has observed that her daughter has abruptly experienced an impairment of consciousness associated with clonic jerking of the eyelids and staring into space lasting approximately 30 s.

146. A 48-year-old woman has had difficulty swallowing for 6 months. She requires premedication (sedation, but conscious) for an endoscopic examination.

147. A 12-year-old boy develops uncontrollable panic while camping with his parents in the Mojave Desert.

148. A 20-year-old man with absence seizures is treated with ethosuximide. Which of the following is the principal mechanism of action of ethosuximide?

a. Sodium channel blockade
b. Increase in the frequency of the chloride channel opening
c. Increase in GABA
d. Calcium channel blockade
e. Increased potassium channel permeability
.f. NMDA receptor blockade

149. A 30-year-old woman with partial seizures is treated with vigabatrin. Which of the following is the principal mechanism of action of vigabatrin?

a. Sodium channel blockade
b. Increase in frequency of chloride channel opening
c. Increase in GABA
d. Calcium channel blockade
e. Increased potassium channel permeability
f. NMDA receptor blockade

150. Of the following antiepileptic agents, which is associated with the highest risk of causing psychosis?

a. Ethosuximide
b. Phenobarbital
c. Phenytoin
d. Valproic acid
e. Vigabatrin

Questions 151–152

A 24-year-old woman has a history of epilepsy that is well controlled with therapeutic doses of phenytoin. She is healthy otherwise. She becomes pregnant.

151. Proper prenatal care, to be implemented for the entire duration of pregnancy, would include which of the following?

a. Adding valproic acid
b. Discontinuing all anticonvulsant medication
c. Increasing daily dietary iron intake
d. Prescribing daily folic acid supplements
e. Switching from the phenytoin to phenobarbital

152. Given the information presented above, which of the following should be administered to this woman starting a couple of weeks before anticipated parturition *and* as a single dose to the newborn immediately upon delivery?

a. A β-adrenergic blocker
b. Heparin
c. Lidocaine
d. Lorazepam
e. Vitamin K

153. Which comorbidity or element of a patient's history is regarded as posing the greatest risk from the administration of valproic acid?

a. Concomitant use of phenobarbital or phenytoin
b. Congestive heart failure
c. History of absence seizures
d. Pregnancy
e. Three or more prior episodes of status epilepticus in the last year

154. A 19-year-old woman whose roommate is being treated for depression decides that she is also depressed and surreptitiously takes her roommate's pills "as directed on the bottle" for several days. One night, she makes herself a snack of chicken liver paté and bleu cheese, accompanied by a glass of red wine. She soon develops headache, nausea, and palpitations. She goes to the ED, where her blood pressure is found to be 200/110 mmHg. What antidepressant did she take?

a. Fluoxetine
b. Nortriptyline
c. Phenelzine
d. Sertraline
e. Trazodone

155. A 41-year-old woman is seen in the psychiatric clinic for a follow-up appointment. She has been taking an antidepressant for 3 weeks with some improvement in mood. However, she complains of drowsiness, palpitations, dry mouth, and feeling faint on standing. Which of the following antidepressants is she most likely taking?

a. Amitriptyline
b. Bupropion
c. Fluoxetine
d. Trazodone
e. Venlafaxine

156. A 31-year-old woman has been treated with fluoxetine for 5 months. She is diagnosed with another medical problem and receives one or more drugs that, otherwise, would be suitable and problem-free. She is rushed to the ED with unstable vital signs, muscle rigidity, myoclonus, CNS irritability and altered consciousness, and shivering. What add-on drug most likely caused these responses?

a. Codeine for cough
b. Loratadine for seasonal allergies
c. Midazolam and fentanyl, used to ease an endoscopic procedure
d. Sumatriptan for migraine
e. Zolpidem for short-term insomnia

157. A 36-year-old unemployed dishwasher with no history of seizures presents with difficulty thinking coherently and claims he is an astronaut. Following treatment, he suddenly has a grand mal seizure. Which of the following neuroleptic agents was the most likely cause?

a. Clozapine
b. Fluphenazine
c. Haloperidol
d. Loxapine
e. Molindone

158. A 31-year-old woman is treated with an antipsychotic agent because of a recent history of spontaneously removing her clothing in public places and claiming she hears voices telling her to do so. Her blood pressure is normally 130/70 mmHg. Since being treated with a drug, she has had several bouts of syncope. Orthostatic hypotension was noted on physical examination. Which of the following drugs most likely caused this?

a. Chlorpromazine
b. Fluphenazine
c. Haloperidol
d. Olanzapine
e. Sertindole

159. A 29-year-old man uses secobarbital to satisfy his addiction to barbiturates. During the past week, he is imprisoned and is not able to obtain the drug. He is brought to the prison medical ward because of the onset of severe anxiety, increased sensitivity to light, dizziness, and generalized tremors. On physical examination, he is hyperreflexic. Which of the following agents should he be given to diminish his withdrawal symptoms?

a. Buspirone
b. Chloral hydrate
c. Chlorpromazine
d. Diazepam
e. Trazodone

160. A 72-year-old woman with a long history of anxiety that is treated with diazepam decides to triple her daily dose because of increasing fearfulness about "environmental noises." Two days after her attempt at self-prescribing, she is found extremely lethargic and nonresponsive. On examination, she is found to be stuporous and have diminished reaction to pain and decreased reflexes. Respirations are 8/min and shallow. Which of the following drugs should we give specifically to reverse these signs and symptoms?

a. Dextroamphetamine
b. Flumazenil
c. Naltrexone
d. Physostigmine
e. Pralidoxime

161. A woman receives a drug, and little else in the way of proper perinatal care, throughout pregnancy. Her child is born with disabling neural tube defects. Which of the following is the most likely cause of the infant's defects?

a. Ethosuximide
b. Phenobarbital
c. Primidone
d. Valproic acid
e. Vigabratin

162. A 29-year-old man requires suturing for a deep laceration in his palm. He is allergic to benzocaine. Which other local anesthetic could be used, posing the lowest risk of another allergic response?

a. Cocaine
b. Tetracaine
c. Lidocaine
d. Procaine

163. A patient who has been treated for Parkinson's disease for about a year presents with purplish, mottled changes to her skin. Which of the following is the most likely cause?

a. Amantadine
b. Bromocriptine
c. Levodopa (alone)
d. Levodopa combined with carbidopa
e. Pramipexole

164. A patient who has stable serum levels begins taking a very efficacious nonsteroidal anti-inflammatory drug (NSAID) for arthritis. There is likely to be an interaction such that the NSAID will increase which of the following?

a. Lithium absorption from the gut
b. Renal tubular lithium reabsorption
c. Lithium plasma protein binding
d. Lithium sensitivity at its site of action

165. A young boy who has been treated for epilepsy for a year is referred to an oral surgeon for evaluation and probable treatment of massive overgrowth of his gingival tissues. Some teeth are almost completely covered with hyperplastic tissue. Which of the following drugs is associated with this finding?

a. Carbamazepine
b. Lorazepam
c. Phenobarbital
d. Phenytoin
e. Valproic acid

166. A patient with undiagnosed coronary artery disease is given a medication. Shortly thereafter she develops intense tightness and "crushing discomfort" of her chest. An EKG reveals ST-segment changes indicative of acute myocardial ischemia. The patient suffered acute myocardial ischemia and angina pectoris. Which of the following drugs is most likely to have caused this reaction?

a. Clozapine
b. Pentazocine
c. Phenytoin
d. Sumatriptan
e. Zolpidem

167. In the setting of drug therapy for status epilepticus, the main advantage(s) of fos-phenytoin over phenytoin is that fos-phenytoin:

a. Has a mechanism of anticonvulsant action that is different from and more effective than plain phenytoin
b. Causes less vascular/venous irritation, can be injected at a faster rate
c. Acts so quickly that it eliminates the need for administering a faster-acting anticonvulsant first
d. Works so long that oral anticonvulsant therapy is not needed once the acute seizure has been stopped
e. Directly stimulates ventilation (action in brain's medulla) that is compromised during status epilepticus

168. A main limitation to using nitrous oxide as the sole agent for surgical anesthesia is which of the following?

a. Almost total lack of analgesic activity, regardless of concentration
b. Inspired concentrations >10% tend to profound cardiac negative inotropic effects
c. MAC (minimum alveolar concentration) is >100%
d. Methemoglobinemia occurs even with low inspired concentrations
e. Such great solubility in blood that its effects take an extraordinarily long time to develop
f. Very high frequency of bronchospasm

169. A patient has a history of cardiac arrhythmias due to a prolonged QT-interval ("long QT syndrome"). Which CNS drug should be avoided in this patient because it can cause further QT-prolongation, with an associated and high risk of serious ventricular arrhythmias including torsades de pointes?

a. Diazepam
b. Fluoxetine
c. Phenobarbital
d. Phenytoin
e. Thioridazine

170. Prompt administration of antipyretics, IV hydration, and bromocriptine or dantrolene, is necessary to combat a relatively rare but potentially fatal adverse response that is characteristically associated with which of the following?

a. Benzodiazepines, especially those used as hypnotics
b. Chlorpromazine
c. Levodopa
d. Phenytoin
e. SSRIs

171. A 66-year-old woman meets diagnostic criteria for Alzheimer's disease, with symptoms being described as mild-to-moderate. The current recommended approach for attempting to slow disease progression and improve cognition, behavior, and daily function, is to use drugs that centrally:

a. Activate a population of serotonin receptors
b. Block dopamine release or receptor activation
c. Inhibit acetylcholinesterase
d. Inhibit MAO
e. Reduce oxidative neuronal damage
f. Dissolve cerebral vascular thrombi

172. A 34-year-old man with anxiety has heard about buspirone and asks whether it might be suitable for him. According to the latest diagnostic criteria, the drug would be appropriate. However, before prescribing it you should know that buspirone does which of the following?

a. Causes a withdrawal syndrome that, if unsupervised, is frequently lethal
b. Requires almost daily dosage titrations in order to optimize the response
c. Seldom causes drowsiness
d. Has a significant potential for abuse
e. Is likely to potentiate the CNS depressant effects of alcohol, benzodiazepines, and sedative antihistamines (e.g., diphenhydramine), so such interactants must be avoided at all cost

Central Nervous System

Answers

100. The answer is c. (*Craig, pp 324–326; Hardman, pp 546–548; Katzung, pp 499, 505, 511–512.*) Pentazocine is a mixed agonist-antagonist on opioid receptors. When a partial agonist, such as pentazocine, displaces a full agonist, such as methadone, the receptor is less activated; this leads to withdrawal syndrome in an opioid-dependent person.

101. The answer is e. (*Craig, pp 379–380; Hardman, pp 476–477; Katzung, pp 392–393.*) You would be safe (and generally accurate) in coming to this general conclusion: valproic acid is the only common anticonvulsant that is a drug metabolism inhibitor; all the rest are either inducers, or have no significant effect on the metabolism of other drugs.

Valproic acid has been cited as an important *inhibitor* of the metabolism of many other drugs, including phenytoin, phenobarbital, and carbamazepine. The outcome is increased serum levels of these other agents (unless dosages are reduced), leading to an increased frequency or severity of expected side effects (or increased risk of toxicity). Valproate may also interact with phenytoin by displacing the latter from plasma protein binding sites, thereby increasing serum levels of free (active) phenytoin. And, at high serum levels valproic acid may actually inhibit its own hepatic metabolism.

Carbamazepine induces the hepatic metabolism of several other drugs (warfarin and oral contraceptives are good examples). It is also a target of drug interactions in which its metabolism is inhibited (e.g., by coadministration of a macrolide antibiotic or azole antifungal). Ethosuximide (or other succinimide anticonvulsants such as methsuximide) tends not to cause clinically significant interactions by altering drug metabolism. Phenytoin and phenobarbital are, of course, classic examples of drugs that induce the P450 system and interact with many other drugs by that mechanism.

102. The answer is d. (*Craig, pp 334–335; Hardman, p 340; Katzung, p 419.*) Nearly all local anesthetics contain a lipophilic functional group, and most have a hydrophilic (amine) group. Benzocaine does not contain the terminal hydrophilic amine group; thus, it is only slightly soluble in water and is slowly absorbed with a prolonged duration. It is, therefore, only useful as a topical anesthetic (e.g., on mucous membranes).

103. The answer is c. (*Craig, pp 364–366, 399–402; Hardman, pp 490–496, 552–555; Katzung, pp 472–475.*) Unwanted side effects produced by phenothiazine antipsychotic drugs (e.g., perphenazine) include Parkinson-like syndrome, akathisia, dystonias, galactorrhea, amenorrhea, and infertility. These side effects are due to the ability of these agents to block dopamine receptors. The phenothiazines also block muscarinic and α-adrenergic receptors, which are responsible for other effects.

104. The answer is b. (*Craig, pp 369–370; Hardman, p 512; Katzung, p 454–455.*) Diphenhydramine, arguably the prototype of all the older ("first generation") antihistamines, causes significant antimuscarinic (atropinelike) actions; because of its liphophilicity it enters the CNS well (this accounts for the drug's marked sedative effects, too) and blocks muscarinic receptors there. That helps adjust the dopamine-ACh imbalance that appears to be the main biochemical underpinning of parkinsonism. Diphenhydramine can be used—has been used—instead of the "traditional" centrally acting antimuscarinic drugs for parkinsonism: benzotropine and trihexyphenidyl.

Diphenhydramine does help alleviate cutaneous allergy symptoms (e.g., urticaria), but those are rare with any of the common antiparkinson drugs (and we did not specify which "other" drug was given). It has no ability to affect manic/hypomanic episodes that might occur with, say, high doses of levodopa. It does not reverse antipsychotic-induced tardive dyskinesias; no drug does that effectively.

105. The answer is e. (*Craig, pp 386–388, 390; Hardman, pp 443–445; Katzung, p 493–494.*) Fatalities have been reported when fluoxetine and MAO inhibitors (MAOIs) such as tranylcypromine have been given simultaneously. The MAOIs should be stopped at least 2 weeks before the administration of fluoxetine or paroxetine. Note that a similar severe interaction can occur between tricyclic antidepressants (e.g., imipramine, amitriptyline) and MAOIs; the same warning against "overlapping" the two classes of drugs, and allowing one to "clear" the system completely before starting the other, applies.

106. The answer is c. (*Craig, pp 386–388; Hardman, pp 434, 436–439; Katzung, pp 483–484, 486, 490.*) Fluoxetine (and related drugs such as sertraline, fluvoxamine, and citalopram) selectively inhibits neuronal serotonin uptake, with minimal effects on other monoamines. The tricyclics (imipramine) and venlafaxine inhibit serotonin and norepinephrine (re)uptake (and, apparently to a small degree, dopamine). And, to add another important drug and action: bupropion affects reuptake of both norepinephrine and dopamine.

107. The answer is b. (*Craig, pp 292t, 297; Hardman, pp 326–327; Katzung, pp 411–412, 415–416.*) The scenario describes most of the classic responses to ketamine, a "dissociative anesthetic": analgesia; an ostensibly light sleep-like state; a trance-like and cataplectic state (including increased muscle tone); and activation of most cardiovascular parameters (in patients with normal cardiovascular status to begin with). The various psychosis-like emergence reactions are the main disadvantages to using a drug that, otherwise, causes many of the desired elements of complete anesthesia, usually without the need for complicated and expensive anesthesia administration devices or personnel. Ketamine undergoes significant metabolism in humans, with about 20% of the absorbed dose recovered as metabolites. Halothane can cause postoperative jaundice and hepatic necrosis with repeated administration in rare instances.

108. The answer is d. (*Craig, pp 366–369; Hardman, pp 509–511; Katzung, pp 448–451.*) When levodopa is administered orally, the vast majority of the administered dose is metabolized in the gut to dopamine by DOPA decarboxylase. However dopamine cannot cross the blood-brain barrier, and so only a fraction of the parent drug gets into the CNS, to be metabolized and cause its desired effects there. Carbidopa inhibits DOPA decarboxylase in the periphery (it cannot cross the blood-brain barrier), reducing peripheral metabolism of levodopa to dopamine and "sparing" a bigger fraction of the dose so it can be metabolized in the nigrostriatum. By reducing peripheral conversion of levodopa to dopamine, the adjunctive use of carbidopa may also allow management of parkinsonian signs and symptoms with lower doses of levodopa. One additional benefit of that is a reduction in the number and severity of peripheral side effects of the levodopa (or, more precisely, its metabolite, dopamine). Adding carbidopa to a regimen involving levodopa only may also help (at least transiently) combat such problems as dopamine's "on-off" phenomenon and "end-of-dose" failure.

109. The answer is b. *(Craig, pp 296, 357t; Hardman, pp 364–365, 372–374; Katzung, pp 357, 359–360, 364.)* Flumazenil is a competitive benzodiazepine receptor antagonist. The drug reverses the CNS sedative effects of benzodiazepines and is indicated where general anesthesia has been induced by or maintained with benzodiazepines such as diazepam, lorazepam, or midazolam.

110. The answer is c. *(Craig, pp 294–295, 381, 411–412; Hardman, pp 376, 380, 472; Katzung, pp 361–363.)* There should be little argument that phenobarbital is used appropriately, long-term, for managing certain epilepsies (mainly as an alternative to phenytoin). Benzodiazepines are almost always preferred, and used, for managing alcohol withdrawal and anxiety management. Benzodiazepines, or the benzodiazepine-like agents zalpelon or zolpidem, are almost always turned to for insomnia. Major reasons for selecting a benzodiazepine over a barbiturate include fewer drug-drug interactions (phenobarbital is a classic P450 inducer), a lower risk of dependence; withdrawal syndromes that are typically less severe or dangerous; lower risk of fatal ventilatory depression with oral overdoses (and the availability of a specific benzodiazepine antagonist to treat them, should they occur); and less narrowing between lethal and effective doses as use continues.

Note that even though benzodiazepines may be preferred, treatment for such problems as anxiety and insomnia should be kept as short as possible. Phenobarbital (or other barbiturates) and benzodiazepines are not indicated for treating endogenous depression.

111. The answer is b. *(Craig, p 383; Hardman, p 484; Katzung, pp 394–395, 397–398.)* Intravenously administered lorazepam is the drug of choice for treatment of status epilepticus. (It has surpassed diazepam because of a faster onset of action and less venous irritation, among other things.) Lorazepam, like the benzodiazepines in general, increases the apparent affinity of the inhibitory neurotransmitter GABA for binding sites on brain cell membranes. The effects of lorazepam (or diazepam) are short-lasting. Immediately after giving the benzodiazepine either phenytoin or fos-phenytoin should be given to provide longer seizure suppression and "coverage" because the effects of lorazepam wear off in a comparatively short time. Other drugs that can be used for status epilepticus include phenobarbital (not a drug of choice) and (paradoxically) lidocaine for refractory seizures (mainly a drug of last resort). None of the other drugs listed in the question are appropriate for status epilepticus, despite their widespread use for oral therapy of seizure disorders long-term.

112. The answer is a. (*Craig, pp 388t, 389–391; Hardman, pp 433, 439, 442; Katzung, pp 483, 486, 488–490, 493.*) The most common side effects associated with tricyclic antidepressants are their antimuscarinic effects, which may be evident in over 50% of patients. Clinically, the antimuscarinic effects may manifest as dry mouth, blurred vision, constipation, tachycardia, dizziness, and urinary retention. At therapeutic plasma concentrations, these drugs usually do not cause changes in the EKG. Direct cardiac effects of the tricyclic antidepressants are important in overdosage.

113. The correct answer is e. (*Craig, pp 53, 377–378; Hardman, pp 468–469; Katzung, pp 380–382.*) The hepatic enzymes responsible for phenytoin metabolism become saturated at blood concentrations in what is generally considered to be the therapeutic (or high-therapeutic) range. While blood concentrations are below what might be considered the metabolic V_{max} for the drug, typical first-order kinetics applies (a constant fraction of the drug is eliminated with the passing of each plasma half-life). Once the metabolic capacity is exceeded, small increases in dosage lead to disproportionately large increases of serum concentrations (and effects) because, in essence, "drug in greatly exceeds drug out"; once the drug is stopped, elimination is slower and follows zero-order kinetics (constant amount of drug eliminated per half-life), until the P450 system is no longer saturated.

114. The answer is d. (*Craig, p 369; Hardman, p 512; Katzung, pp 83, 453.*) Two types of MAO have been found: (1) MAO-A, which metabolizes norepinephrine and serotonin, and is the predominant hepatic form of the enzyme; and (2) MAO-B, which metabolizes dopamine. Selegiline is a selective inhibitor of MAO-B. It therefore inhibits the breakdown of dopamine and prolongs the therapeutic effectiveness of levodopa in parkinsonism. The risks of serious drug interactions in patients taking nonselective MAO inhibitors (e.g., phenelzine, tranylcypromine), such as hypertensive crisis in response to mixed- and indirect-acting sympatho-mimetics (tyramine, pseudoephedrine, amphetamines) are much less (but still possible) with selegiline.

Bromocriptine is a dopamine receptor agonist. Carbidopa inhibits the peripheral metabolism of levodopa. Both are useful in the treatment of parkinsonism. Phenelzine and tranylcypromine are nonselective MAOIs. Combining them with L-dopa may lead to hypertensive crises, and thus they are not used in the therapy of parkinsonism.

115. The answer is b. (*Craig, pp 319–321; Hardman, pp 530–531, 536; Katzung, pp 504–505, 509.*) Unless the patient can be put on a ventilator to control blood gases (and perhaps have intracranial pressure surgically reduced), closed head injury contraindicates morphine use. Cerebral vasodilation occurs in response to expected morphine-induced ventilatory depression. That increases intracranial pressure. This is precisely what one doesn't want to do with closed head injuries (brain swelling) or with, for example, the presence of a large brain tumor—two situations in which intracranial pressure is already (likely) increased.

Parenteral morphine is a routine part of the approach to acute pul-monary edema and myocardial infarction. The drug is apt to lower blood pressure in some patients, and so there is little specific concern with respect to hypertension. Opioid abuse of recent history poses a problem: the patient may be tolerant to opioids, and so higher than usual doses of morphine may be needed to get adequate pain control and other subjective responses. However, that does not pose a risk and certainly doesn't consti-tute a contraindication to using the drug.

116. The answer is e. (*Craig, pp 322–323; Hardman, pp 540–542; Katzung, p 511.*) High or frankly toxic serum levels of meperidine can cause seizures in addition to typical morphine-like effects including analgesia and ventila-tory depression, or hypertension and a psychosis-like state. It appears that administration of naloxone to combat excessive effects of meperidine may increase the risk of seizures. Meperidine causes less biliary tract spasm than morphine, so when bile duct disease is present and only short-term analge-sia is indicated, meperidine may be preferred. Because of the toxicity risk, meperidine should not be used for more than brief analgesic effects.

The rather unique adverse effects attributed to meperidine are probably due to a major metabolite, normeperidine. A weak opioid analgesic, propoxyphene (structurally related to methadone), can produce similar toxic reactions. One of its metabolite, norpropoxyphene, is thought to be the cause.

117. The answer is b. (*Craig, p 369; Hardman, p 512; Katzung, pp 453.*) Selegiline inhibits MAO-B, thus delaying the metabolic breakdown of dopamine. It is effective alone in parkinsonism and increases the effectiveness of L-dopa. Benztropine and trihexyphenidyl are cholinergic antagonists in the brain. Bromocriptine is a dopamine receptor agonist. Chlorpromazine is an antipsychotic drug with antiadrenergic properties.

118. The answer is b. (*Craig, p 369; Hardman, pp 278t, 511–512; Katzung, pp 452.*) Bromocriptine mimics the action of dopamine in the brain but is not as readily metabolized. It is especially useful in parkinsonism that is unresponsive to L-dopa. Apomorphine is also a dopamine receptor agonist, but its side effects preclude its use for parkinsonism. Selegiline is an MAO-B inhibitor, atropine is a belladonna preparation, and amantadine is an antiviral agent that probably affects the synthesis or uptake of dopamine.

119. The answer is c. (*Craig, pp 400–401; Hardman, pp 407–412; Katzung, p 469.*) Chlorpromazine, the prototype phenothiazine antipsychotic drug, is also indicated for managing nausea and vomiting, in both adults and children, from a number of causes. The drug can be administered orally, rectally, or intramuscularly for this purpose. (Some phenothiazines with better antiemetic activity, such as prochlorperazine or promethazine, are usually used instead.) Regardless, the antiemetic mechanism appears to involve blockade of dopaminergic receptors in the chemoreceptor trigger zone of the brain's medulla.

Chlorpromazine (and most other antipsychotics) can lower the brain's seizure threshold, thereby potentially increasing the risk of seizures in susceptible patients with epilepsy. It tends to lower blood pressure (probably via blocking α-adrenergic receptors in the vasculature) and so may aggravate preexisting hypotension. Most of the phenothiazines also cause significant antimuscarinic effects, which would aggravate xerostomia (and other conditions involving reduced exocrine gland secretions). The antimuscarinic effects would inhibit activation of the bladder's detrusor muscle and inhibit relaxation of the sphincter, thereby aggravating problems with micturition in such patients as the elderly man with an enlarged prostate.

Note: In general, phenothiazines are not used often for managing emesis or nausea. That is, in part, because of the risk of excessive sedation, extrapyramidal reactions, orthostatic hypotension, and occasional cholestatic jaundice (hepatitis) or blood dyscrasias. Far more often we turn to other dopamine antagonists (e.g., metoclopramide), a cannabinoid (tetrahydrocannabinol), or a serotonin receptor blocker (ondansetron; a 5-HT$_3$-selective blocker).

120. The answer is c. (*Craig, pp 317–321; Hardman, pp 527–534; Katzung, pp 497–498.*) Morphine is a pure agonist opioid drug with agonist activity toward all the opioid subtype receptor sites. In high doses, deaths associated with morphine are related to the depression of the respiratory center in the medulla. Morphine has a high addiction potential related to the activity of heroin or dihydromorphine. Codeine has a significantly lower addiction potential.

121. The answer is d. (*Craig, pp 407–410; Hardman, pp 133, 135, 337, 570; Katzung, pp 78, 137, 425, 521–523.*) Cocaine, an ester of benzoic acid, has local anesthetic properties; it can block the initiation or conduction of a nerve impulse. It is metabolized by plasma esterases to inactive products. In addition, cocaine blocks the reuptake of norepinephrine. This action produces CNS stimulant effects including euphoria, excitement, and restlessness. Peripherally, the blocked norepinephrine reuptake cause sympathomimetic effects including tachycardia and vasoconstriction. Death from acute overdose can be from cardiac failure, stroke, seizures, or apnea during the seizures.

122. The answer is b. (*Craig, p 369; Hardma, pp 507–508, 511–512; Katzung, p 451–453.*) Central dopamine receptors are divided into D$_1$ and D$_2$ receptors. Antipsychotic activity is better correlated to blockade of D$_2$ receptors. Haloperidol, a potent antipsychotic, selectively antagonizes the actions of dopamine on D$_2$ receptors. Phenothiazine derivatives, such as chlorpromazine, fluphenazine, and promethazine, are not selective for D$_2$ receptors. Bromocriptine, a selective D$_2$ agonist, is useful in the treatment of parkinsonism and hyperprolactinemia. It produces fewer adverse reactions than do nonselective dopamine receptor agonists.

123. The answer is a. *(Craig, pp 399–400; Hardman, pp 404–405; Katzung, pp 462–463, 466–467, 471.)* Although some may disagree, it is common to classify chlorpromazine and other phenothiazine antipsychotics as "low potency" agents, in comparison with haloperidol (butyrophenone class), which has been called "high potency." Potency, of course, usually refers to the dose needed to cause a stated effect of a certain intensity. In that regard, haloperidol is more potent than phenothiazines and is more selective for blocking dopamine D_2 receptors. But another implied meaning of using this term is that chlorpromazine and other "low potency" agents tend to cause a higher incidence of peripheral autonomic side effects (from α blockade and antimuscarinic effects) than haloperidol; and a lower incidence of extrapyramidal reactions, which can be severe and of sudden onset with haloperidol—a very rapidly acting drug, especially when given parenterally (as for acute psychosis).

124. The answer is c. *(Craig, p 402; Hardman, pp 415–417; Katzung, p 474.)* Neuroleptic malignant syndrome is thought to be a severe form of an extrapyramidal syndrome that can occur at any time with any dose of a neuroleptic agent. However, the risk is higher when high-potency agents are used in high doses, especially if given parenterally. Mortality from NMS is greater than 10%.

125. The answer is c. *(Craig, pp 417–418; Hardman, pp 638–640; Katzung, pp 523–525.)* Phencyclidine is a hallucinogenic compound with no opioid activity. Its mechanism of action is amphetamine-like. A withdrawal syndrome has not been described for this drug in human subjects. In overdose, the treatment of choice for the psychotic activity is the antipsychotic drug haloperidol.

126. The answer is b. *(Craig, pp 399–403; Hardman, pp 407–412, 414–417; Katzung, pp 466, 472–473.)* Haloperidol, a butyrophenone, is by far the most likely antipsychotic to cause extrapyramidal responses. Other agents, such as piperazine (an aromatic phenothiazine), thiothixene (a thioxanthene), or pimozide (a diphenylbutyropiperidine), less likely to produce extrapyramidal toxicity than haloperidol. The antagonism of dopamine in the nigrostriatal system might explain the Parkinson-like effects. Both haloperidol and pimozide act mainly on D_2 receptors, whereas thioridazine and piperazine act on α-adrenergic receptors, and have a less potent but definite effect on D_2 receptors.

127. The answer is a. (*Craig, pp 399–403; Hardman, pp 404–405; Katzung, pp 466–468.*) The signs and symptoms described in the question are antimuscarinic side effects, and of all the antipsychotics the incidence and severity of these is highest with the phenothiazines. [See Question 123 for more on fundamental differences between "high potency" and "low potency" antipsychotics, especially as they predict the relative incidence of peripheral autonomic and central (extrapyramidal) side effects.]

128. The answer is b. (*Craig, p 401; Hardman, p 420; Katzung, p 469.*) We are describing some of the symptoms and signs of Tourette's syndrome. It is effectively treated with haloperidol, a high-potency antipsychotic. If patients are unresponsive or do not tolerate haloperidol, they might be switched to pimozide.

129. The answer is d. (*Craig, pp 393–395; Hardman, pp 448–449; Katzung, pp 477–478.*) Lithium treatment frequently causes polyuria and (as a consequence of extreme renal fluid loss) polydipsia. The collecting ducts of the kidney lose the capacity to conserve water via antidiuretic hormone. This results in significantly increased free-water clearance, which is referred to as *nephrogenic diabetes insipidus.*

130. The answer is e. (*Craig, pp 325–326; Hardman, pp 546–548; Katzung, pp 505–507, 509.*) Adding pentazocine to an analgesic regimen involving morphine will counteract key effects of morphine. In this case, the patient's pain will grow worse, not become less. Pentazocine is classified as a partial agonist (or mixed agonist-antagonist). Recall that morphine causes the following effects by acting as a "pure" agonist on μ receptors: analgesia, respiratory depression, euphoria, sedation, physical dependence, and decreased gut motility. Pentazocine, given alone, causes analgesia, sedation, and decreased gut motility by acting as an agonist on κ receptors. However, it is a weak agonist. But it antagonizes the actions of morphine on μ receptors in a concentration-dependent fashion, and so pain returns in this patient.

131. The answer is b. (*Craig, pp 323–324, 409–412; Hardman, pp 544–545; Katzung, p 510.*) Methadone is a slow, long-acting opioid receptor agonist. It is used as an analgesic (for long-term pain control when an opioid is indicated) and for maintenance therapy of individuals dependent on stronger opioids such as heroin or morphine. Methadone has greater oral efficacy than morphine, especially when oral therapy is started. (Recall that morphine is subject to extensive first-pass hepatic metabolism, and only with repeated oral administration can we saturate its drug-metabolizing enzymes such that bioavailability is improved enough to get good analgesia.) The long biologic half-life accounts for the milder but more protracted abstinence syndrome associated with methadone. Methadone does not possess opioid antagonist properties (whether κ or μ) and, thus, would not precipitate withdrawal symptoms in a heroin addict, as would naloxone or naltrexone.

132. The answer is d. *(Craig, pp 386–388; Hardman, pp 432–437; Katzung, pp 483–486.)* Fluoxetine is a highly selective serotonin reuptake inhibitor (SSRI), acting on the 5-HT transporter. It forms an active metabolite that is effective for several days. Selective serotonin reuptake inhibitors are, in general, inhibitors of cytochrome P450 isoenzyme. This is the basis of potential drug-drug interactions.

133. The answer is b. *(Craig, pp 389–391; Hardman, pp 432–437; Katzung, pp 483–486.)* Amitriptyline is a tertiary amine tricyclic antidepressant. It functions as a norepinephrine reuptake inhibitor. Brain levels of amines are increased. This results in increased vesicular stores of norepinephrine and serotonin. Amitriptyline is a prototypical tricyclic antidepressant that has proved useful in patients with sleep and appetite disorders.

134. The answer is a. *(Craig, pp 399–402; Hardman, pp 416–417; Katzung p 470.)* Clozapine causes agranulocytosis in 1 to 2% of treated patients. It is generally reversible on discontinuation of the drug, but this, of course, depends on frequent blood tests to detect the problem early on. Monitoring for this adverse response is so critical that prescriptions for refills cannot be filled without proof of blood counts that are within "acceptable" levels.

135. The answer is d. *(Craig, pp 399–402; Hardman, pp 504–506; Katzung p 466, 469–471.)* In addition to its antipsychotic action, olanzapine diminishes emotional bluntness and social withdrawal that are seen in schizophrenic patients, without significant anticholinergic and extrapyramidal effects.

136. The answer is a. *(Craig, pp 389–391; Hardman, pp 457, 468–472; Katzung p 484, 488–490.)* Amoxapine, a tricyclic antidepressant, effectively blocks neuronal norepinephrine reuptake, is somewhat less potent in terms of blocking serotonin uptake, and is far less potent in terms of blocking dopamine reuptake.

A metabolite of amoxapine *blocks* dopamine receptors quite well, and that effect makes it the most likely choice as the drug that caused the patient's menstrual irregularities and galactorrhea. You should recall that such drugs as the phenothiazines, which exert their main antipsychotic effects via blockade of dopamine receptors, may also cause amenorrhea-galactorrhea by the same mechanism, and drugs that activate dopamine receptors (e.g., bromocriptine) can be used to manage this endocrine dysfunction.

Amoxapine's dopamine receptor blockade also seems to account for why the drug exerts some antipsychotic properties, theoretically making it useful for patients with both psychosis and depression.

137. The answer is a. (*Craig, pp 106, 349–350, 407; Hardman, pp 220–221; Katzung, pp 521–523, 990.*) Methylphenidate, which is widely used to manage ADD-ADHD, has amphetamine-like sympathetic and CNS-stimulating effects.

Peripheral sympathetic (adrenergic) effects arise from the drug's ability to release neuronal norepinephrine. Related findings would include increased vasoconstriction (α-receptor activation on vascular smooth muscle), and therefore increased blood pressure, and tachycardia (plus increased cardiac contractility and electrical impulse conduction rates, probably accompanied by tachyarrhythmias and β_1 activation).

At toxic doses, the CNS effect of the drug probably would lead to seizures.

There is no mechanism by which direct effects of methylphenidate (whether at normal or toxic doses) would cause bronchospasm, bronchoconstriction, or even bronchodilation (because norepinephrine that is released has no ability to activate or block β_2 receptors on airway smooth muscle). Miosis (which occurs with either muscarinic activation of α blockade) would be the opposite of what you would predict in terms of ocular effects.

In terms of autonomic effects, skeletal muscle weakness or paralysis are findings you would expect from drugs that either blocked nicotinic cholinergic receptors (e.g., tubocurarine or another similar nondepolarizing neuromuscular blocker) or stimulated them in excessive and prolonged fashion (e.g., succinylcholine).

138. The answer is c. (*Craig, p 331; Hardman, pp 333–336; Katzung, pp 422–423.*) For the key to the simple answer, consider the British term for local anesthetics: regional analgesics. Pain is typically the first sensation to go, the last to return. For a more detailed explanation: The primary effect of local anesthetics is blockade of voltage channel-gated Na channels. Progressively increasing concentrations of local anesthetics result in an increased threshold of excitation, a slowing of impulse conduction, a decline in the rate of rise of the action potential, a decrease in the height of the action potential, and eventual obliteration of the action potential. Local anesthetics first block small unmyelinated or lightly myelinated fibers (pain), followed by heavily myelinated but small-diameter fibers, and then larger-diameter fibers (proprioception, pressure, motor). At high serum concentrations autonomic nerve function can be affected. At toxic concentrations other excitable tissues (cardiac, smooth, skeletal muscle) can be affected.

139. The answer is b. (*Craig, pp 342, 344; Hardman, pp 188, 312–316; Katzung, pp 410–411.*) Although a rare occurrence, halothane and other inhaled volatile liquid anesthetics may cause malignant hyperthermia, the signs and symptoms of which we have described in the question. Apparently, this occurs mainly in genetically susceptible individuals (whether a personal or familial history, as the predisposition seems to be heritable). The prevalence of the reaction is increased by concomitant use of succinylcholine.

140. The answer is d. (*Craig, p 344; Hardman, p 416; Katzung, pp 443–444.*) Skeletal muscle (myocyte) dysfunction seems to be at the core of malignant hyperthermia signs and symptoms. It appears to involve sustained increases in the availability and concentration of free calcium (Ca^{2+}) ions in the myocytes, such that contractile proteins are continually activated (and unable to relax). Dantrolene, which interferes with release of Ca^{2+} from the sarcoplasmic reticulum, is indicated in treatment of the disorder (and for neuroleptic malignant syndrome). Baclofen, diazepam (and certain other benzodiazepines, e.g., chlordiazepoxide), and cyclobenzaprine are centrally acting skeletal muscle relaxants. They are not useful in treating malignant hyperthermia.

141. The answer is d. (*Craig, pp 298–302; Hardman, pp 301–302, 308–311; Katzung, pp 402–405.*) MAC (minimum alveolar concentration) is an expression of inhaled anesthetic "potency." It is defined as the minimum inspired concentration needed to abolish a specified painful response in 50% of treated patients. (Thus, it is much like the ED_{50}, measured in a population dose-response curve, for most other drugs.) Obviously, giving a drug at a dose that suppresses a response in only half the treated patients is not desirable, so inhaled anesthetics are typically given at a dose more than the MAC. (Recall, too, that MAC is not absolute: it can change depending on the use of other anesthesia adjuncts and such other factors as body temperature, ventilatory rate, presence of other diseases, etc.)

A drug's MAC gives us no useful information about onsets or durations of action. We cannot state correctly that Drug B (MAC = 100%) causes greater analgesia and/or skeletal muscle relaxation than another drug any more than we can say that a drug with an ED_{50} of 5 mg causes a greater response than one with ED_{50} = 1 mg. It all depends on the dose given, not the MAC or ED_{50}.

142. The answer is d. *(Craig, pp 358–360, 383, 414–415; Hardman, pp 478–480, 562–563; Katzung, pp 373–375.)* Long-acting benzodiazepines such as diazepam are useful in alcohol withdrawal. One of diazepam's active metabolites is eliminated slowly, thereby increasing its duration of action. [In patients with liver disease, short-acting benzodiazepines might prove better if they are metabolized to inactive water-soluble metabolites (e.g., oxazepam).]

Amitriptyline, carbamazepine, or valproic acid would not be nearly as effective (or appropriately used) as a benzodiazepine. Although one could envisage this patient developing status epilepticus, even in that situation the anticonvulsants (carbamazepine, valproic acid) would not be indicated. Dextroamphetamine, a powerful cortical stimulant, would worsen signs and symptoms and increase the risk of seizures. Disulfiram would be a poor choice. If the patient still had ethanol in the bloodstream the interference of alcohol metabolism (the "acetaldehyde syndrome") would make matters worse. Even if there was no residual blood alcohol, disulfiram would provide no symptom relief.

143. The answer is c. *(Craig, p 415; Hardman, pp 391–393; Katzung, pp 375.)* Disulfiram is used in controlling alcohol consumption. The onset of symptoms is almost immediately following ingestion of alcohol and may last for several hours in some patients. Disulfiram acts by inhibition of aldehyde dehydrogenase, resulting in the accumulation of acetaldehyde. Central nervous system depression can occur with centrally acting sedative agents such as diazepam and phenobarbital.

144. The answer is e. (*Craig, p 388; Hardman, pp 433–435, 442; Katzung, pp 492–493.*) Sexual dysfunction (probably of CNS origin) and weight gain (sometimes significant) are relatively common problems associated with SSRI therapy. Orthostatic hypotension and reflex tachycardia sometimes occur with older antidepressants (tricyclics, e.g., imipramine), but are rare with SSRIs. Migraine is not likely; blockade of serotonin reuptake might actually reduce the risk (note that triptans exert antimigraine actions by acting as serotonin agonists). Lithium is the drug likely to cause polyuria and polydipsia. None of the other side effects or adverse responses listed in the question are likely with an SSRI.

145. The answer is c. (*Craig, pp 292, 295–296, 357; Hardman, pp 482–485; Katzung, pp 390–391, 396–397.*) The symptoms describe absence seizures, for which ethosuximide is very effective (and, according to many, the drug of choice). None of the other drugs are effective or indicated, and phenytoin may *aggravate* absence seizures.

146. The answer is d. (*Craig, pp 292, 295–296, 357; Hardman, pp 482–485; Katzung, pp 358, 413.*) Midazolam is useful for "conscious sedation" because, in part, it produces a higher incidence of amnesia and has a more rapid" onset of action and a shorter half-life than other benzodiazepines used in anesthesia.

147. The answer is a. (*Craig, pp 292, 295–296, 357; Hardman, pp 482–485; Katzung, pp 361–362.*) Compared with other benzodiazepines, alprazolam is selective for treating agoraphobia and panic disorders.

148. The answer is d. (*Craig, pp 381–382; Hardman, pp 475–476; Katzung, pp 390–391.*) Ethosuximide is especially useful in the treatment of absence seizures. Although it may act at several sites, the principal mechanism of action is on T-type Ca currents in thalamic neurons at relevant concentrations. This action blocks the pacemaker current that effects the generation of rhythmic cortical discharge associated with an absence attack.

149. The answer is c. (*Craig, p 381; Hardman, p 481; Katzung, pp 387.*) Vigabatrin (γ-vinyl GABA) is useful in partial seizures. It is an irreversible inhibitor of GABA aminotransferase, an enzyme responsible for the termination of GABA action. This results in accumulation of GABA at synaptic sites, thereby enhancing its effect.

150. The answer is e. (*Hardman, p 481; Katzung, pp 387.*) Vigabatrin can induce psychosis. It is recommended that it not be used in patients with preexisting depression and psychosis.

151. The answer is d. (*Craig, pp 382–383; Hardman, p 484; Katzung, p 398.*) Folic acid supplementation is generally thought to be important for all pregnant women, but it is particularly important during therapy with such anticonvulsants as phenytoin. The purpose is to reduce the risk of spina bifida and other neural tube defects (and some other teratogenic consequences). The scenario describes no reason to add valproic acid (or add or switch to any other anticonvulsant, including phenobarbital) if the mother is kept seizure-free during pregnancy (pregnancy class D; most others are C), in particular, might be a poor choice because it appears to carry the highest risk of teratogenic effects of all the common anticonvulsants. Discontinuing all anticonvulsants during pregnancy is inappropriate in this and most circumstances, as it carries the risk of seizure recurrence than can be more dangerous to the mother and the fetus than continuing effective therapy and providing good holistic prenatal care.

152. The answer is e. (*Craig, pp 382–383; Hardman, p 484; Katzung, pp 556–557.*) The use of phenytoin, phenobarbital, or several other anticonvulsants is associated with a risk of bleeding tendencies in the newborn. It centers on inadequate fetal levels of vitamin K–dependent clotting factors. Given this information, heparin certainly would increase the risk of peripartum bleeding (even in the absence of anticonvulsant therapy). There is no rational basis for prescribing lidocaine. Lorazepam might be suitable for controlling acute seizures in the mother or newborn. However, the scenario describes no such event, and one should not expect acute maternal or neonatal seizures upon delivery when the mother has received proper anticonvulsant therapy and other elements of care during pregnancy.

153. The answer is d. (*Craig, pp 379–380; Hardman, p 484; Katzung, pp 392–393, 398.*) Pregnancy poses the greatest risk with valproic acid [it is in the FDA's pregnancy category D, which basically means don't use the drug unless the benefits are likely to outweigh (fetal) risks, and no safer alternatives are available]. To be sure there will be interactions between valproic acid and phenobarbital or phenytoin (or many other drugs), but with careful monitoring of serum concentrations and dosage adjustments, this is not a great "risk." A history of CHF does not rule out using valproic acid. The drug is indicated for a variety of seizure types, including absence seizures, and episodes of status epilepticus argue in favor of using valproic acid if current therapies have been ineffective in preventing this life-threatening seizure.

Valproic acid has been associated with severe hepatotoxicity; it appears to be an idiosyncratic reaction, with the risk much higher in pediatric patients (especially <2 years old). Fatalities generally occur within 4 months of treatment, but for some patients the liver damage is reversible after stopping the drug.

154. The answer is c. (*Craig, pp 391–392; Hardman, p 444; Katzung, pp 486, 490, 494.*) This patient ate tyramine-rich foods while taking an MAOI, and went into hypertensive crisis. Tyramine causes release of stored catecholamines from presynaptic terminals, which can cause hypertension, headache, tachycardia, arrhythmias, nausea, and stroke. In patients who do not take MAOIs, tyramine is inactivated in the gut by MAO, and patients taking MAOIs must be warned about the dangers of eating tyramine-rich foods.

155. The answer is a. (*Craig pp 385–386, 389–391; Hardman, pp 453, 456–458, 466–468.*) Of the listed antidepressants, only amitriptyline, a tricyclic, causes adverse effects related to blockade of muscarinic acetylcholine receptors. Both trazodone and amitriptyline cause adverse effects related to α-adrenoreceptor blockade.

156. The answer is d. (*Craig, pp 386–388; Hardman, pp 444–445, 497; Katzung, pp 271, 493–494, 991.*) This patient has the serotonin syndrome. Serotonin is already present in increased amounts in synapses because of blockade of its reuptake by the SSRIs. When sumatriptan (or other triptans used for migraine therapy; they are 5-HT$_{1B/2D}$ agonists) is added, rapid accumulation of serotonin and/or the triptan in the brain can occur.

The risk of the serotonin syndrome in SSRI-treated patients is much higher when MAO inhibitors are used concomitantly. Nonetheless, such severe reactions from an SSRI-triptan interaction have been reported. In addition, do not forget that MAO inhibitors can also cause an acute and potentially fatal hypertensive crisis when co-administered with tricyclic/tetracyclic antidepressants (e.g., imipramine); such combined use should be avoided.

157. The answer is a. (*Hardman, pp 457, 503; Katzung, pp 466–471.*) Clozapine differs from other neuroleptic agents in that it can induce seizures in nonepileptic patients. In patients with a history of epileptic seizures for which they are not receiving treatment, stimulation of seizures can occur following the administration of neuroleptic agents because they lower seizure threshold and cause brain discharge patterns reminiscent of epileptic seizure disorders.

158. The answer is a. (*Craig, pp 399–403; Hardman, pp 497–498; Katzung, pp 472–474.*) Although many antipsychotic agents can cause orthostatic hypotension, chlorpromazine has the highest risk (as do nearly all the other phenothiazines) in general. Recall: phenothiazines are called low-potency antipsychotics, and one inference of that is that compared with other (high potency) agents such as haloperidol they cause a relatively greater incidence of autonomic side effects: orthostatic hypotension (from α-adrenergic blockade) and a host of other side effects from blocking muscarinic-cholinergic receptors.

159. The answer is d. (*Craig, pp 359–408, 411–412; Hardman, pp 412–419, 628–630; Katzung, pp 520–521.*) A long-acting benzodiazepine, such as diazepam, is effective in alleviating barbiturate withdrawal symptoms. The anxiolytic effects of buspirone take several days to develop, obviating its use for acute, severe anxiety.

160. The answer is b. (*Craig, pp 296, 357; Hardman, pp 364–365, 372–374; Katzung, pp 357–360, 364, 989.*) Flumazenil is a competitive antagonist of benzodiazepines at the GABA receptor. Repeated administration is necessary because of its short half-life relative to that of most benzodiazepines—especially diazepam, which forms many long-lasting active metabolites.

161. The answer is d. (*Craig, pp 382–383; Hardman, p 484; Katzung, p 398.*) An increased incidence of spina bifida may occur with the use of valproic acid during pregnancy. Cardiovascular, orofacial, and digital abnormalities may also occur. The main issue with the use of phenobarbital or primidone (metabolite is phenobarbital) for the fetus is neonatal dependence on barbiturates.

162. The answer is c. (*Craig, pp 330–335; Hardman, pp 337–338; Katzung, pp 419, 427.*) Of the listed agents, only lidocaine is an amide. Allergy to amide-type local anesthetics is much less frequent than with ester-type local anesthetics, such as lidocaine or benzocaine. The reaction with esters appears to be due to a metabolite, probably *p*-aminobenzoic acid, which forms a hapten. PABA is not formed with amide metabolism. (Be sure you remember that esters are hydrolyzed by esterases in the plasma; amides are metabolically inactivated in the liver.) Patients who have had a true allergic response to one ester is likely to react to another (cross-allergenicity). However, there is no cross-allergenicity such that patients who have had an anaphylactoid reaction to an ester will react similarly to an amide.

163. The answer is a. (*Craig, p 370; Hardman, p 513; Katzung, p 454.*) This cutaneous response, called livedo reticularis, is characteristically associated with amantadine. Recall that this seldom-used antiparkinson drug probably works by releasing endogenous dopamine and blocking its neuronal reuptake. Livedo reticularis is not associated with levodopa (used alone or with carbidopa), nor with the dopamine agonists bromocriptine or pramipexole (a newer and generally preferred drug for starting treatment of mild parkinsonian signs and symptoms).

164. The answer is b. (*Craig, pp 393–395; Hardman, p 449; Katzung, p 477–478.*) Some NSAIDs can increase proximal tubular reabsorption of lithium salts, which can create toxic levels of lithium in the plasma.

165. The answer is d. (*Craig, p 378; Hardman, p 530; Katzung, p 383.*) For many years, phenytoin has been cited as a classic example of a drug that can cause gingival hyperplasia. (Among oral surgeons and dentists, it is often referred to as Dilantin hyperplasia, in recognition of phenytoin's main proprietary name.) The mechanism is unknown, but we suspect the drug alters collagen metabolism in the gingival tissues. Although phenytoin isn't the only drug associated with potential gingival hyperplasia (verapamil is another common one), it is the only one listed as a choice. Note that phenobarbital, which is often used as an alternative to phenytoin, does not cause gingival hyperplasia. It is precisely for that reason that phenobarbital is often prescribed for children with responsive seizure disorders in lieu of phenytoin.

166. The answer is d. (*Hardman, p 479; Katzung, pp 271, 493–494, 991.*) The serotonin receptor agonist actions of the "triptans," including the prototype, sumatriptan, can trigger intense vasoconstriction in various vascular beds. The cerebral vasoconstrictor effects of these drugs contribute importantly to the relief they afford in migraine headaches. However, coronary vasospasm can occur also, and these drugs are therefore contraindicated for patients with coronary artery disease.

None of the other drugs listed have any coronary (or other) vasoconstrictor effects. Indeed, some such as phenytoin and zolpidem (a benzodiazepine-like hypnotic) actually cause slight cardiovascular changes that would actually reduce the risk of myocardial ischemia and angina.

167. The answer is b. (*Craig, p 383; Katzung, pp 380, 397–398.*) Fosphenytoin is the prodrug form of phenytoin. It is the metabolite (the phenytoin itself) that is responsible for anticonvulsant effects, and so the mechanism of actions are identical. Using fos-phenytoin does not: have a faster onset of action than its metabolite; eliminate the need for giving such drugs as lorazepam first; or giving oral agents for chronic seizures; or stimulate ventilation. The main advantages of fos-phenytoin are less vascular irritability, the ability to be injected faster, and greater physical compatibility with IV solutions that might be used to dilute or administer it (e.g., phenytoin must be diluted before injection, but it is physically incompatible with glucose-containing solutions that so often are used as a vehicle for many IV drugs).

168. The answer is c. (*Craig, p 305; Hardman, pp 307–308, 319–321; Katzung, pp 402–404.*) Recall that nitrous oxide has a MAC (minimum alveolar concentration) of about 105%. Achieving that concentration in an inspired gas mixture is physically impossible at normal atmospheric pressure. Even if pure nitrous oxide were given, and the MAC was 100%, the drug would (1) cause abolition of a painful response in only 50% of subjects (this is one element of the definition of MAC), and (2) be lethal, since

100% nitrous oxide means no (0%) oxygen. This very effective analgesic gas is poorly soluble in the blood, so equilibration between alveolar and blood concentration and the onset of its central effects are quite rapid.

Even at the usual concentrations, and whether used only with air (as in dental practice) or with other inhaled anesthetics (common in surgery), nitrous oxide causes little or no bronchospasm nor significant cardiac depression.

169. The answer is e. (*Craig, pp 195, 400; Hardman, p 412; Katzung, p 473.*) The long QT syndrome is not at all uncommon, and thioridazine (a phenothiazine antipsychotic drug) is often cited as a drug that can cause further prolongation of the QT interval (further prolongation of ventricular repolarization) and lead to rapidly worsening and serious arrhythmias such as torsades de pointes (which can deteriorate to ventricular fibrillation rather quickly). This risk is not shared by most other phenothiazines, but it is a problem with haloperidol, a butyrophenone antipsychotic.

170. The answer is b. (*Craig, p 402; Hardman, pp 414–416; Katzung, p 474.*) The question described common and necessary interventions for managing neuroleptic malignant syndrome, which is characteristically associated with older antipsychotics—chlorpromazine and other "low potency" antipsychotics to a degree, but occurs moreso with haloperidol (butyrophenone). Signs and symptoms include muscle tetany/rigidity ("lead pipe rigidity"), profound fever, rapid swings of heart rate, rhythm, blood pressure (autonomic instability), electrolyte abnormalities and dehydration. None of the other agents are associated with this syndrome, whether acutely or with long-term therapy or at therapeutic or toxic serum levels.

171. The answer is c. (*Craig, p 371; Hardman, pp 513–514; Katzung, pp 1010–1011.*) Initial, recommended therapy involves use of acetylcholinesterase inhibitors such as tacrine, donepezil, galantamine (which are reversible cholinesterase inhibitors), or rivastigmine (irreversible). These drugs are not cures; they do not halt disease or symptom progression, but they appear to slow symptoms of brain pathology in some patients. None appears to be invariably superior to any other. Their actions almost certainly involve activation of central muscarinic receptors (indirectly, by inhibiting metabolism of ACh released from viable nerves, of course), because drugs with central antimuscarinic actions reduce their efficacy. Selegiline (MAO inhibitor) and high doses of vitamin E (antioxidant) apparently slow neu-rodegenerative processes, but so far there are no convincing data that they slow cognitive decline. They are not first-line therapies.

172. The answer is c. *(Craig, pp 356–357t; Hardman, pp 425–426; Katzung, pp 272, 360.)* Buspirone is an attractive drug for managing short-term anxiety. Among the reasons (and especially when compared with more traditional anxiolytics, such as benzodiazepines) are a lack of seda-tion (buspirone is not a CNS depressant) and virtually no potentiation of the effects of other CNS depressants, including alcohol; no known abuse potential (it is not regulated by the Controlled Substances Act) or ten-dency for development of tolerance; and no major withdrawal syndrome. One major drawback to the drug is a very slow onset of symptom relief (a week or two), and typically it takes about a month from the onset of ther-apy for antianxiety effects to peak. (This slow time course, obviously, does not warrant "almost daily" dosage titrations.)

You should recall that long-term benzodiazepine administration is associated with withdrawal phenomena (and, depending on the use, the syndrome can be severe). Thus, one can envisage a switch from a benzo-diazepine to buspirone. Because buspirone lacks CNS depressant effects and its effects take some time to develop, one should start the buspirone several weeks before stopping the benzodiazepine and also taper the ben-zodiazepine dose once it's time to stop the drug.

Cardiovascular System

Agents for heart failure
Antianemics
Antianginals
Antiarrhythmics
Anticoagulants

Antihyperlipidemics
Antihypertensives
Antiplatelet agents
Thrombolytics/Fibrinolytics

Questions

DIRECTIONS: Each item contains a question or incomplete statement that is followed by possible responses. Select the **one best** response to each question.

173. The figure below shows typical cardiovascular responses to the intravenous injection of four adrenergic drugs into a *normal, resting* subject. Assume the doses of each are high enough to cause expected effects, but not so high that toxic effects occur. No other drugs are present, and sufficient time has been allowed to enable complete dissipation of the effects of any prior drugs. The dashed line between the systolic and diastolic pressure traces represents mean arterial pressure.

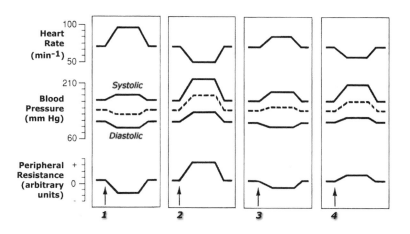

Select the letter that indicates the drugs that are ordered in the correct sequence (1, 2, 3, 4) on the previous page.

Abbreviations used, and potential answer choices, are

EPI, epinephrine
ISO, isoproterenol
NE, norepinephrine
PHE, phenylephrine
PHN, phentolamine
PRO, propranolol

a. EPI, NE, PHE, ISO
b. ISO, EPI, NE, PHE
c. ISO, PHE, EPI, NE
d. NE, ISO, PHE, EPI
e. PHE, EPI, NE, PRO
f. PHE, ISO, NE, EPI
g. PRO, PHN, PHE, ISO

174. A 75-year-old woman with congestive heart failure (CHF) is unable to climb a flight of stairs without experiencing shortness of breath. Digoxin is administered to improve cardiac muscle contractility. Within 2 weeks, she has a marked improvement in her symptoms. The direct cellular action of digoxin that accounts for its ability to improve cardiac output is inhibition of which of the following?

a. β_1-adrenergic receptor activation
b. Cyclic adenosine 5'-monophosphate (cAMP) synthesis
c. GTP binding to specific G proteins
d. Mitochondrial calcium (Ca^{2+}) release
e. Na^+-K^+-ATPase

175. A patient has periodic episodes of paroxysmal supraventricular tachycardia. Which of the following would be suitable for outpatient prophylaxis?

a. Adenosine
b. Lidocaine
c. Nifedipine
d. Nitroglycerin
e. Verapamil

176. The therapeutic actions of β-adrenergic receptor blockers in chronic-stable angina pectoris are primarily the result of which of the following?

a. Antiplatelet/antithrombotic effects
b. Coronary vasodilation
c. Decreased myocardial oxygen demand
d. Reduced total peripheral resistance
e. Slowed A-V nodal conduction velocity

Questions 177–186

Listed below are short descriptions of various patients, all of whom have recently diagnosed Stage II essential hypertension and a stated comorbidity or other pertinent finding.

You are to start oral therapy for the hypertension. Your goal is to select the antihypertensive drug with a profile that makes it the best choice—or, in other stated instances, the poorest or worst choice—for the patient described.

A letter may be used once, more than once, or not at all.

a. Angiotensin-converting enzyme (ACE) inhibitor or angiotensin receptor blocker
b. β-adrenergic blocker
c. Nifedipine
d. Thiazide diuretic
e. Verapamil or diltiazem

177. Best choice for a 50-year-old man with well-controlled type 2 diabetes and normal renal function (and no microalbuminuria)

178. Most likely to trigger a gout attack or worsen asymptomatic hyperuricemia

179. Best choice for a patient who is tachycardic and has chronic open-angle glaucoma

180. Best choice for a patient who has a history of vasospastic (variant, or Prinzmetal's) angina pectoris

181. Worst choice for a patient with vasospastic angina because it may worsen the condition

182. Worst choice for a pregnant woman

183. Most likely to exacerbate tachycardia in a patient who is already taking sublingual nitroglycerin for chronic-stable (exercise-induced) angina pectoris

184. Most likely to exacerbate asthma by facilitating or causing bronchoconstriction

185. May cause breathing difficulty for an asthmatic by thickening airway mucus secretions and so obstructing the airways with viscous mucus

186. Poorest choice for a patient with poorly controlled insulin-dependent diabetes mellitus because it will mask a symptom of severe hypoglycemia and delay recovery from a hypoglycemic episode

187. Quinidine is ordered for a patient with recurrent atrial fibrillation. This drug

a. Is likely to increase blood pressure via a direct vasoconstrictor effect
b. Is contraindicated if the patient also requires anticoagulant therapy
c. Slows spontaneous S-A nodal depolarization as its predominant effect
d. Tends to slow electrical impulse conduction velocity through the A-V node
e. Will increase cardiac contractility (positive inotropic effect) independent of its antiarrhythmic effects

188. A patient who has been taking an oral antihypertensive drug for about a year develops a positive Coombs' test. Which of the following is the most likely cause?

a. Captopril
b. Clonidine
c. Labetalol
d. Methyldopa
e. Prazosin

189. Which antiarrhythmic has relatively few electrophysiologic effects on normal myocardial tissue, but suppresses the arrhythmogenic properties of ischemic tissues?

a. Disopyramide
b. Lidocaine
c. Procainamide
d. Propranolol
e. Quinidine

190. We want to compare and contrast the cardiac and hemodynamic profiles of immediate-acting dihydropyridine-type calcium channel blockers (CCBs) and the nondihydropyridines, verapamil and diltiazem (benzothiazepines). A most striking difference is that compared with nifedipine, verapamil and diltiazem:

a. Are suitable for use in conjunction with a β blocker or digoxin
b. Cause a much higher incidence of reflex tachycardia
c. Cause significant dose-dependent slowing of A-V nodal conduction velocity
d. Cause significant venodilation, leading to profound orthostatic hypotension
e. Have significant positive inotropic effects

191. Digoxin affects a host of cardiac electrophysiologic properties. Some of its effects are caused directly by the drug. Others are indirect: they may involve increasing "vagal tone" to the heart or other compensations that arise when cardiac output is improved in a patient with heart failure. For some parameters the direct and indirect effects may be qualitatively (but not quantitatively) opposing, but one will predominate over the other. Which of the following is an expected, predominant effect of the drug?

a. Increased rate of S-A nodal depolarization
b. Reduced atrial automaticity
c. Reduced ventricular automaticity
d. Slowed A-V nodal conduction velocity
e. Slowed conduction velocity through the atrial myocardium and His-Purkinje system

192. A patient has Stage III essential hypertension but normal ventricular function. After evaluating the responses to several other antihypertensive drugs, alone and in combination, the physician places the patient on oral hydralazine. Which of the following adjunct(s) is/are likely to be needed to manage the expected and unwanted cardiovascular side effects of the hydralazine?

a. Captopril plus nifedipine
b. Digoxin plus spironolactone
c. Digoxin plus vitamin K
d. Hydrochlorothiazide and a β blocker
e. Nitroglycerin
f. Triamterene plus amiloride

193. Which of the following drugs, recommended for lowering of serum cholesterol (total and LDL), inhibits cholesterol synthesis by inhibiting 3-hydroxy-3-methylglutaryl-coenzyme A [better known as (HMG-CoA) reductase]?

a. Clofibrate
b. Gemfibrozil
c. Lovastatin
d. Nicotinic acid (niacin)
e. Probucol

194. Drugs that block neuronal catecholamine reuptake (e.g., tricyclic antidepressants) are likely to block the antihypertensive action of which of the following drugs?

a. Diazoxide
b. Guanethidine
c. Hydralazine
d. Prazosin
e. Propranolol

Questions 195–196

Given the preeminent role (usually the #1 choice) of nitroprusside sodium as the main intravenous agent for managing most hypertensive emergencies, for causing "controlled" hypotension in some surgical settings, and for being an adjunct for managing some cases of acute heart failure, it is important to know the following.

195. When nitroprusside doses are too high or the drug has been administered too long, refractoriness (loss of blood pressure control) plus other signs and symptoms of potentially severe toxicity develop. These manifestations of toxicity arise because nitroprusside is metabolized to which of the following?

a. A highly efficacious α-adrenergic blocker
b. An extraordinarily potent and irreversible Na-K-ATPase inhibitor
c. An irreversible agonist for angiotensin II receptors
d. Cyanide
e. Nitric oxide

196. Which of the following can be administered concomitant with nitroprusside to prevent or minimize metabolism of the drug to the toxic metabolite responsible for refractoriness and other manifestations of nitroprusside toxicity?

a. Epinephrine
b. Sodium thiosulfate
c. Thrombin
d. Vitamin C
e. Vitamin E
f. Vitamin K

197. In a hypertensive patient who is taking insulin to treat diabetes, which of the following drugs is to be used with extra caution and advice to the patient?

a. Hydralazine
b. Prazosin
c. Guanethidine
d. Propranolol
e. Methyldopa

198. Which of the following is appropriate and generally regarded as most effective for relieving and preventing ischemic episodes in patients with variant angina?

a. Aspirin
b. Atorvastatin
c. Diltiazem
d. Nitroglycerin
e. Propranolol

199. Compared with captopril or another angiotensin-converting enzyme (ACE) inhibitor, drugs such as losartan:

a. Are associated with a higher incidence of bronchospasm and hyperuricemia
b. Are preferred for managing hypertension during pregnancy
c. Do not inhibit synthesis of angiotensin II
d. Effectively block catecholamine-mediated vasoconstriction
e. Exert many more actions, at more sites of action, to lower blood pressure
f. Should only be tried after β blockers, diuretics, calcium channel blockers, and ACE inhibitors have been tried first and proven ineffective
g. Usually cause hyperkalemia

200. A 55-year-old man has heart failure. He is being treated with digoxin, furosemide, and triamterene. He presents with atrial fibrillation. Serum electrolyte levels are normal; serum digoxin concentrations are at the high end of the normal range. The arrhythmia is electrically converted. In addition to beginning anticoagulant therapy for prophylaxis of thromboembolism, the physician starts oral quinidine, at a usually effective dose.

Which of the following is the most likely outcome of adding the quinidine?

a. Development of signs and symptoms of quinidine toxicity (cinchonism)
b. Hyponatremia due to quinidine's ability to enhance diuretic-induced sodium loss
c. Onset of signs and symptoms of digoxin toxicity
d. Precipitous development of hypokalemia
e. Prompt suppression of cardiac contractility, onset of acute heart failure

201. A key point to know about antiarrhythmics in Vaughn-Williams Class I-C (e.g., flecainide, propafenone) is that they:

a. Are only given for arrhythmias during acute myocardial infarction
b. Are particularly suited for patients with low ejection fractions
c. Are preferred drugs (drugs of choice) for relatively innocuous ventricular arrhythmias
d. Cause pulmonary fibrosis and a hypothyroid-like syndrome when given long term
e. Have a significant pro-arrhythmic effect (induction of lethal arrhythmias)

202. A 44-year-old obese man has extremely high plasma triglyceride levels. Following treatment with a drug triglyceride levels decrease to almost normal. Which of the following agents is most likely to have caused this desired change?

a. Atorvastatin
b. Cholestyramine
c. Colestipol
d. Ezetemibe
e. Gemfibrozil

203. A 64-year-old man with arteriosclerotic heart disease (AHD) and CHF who has been treated with digoxin complains of nausea, vomiting, and diarrhea. His EKG reveals a bigeminal rhythm. The symptoms and EKG findings occurred shortly after another therapeutic agent was added to his regimen. A drug-drug interaction is suspected. Which of the following add-on agents most likely provoked the problem?

a. Lovastatin
b. Hydrochlorothiazide
c. Phenobarbital
d. Nitroglycerin
e. Captopril

204. Nicotinic acid in large doses used to treat hyperlipoproteinemia causes a cutaneous flush. The vasodilatory effect is due to which of the following?

a. Release of histamine
b. Production of local prostaglandins
c. Release of platelet-derived growth factor (PDGF)
d. Production of NO
e. Ca channel blockade

205. A patient with Stage 2 essential hypertension is treated with usually effective therapeutic doses of an angiotensin-converting enzyme inhibitor. After a suitable period of time blood pressure has not been lowered satisfactorily. The patient has been compliant with drug therapy and other recommendations (e.g., weight reduction, exercise).

A thiazide is added to the ACE inhibitor regimen. Which of the following is the most likely and earliest untoward outcome of this drug add-on, for which you should monitor closely?

a. Fall of blood pressure sufficient to cause syncope
b. Hypokalemia due to synergistic effects of the ACE inhibitor and the thiazide on renal potassium excretion
c. Onset of acute heart failure from depression of ventricular contractility
d. Paradoxical hypertensive crisis
e. Sudden prolongation of the P-R interval and increasing degrees of heart block

206. A 52-year-old woman with essential hypertension, hypercholesterolemia, and chronic-stable angina develops severe constipation. It is attributed to one of her medications. Which was the most likely cause?

a. Atorvastatin
b. Captopril
c. Labetalol
d. Nitroglycerin
e. Verapamil

207. Angiotensin-converting enzyme (ACE) inhibitors are associated with a relatively high incidence of which of the following adverse reactions?

a. Hepatitis
b. Hypokalemia
c. Agranulocytosis
d. Proteinuria
e. Hirsutism

208. A 45-year-old man postmyocardial infarction (MI) for 1 week is being treated with intravenous (IV) heparin. Stool guaiac on admission was negative, but is now 4+, and he has had an episode of hematemesis. We stop the heparin. Which of the following should be administered to counteract the effects of excessive heparin remaining in the circulation?

a. Aminocaproic acid
b. Dipyridamole
c. Factor IX
d. Protamine
e. Vitamin K

Questions 209–210

Two patients with multiple cardiovascular disorders present in your clinic. They are taking the following medications, for the indications listed.

   For both patients, the medications are

a. Captopril for hypertension and heart failure
b. Carvedilol for hypertension, heart failure, and angina prophylaxis
c. Nitroglycerin, sublingual, for acute angina
d. Procainamide for atrial fibrillation
e. Atorvastatin for primary prevention of CAD
f. Warfarin for prophylaxis of thromboembolism
g. Furosemide as adjunctive management of CHF

209. Patient 1 complains of fever and arthralgia (joint aches and pains) and other "flu-like symptoms." These findings, plus a facial "rash" and results of blood work, all point to a drug-induced lupus-like syndrome. Heart rate, BP, and all other cardiovascular findings are completely normal. Which of the above drugs is the most likely cause of these findings?

210. Patient 2, 67-years-old, complains of muscle aches, pain, and tenderness. These affect the legs and trunk. There is no fever, bruising, or any recent history of muscle trauma or strains (as from excessive exercise). There is myoglobinuria, a clinically significant fall of creatinine clearance, and a rise of serum creatine kinase (CK) to levels nearly 10 times the upper limit of normal. Which of the above drugs is the most likely cause of these findings?

Questions 211–212

A physician is preparing to administer a drug for which there is a label warning: "do not administer this drug to patients with second-degree or greater heart block, or give with other drugs that may cause heart block."

211. Which of the following findings would be indicative of heart block, and second-degree heart block in particular?

a. Auscultation of the precordium reveals an irregular rhythm
b. Blood pressure is low
c. Heart rate is abnormally low (bradycardia), but there is normal sinus rhythm
d. The EKG reveals ventricular ectopic beats
e. The EKG shows a prolonged PR interval, and some P waves are not followed by a normal QRS complex
f. The EKG shows abnormally widened QRS complexes

212. Which of the following drugs might carry the above warning against use in patients with heart block or in conjunction with other drugs that might cause it?

a. Captopril
b. Losartan
c. Nifedipine
d. Nitroglycerin
e. Prazosin
f. Verapamil

213. A 45-year-old man asks his physician for a prescription for sildenafil to improve his sexual performance. Because of risks from a serious drug interaction, this drug should not be prescribed, and the patient should be urged not to try to obtain it from other sources, if he is also taking which of the following drugs?

a. An angiotensin-converting enzyme inhibitor
b. A β-adrenergic blocker
c. A nitrovasodilator (e.g., nitroglycerin)
d. A statin-type antihypercholesterolemic drug
e. A thiazide or loop diuretic

214. Significant relaxation of both venular and arteriolar smooth muscle occurs in response to which of the following?

a. Hydralazine
b. Minoxidil
c. Diazoxide
d. Sodium nitroprusside
e. Nifedipine

215. Which of the following precautions is advisable when using lovastatin?

a. Serum transaminase measurements
b. Renal function studies
c. Acoustic measurements
d. Monthly complete blood counts
e. Avoidance of bile acid sequestrants

216. Which of the following is generally considered to be the first-line drug for treating an acute attack of reentrant supraventricular tachycardia (SVT)?

a. Adenosine
b. Digoxin
c. Edrophonium
d. Phenylephrine
e. Propranolol

Questions 217–219

For each patient, select the drug most likely to have caused the changes described in the scenario.

a. Acetazolamide
b. Amiloride
c. Furosemide
d. Hydrochlorothiazide
e. Mannitol

217. An 83-year-old man has been effectively treated with hydrochlorothiazide to control his elevated blood pressure. He has had a recent onset of weakness. Blood chemistry analysis reveals a K^+ of 2.5 mEq/L. Another drug is added, and 1 month later his serum K^+ is 4.0 mEq/L.

218. A 76-year-old man with a combined history of bronchogenic carcinoma and CHF is maintained on a diuretic to control pulmonary and peripheral edema. Recent measurement of blood electrolytes reveals an elevated serum Ca^{2+}.

219. A 66-year-old woman with CHF and hearing loss is given a diuretic as part of a regimen that includes digoxin and an ACE inhibitor. In the course of treatment, she develops an AV conduction defect and is found to be hypomagnesemic. She also reports what she describes as some hearing loss, which is reversed when the drug is stopped.

220. A 60-year-old man, following hospitalization for an acute myocardial infarction, is treated with warfarin. What is the main mechanism by which warfarin is exerting the effects for which it is given?

a. Increase in the plasma level of Factor IX
b. Inhibition of thrombin and early coagulation steps
c. Inhibition of synthesis of prothrombin and coagulation Factors VII, IX, and X
d. Inhibition of platelet aggregation in vitro
e. Activation of plasminogen
f. Binding of Ca^{2+} ion cofactor in some coagulation steps

221. A 39-year-old pregnant woman requires heparin for prophylaxis of thromboembolism. What is the mechanism of action of heparin?

a. Increase in the plasma level of Factor IX
b. Inhibition of thrombin and early coagulation steps
c. Inhibition of synthesis of prothrombin and coagulation Factors VII, IX, and X
d. Inhibition of platelet aggregation in vitro
e. Activation of plasminogen
f. Binding of Ca^{2+} ion cofactor in some coagulation steps

222. A 42-year-old man with an acute MI is treated with alteplase. This drug exerts its main desired effects via which of the following?

a. Inhibition of platelet thromboxane production
b. Antagonism of ADP receptor
c. Glycoprotein IIb/IIIa antagonist
d. Inhibition of the synthesis of vitamin K–dependent coagulation factors
e. Activation of plasminogen from plasmin

223. A 65-year-old man with a previous history of a stroke is treated with clopidogrel to guard against another stroke. What is the mechanism of action by which the drug works prophylactically?

a. Inhibition of platelet thromboxane production
b. Antagonism of ADP receptor
c. Antagonism of glycoprotein IIb/IIIa
d. Inhibition of the synthesis of vitamin K–dependent coagulation factors
e. Activation of plasminogen to plasmin

224. A patient with atrial fibrillation is placed on long-term arrhythmia control with amiodarone. In addition to "standard" monitoring, periodic assessments of which of the following should be made in order to detect adverse effects that are unique to this drug?

a. Blood glucose, triglyceride, cholesterol, and sodium concentrations
b. Hearing thresholds (audiometry) and serum albumin concentration
c. Prothrombin time and antinuclear antibody (ANA) titers
d. Pulmonary function and thyroid hormone status
e. White cell counts and serum urate concentration

225. A 64-year-old woman has had several episodes of transient ischemic attacks (TIAs). Aspirin would be a preferred treatment, but she has a history of severe "aspirin sensitivity" manifest as intense bronchoconstriction. What would be a suitable alternative to the aspirin?

a. Acetaminophen
b. Aminocaproic acid
c. Clopidogrel
d. Dipyridamole
e. Streptokinase

226. A 70-year-old woman is treated with sublingual nitroglycerin for her occasional bouts of angina. Which of the following is involved in the action of nitroglycerin?

a. α-adrenergic blockade
b. Phosphodiesterase activity
c. Phosphorylation of myosin light chains in smooth muscle
d. Forms cyanide, which lowers smooth-muscle cell levels of ATP needed for contraction
e. cGMP

227. A patient with CHF, Stage 2 essential hypertension, and hyperlipidemia (elevated LDL cholesterol and abnormally low HDL-C) is taking proper therapeutic doses of digoxin, bumetanide, captopril, and simvastatin (an HMG-CoA reductase inhibitor).

During a scheduled physical exam, about a month after starting all the above drugs, the patient reports a severe, hacking, and relentless cough. Other vital signs, and the overall physical assessment, are consistent with good control of both the heart failure and blood pressure and indicate no other underlying disease or abnormalities. Results of blood tests are not yet available.

Which of the following is the most likely cause of the cough?

a. An expected side effect of the captopril
b. An allergic reaction to digoxin
c. Digoxin toxicity caused by displacement of the digoxin by captopril
d. Dyspnea due to captopril's known and powerful bronchoconstrictor action
e. Hyperkalemia caused by an interaction between the diuretic and captopril
f. An expected adverse response to the simvastatin

228. A 60-year-old woman with deep-vein thrombosis (DVT) is given a bolus of heparin, and a heparin drip is also started. Thirty minutes later, she is bleeding profusely from the intravenous site. The heparin is stopped, but the bleeding continues. You decide to give protamine to reverse the adverse effect of heparin. How does protamine act?

a. It causes hydrolysis of heparin
b. It changes the conformation of antithrombin III to prevent binding to heparin
c. It activates the coagulation cascade, overriding the action of heparin
d. It combines with heparin as an ion pair, thus inactivating it

229. A 47-year-old woman comes to the emergency department (ED) with severe crushing chest pain of 1 hour's duration. Electrocardiogram and blood chemistries are consistent with a diagnosis of acute MI. Streptokinase is chosen as part of the therapeutic regimen. Which of the following is its mechanism of action?

a. It activates the conversion of fibrin to fibrin-split products
b. It activates the conversion of plasminogen to plasmin
c. It inhibits the conversion of prothrombin to thrombin
d. It inhibits the conversion of fibrinogen to fibrin

Questions 230–232

For each patient, select the drug most likely to have caused the adverse effect.

a. Adenosine
b. Captopril
c. Clonidine
d. Digoxin
e. Dobutamine
f. Furosemide
g. Guanethidine
h. Lidocaine
i. Nifedipine
j. Prazosin
k. Procainamide

230. A 36-year-old man is seen in the ED with tachycardia, a respiratory rate of 26 breaths per minute (BPM), and EKG evidence of an arrhythmia. An intravenous bolus dose of an antiarrhythmic agent is administered, and within 30 s, he has a respiratory rate of 45 BPM and complains of a burning sensation in his chest.

231. Following a cardiac triple-bypass operation, a 65-year-old normotensive hospitalized woman has shortness of breath, diffuse rales bilaterally, a pulse of 110/min, an elevated venous pressure, and a blood pressure of 140/85 mmHg. An intravenous dose of drug is given to counteract her findings. However, following administration of this drug, her pulse increases to 150/min and her blood pressure to 180/110 mmHg.

232. A 50-year-old man with a 2-year history of essential hypertension well controlled on hydrochlorothiazide is found on a recent physical examination to have a blood pressure of 160/105 mmHg. The hydrochlorothiazide is substituted with another agent. Two weeks later, he returns for follow-up complaining of a loss of taste.

233. A patient with a history of hypertension, heart failure, and peripheral vascular disease has been on oral therapy with drugs suitable for each for about 3 months. He runs out of the medication and plans to have the prescriptions refilled in a week.

Within a day or two after stopping his medications he experiences an episode of severe tachycardia accompanied by tachyarrhythmias, and an abrupt rise of blood pressure to 240/140 mmHg—well above pretreatment levels. He complains of chest pain, anxiety, and a pounding headache. Soon thereafter he suffers a hemorrhagic stroke.

Abruptly stopping which of the following drugs is most likely to account for these responses?

a. ACE inhibitors
b. Clonidine
c. Digoxin
d. Hydrochlorothiazide
e. Nifedipine (a long-acting formulation)
f. Warfarin

Questions 234–235

The following scenario applies to the next two questions.

Two patients with multiple cardiovascular diseases are being treated long-term with digoxin, furosemide, triamterene, atorvastatin, and nitroglycerin.

234. One patient reports occasional nausea, vomiting, and anorexia, and a "yellowish-greenish tint" to white objects and bright lights. These signs and symptoms are most characteristic of toxicity due to which of the following drugs?

a. Atorvastatin
b. Digoxin
c. Furosemide
d. Nitroglycerin
e. Triamterene
f. The triamterene-furosemide combination (drug interaction)

235. Another patient, treated with the same regimen, reports nonspecific muscle aches and pains. Serum electrolyte profiles are normal. Muscle trauma has been ruled-out. Which of the following is the most likely cause of the symptoms?

a. Atorvastatin
b. Digoxin
c. Furosemide
d. Nitroglycerin
e. Triamterene
f. The triamterene-furosemide combination (drug interaction)

Questions 236–238

For each antiplatelet drug listed below, identify its main mechanism of action.

a. Blocks thrombin receptors selectively
b. Blocks ADP receptors
c. Blocks glycoprotein IIb/IIIa receptor
d. Inhibits cyclooxygenase
e. Inhibits prostacyclin production

236. Clopidogrel

237. Aspirin

238. Abciximab

239. A 56-year-old man presents with NYHA Stage II ("mild") heart failure. He is placed on usual therapeutic doses of digoxin and furosemide. At a follow-up exam 3 months later we find good symptomatic relief of the heart failure. Serum electrolytes and all other lab tests are within normal limits. At this time, which electrocardiographic change would you expect to see in response to the digoxin's expected effects, compared with a baseline (pretreatment) EKG?

a. P waves widened, amplitude increased
b. P-R intervals prolonged
c. QRS complexes widened
d. R-R intervals shortened
e. S-T segments elevated

Questions 240–241

A patient is hospitalized and waiting for coronary angiography. His history includes angina pectoris that is brought on by "modest" exercise (there is no evidence of coronary spasm), accompanied by transient electrocardiographic changes consistent with myocardial ischemia. In the hospital he is receiving nitroglycerine and morphine (slow intravenous infusions), plus oxygen via nasal cannula.

He suddenly develops episodes of chest discomfort. Heart rate during these episodes rises to 170 to 190 beats/min; blood pressure reaches 180–200/110–120 mm Hg, and prominent findings on the EKG are runs of ventricular ectopic beats that terminate spontaneously, plus ST-segment elevation.

240. Although there are several things that need to be done for immediate care, administration of which one of the following is most likely to remedy (at least temporarily) the majority of these signs and symptoms and pose the lowest risk of doing further harm?

a. Aspirin
b. Captopril
c. Furosemide
d. Labetalol
e. Lidocaine
f. Nitroglycerin (increased dose as a bolus)
g. Prazosin

241. A first-year house officer observes the acute changes noted above. They obtain a capsule of immediate-acting nifedipine, open it, and dispense the drug into the patient's mouth. This technique avoids "first-pass" metabolism of the drug and causes rapid absorption and all the effects associated with this calcium channel blocker—intensely. Which of the following is the most likely outcome, given the scenario?

a. A-V nodal block
b. Further rise of heart rate, worsening of the ventricular arrhythmia
c. Hypotension and bradycardia
d. Normalization of heart rate, blood pressure, and the EKG
e. Return of blood pressure toward normal, no significant effect on heart rate or the EKG

Questions 242–244

Look at the ECG below and answer the following three questions.

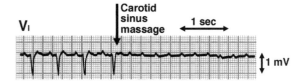

Here you see a continuous (uninterrupted) tracing of V1, before and after carotid sinus massage (at arrow).

242. What is the mechanism by which carotid massage exerted its effect?

a. Activated what is tantamount to the baroreceptor reflex, increasing vagal tone and acetylcholine release considerably
b. Caused catecholamine release
c. Induced atrial fibrillation (atrial rate >> 300/min)
d. Occluded venous return to the heart, thereby interfering with filling and contraction of all heart chambers "downstream" of the right atrium

243. Based on the outcome of carotid sinus massage, what can you say about the origin of the aberrant electrical activity that leads to the tachycardia that you see before the massage?

a. Bundle of Kent (i.e., anomalous or accessory pathway for AV conduction) with retrograde and antegrade conduction
b. Left bundle branch
c. Multiple ectopic ventricular foci
d. Supraventricular

244. What drug, given as an intravenous bolus, might be used as an alternative to carotid massage, causing essentially the same outcome and, therefore, the same interpretation of the origin of the ventricular tachycardia?

a. Adenosine
b. Atropine
c. Epinephrine
d. Isoproterenol
e. Lidocaine

Questions 245–246

Your patient has severe (Stage 4) hypertension that is being controlled with a combination of hydralazine, furosemide, and carvedilol. He also has had bouts of atrial fibrillation that are being managed long term with quinidine and warfarin for prophylaxis of thromboembolism.

245. The patient presents with fever, chills, arthralgia, and a purplish discoloration on the face. The diagnosis is a drug-induced lupus-like syndrome. Which drug in the regimen noted above is most likely to have accounted for this finding?

a. Carvedilol
b. Furosemide
c. Hydralazine
d. Quinidine
e. Warfarin

246. If the patient in the above scenario had a major contraindication to β-adrenergic blockers, which would be the most suitable substitute for the carvedilol?

a. Digoxin
b. Diltiazem
c. Nifedipine
d. Phentolamine
e. Prazosin

247. Your patient has bipolar illness, hypercholesterolemia, chronic-stable angina, and Stage II essential hypertension. He has been taking lithium and an atypical antipsychotic agent for the bipolar illness. Cardiovascular drugs include atorvastatin, diltiazem, sublingual nitroglycerin, captopril, and hydrochlorothiazide. Which of the following outcomes, caused by an important drug-drug interaction, is most likely?

a. Development of acute psychosis from an ACE inhibitor-antipsychotic interaction
b. Development of hypomanic state from antagonism of lithium's action by the nitroglycerine
c. Lithium toxicity because of hyponatremia caused by the hydrochlorothiazide
d. Loss of cholesterol control from antagonism of the HMG Co-A reductase inhibitor by the antipsychotic
e. Worsening of angina because the antipsychotic counteracts the effects of the calcium channel blocker
f. Worsening of angina because the lithium antagonizes the effects of the nitroglycerin

248. A 76-year-old woman with an 8-year history of CHF that has been well controlled with digoxin and furosemide develops recurrence of dyspnea on exertion. On physical examination, she has sinus tachycardia, rales at the base of both lungs, and 4+ pitting edema of the lower extremities. Which of the following agents could be added to her therapeutic regimen?

a. Dobutamine
b. Hydralazine
c. Minoxidil
d. Prazosin
e. Enalapril

249. A patient presents with Stage 3 hypertension. The underlying cause—a pheochromocytoma—is not looked-for nor detected in the work-up. An oral antihypertensive drug is prescribed. We soon find that the patient's blood pressure has gone up to levels above pretreatment levels. Which of the following drugs was most likely administered?

a. Captopril
b. Hydrochlorothiazide
c. Labetalol
d. Losartan
e. Propranolol
f. Verapamil

250. A patient on long-term warfarin therapy arrives at the clinic for her weekly prothrombin time measurement. Her INR is dangerously prolonged, and the physical exam reveals petechial hemorrhages. She's had episodes of long-lasting epistaxis over the last 2 days. Aside from stopping the warfarin (and admitting the patient for follow-up), which of the following should be administered?

a. Aminocaproic acid
b. Epoetin alfa
c. Ferrous sulfate
d. Phytonadione
e. Protamine sulfate

251. The most common cause of digoxin intoxication, when the drug is used long term for managing chronic heart failure, is coadministration of which of the following?

a. Angiotensin-converting enzyme inhibitors (or angiotensin receptor blockers)
b. Cholestyramine or colestipol
c. Hepatic mixed function oxidase inhibitors (cimetidine or any other)
d. Potassium-wasting diuretics (i.e., resulting hypokalemia)
e. Quinidine

252. A patient with hypertension and heart failure has been treated for 2 years with carvedilol and lisinopril. He has just had hip replacement surgery, and because he is not ambulating, is on unfractionated heparin, postoperatively, for prophylaxis of deep venous thrombosis. The ACE inhibitor and β blocker are being given too, and oral antacids and ranitidine (H$_2$ antagonist) have been added for prophylaxis of acute stress ulcers. Five days postop he experiences sudden onset dyspnea and electrocardiographic and other indications of an acute MI. The patient's platelet counts are dangerously low. Which of the following is the most likely underlying problem?

a. Accidental substitution of low-molecular-weight heparins (LMWH) for unfractionated heparin
b. Accidental/inadvertent aspirin administration
c. Hemolytic anemia from a carvedilol-ACE inhibitor interaction
d. Heparin-induced thrombocytopenia
e. Reduced heparin effects by increased metabolic clearance (caused by ranitidine)

253. A 22-year-old varsity hockey player visits you because he has excessive bruising after a game 2 days before. His knee had been bothering him, so he took two aspirin tablets before the game. Other than getting checked 10 times during the game, he denies any excessive or unusual trauma. As you ponder the etiology you order several blood tests. Which test or finding do you expect to be abnormal?

a. Activated partial thromboplastin time (APTT)
b. Bleeding time
c. INR (International Normalized Ratio)
d. Platelet count
e. Prothrombin time

Cardiovascular System

Answers

173. The answer is c. *(Craig, pp 97–98, 100–102; Hardman, p 205; Katzung, pp 129–132.)* ISO, PHE, EPI, NE. Yes, responses to some of these drugs are variable, largely depending on the dose and the speed of administration. Nonetheless, the responses shown are typical.

ISO, a β_1/β_2 agonist, lowers peripheral resistance (and diastolic blood pressure) via β_2-mediated peripheral vasodilator actions. That fall of diastolic pressure is greater than the rise of systolic pressure (which occurs because of a direct cardiac positive inotropic/β_1-activating effect), so mean pressure falls a bit. The combined reflex response to a fall of mean pressure (albeit slight), plus the drug's direct positive chronotropic effect, leads to significant tachycardia.

PHE, which activates only (and all) α-adrenergic receptors, causes only a vasopressor response that accounts for the changes of pressures and peripheral resistance. These changes activate the baroreceptor reflex, leading to reflex bradycardia. The drug has no β agonist activity.

EPI, injected in (reasonably) low doses in normal humans, can cause the effects shown here (and certainly no other drug listed as a possible answer could do the same). The fall of peripheral resistance and diastolic pressure reflects predominant β_2-mediated vasodilation; the rise of systolic pressure is a melding of both peripheral vasoconstriction (α) and direct cardiac stimulation (β_1). Heart rate also reflects direct changes (β_1), as there is no appreciable baroreceptor influence because there is no sudden or significant blood pressure change. Responses to epinephrine are arguably more variable than those of any other drugs listed. Clearly, when large doses are given to a hypotensive patient (e.g., in anaphylaxis), the predominant and wanted vascular effect is a pressor response, much greater than what we see here.

NE, lacking any β_2 activity but being quite effective as an α and β_1 agonist, causes typical responses like those shown here. Peripherally, there is no vasodilation; just constriction. Diastolic, mean, and systolic pressures rise. The rise is sufficient to reflexly slow heart rate; i.e., it is sufficient to overcome NE's direct positive chronotropic effects.

174. The answer is e. (*Craig, p 154; Hardman, pp 810–811; Katzung, pp 205–207.*) Digitalis inhibits the sarcolemmal Na^+, K^+-ATPase ("sodium pump"). This reduces the active (ATP-dependent) extrusion of intracellular Na^+. The excess intracellular Na^+ competes with intracellular Ca^{2+} for sites on a sarcolemmal 2Na-Ca exchange diffusion carrier. The net result is a rise of free $[Ca^{2+}]_i$ and greater actin-myosin interactions (i.e., an increased inotropic state).

175. The answer is e. (*Craig, pp 171t, 183t, 192–193; Hardman, pp 773, 854; Katzung, pp 227–228, 235–236.*) Verapamil, a nondihydropyridine Ca channel blocker (CCB), depresses both the S-A node and the A-V node and would be effective for prophylaxis of paroxysmal atrial or supraventricular tachycardia. Nifedipine, the prototypic dihydropyridine CCB, has little effect on SVT. If we chose a fast-/immediate-acting dosage form of nifedipine, we would probably trigger substantial reflex cardiac stimulation. The increased sympathetic tone to the heart could worsen the PSVT. (And, although nitroglycerin is mainly a venodilator, it too could trigger reflex cardiac activation and worsen matters.) Lidocaine and adenosine are parenteral drugs with short half-lives and, thus, are not suitable for prophylactic therapy.

176. The answer is c. (*Craig, pp 200–203; Hardman, p 774; Katzung, pp 151–157, 197–199.*) β-adrenergic receptor blockers slow resting heart rate and reduce contractility, both of which reduce myocardial oxygen demand. They also blunt the cardiac stimulatory effects, which increase oxygen demand, whenever the sympathetic nervous system is activated (e.g., in response to exercise or drugs that tend to cause reflex sympathetic activation). Recall, too, that coronary blood flow occurs during diastole. By slowing heart rate they prolong diastole, thereby indirectly allowing more time for the myocardium to be perfused.

These drugs have no antiplatelet/antithrombotic effects; they do not cause coronary vasodilation (and may favor constriction, which can become clinically significant in patients with variant angina; see Question 198); and they may increase total peripheral resistance by blocking dilation in some vascular beds (the effect is usually slight and insignificant). The β blockers do slow A-V nodal conduction velocity, but that effect per se contributes little to the reduced oxygen demand that is mainly derived from the drugs' effects on overall rate and contractility.

177. The answer is a. (*Craig, p 212; Hardman, pp 824–8, 893–4; Katzung, pp 177–179.*) ACE inhibitors are generally the preferred drugs for hypertensive patients who also have diabetes mellitus—provided their renal function is satisfactory (specifically, no severe bilateral renal arterial stenosis, or adequate blood flow to one kidney if the other was removed). These drugs do not cause any problems with glucose regulation or the responses to antidiabetic drugs, and they seem to exert some protective effect that slows or delays diabetes-related nephropathy.

β-adrenergic blockers would not be a good choice if hypertension is accompanied only by diabetes mellitus. Should the diabetic patient experience an episode of hypoglycemia (more of a concern with Type I diabetes than with type 2), a β blocker may delay recovery of blood glucose levels, mask tachycardia that is one symptom of hypoglycemia development, and interact with some antidiabetic drugs (even those used for Type II; excessive blood glucose-lowering). (If the diabetes is well controlled, and if the patient has other disorders for which benefits of β blockade may outweigh potential problems, such as mild-moderate heart failure or recent myocardial infarction, then a β blocker may be considered.)

Thiazides can elevate blood glucose levels, or at least antagonize the desired effects of antidiabetic drugs (probably by reducing parenchymal cell responsiveness to insulin). Nonetheless, they usually would not be a first-choice in the setting of diabetes.

Verapamil, diltiazem, and nifedipine seem not to complicate blood glucose regulation or interact with antidiabetic drug therapy. Nonetheless, they lack other benefits offered by ACE inhibitors (especially the renal-protective effects) in the setting of diabetes and so would not be a first choice or of special value.

178. The answer is d. (*Craig, pp 246, 441–442; Hardman, pp 776–777, 874–876; Katzung, pp 178–180, 249–251.*) Thiazide diuretics tend to raise serum uric acid levels. This may be of little concern for patients with no history of hyperuricemia or gout, but for those with such a history it can be a problem that is not associated with any of the other answer choices given. Thiazides *can* be administered to hyperuricemic/gouty patients, but that usually requires another drug (allopurinol; xanthine oxidase inhibitor) to counteract diuretic-induced rises of urate levels. If we can avoid the problems by avoiding the thiazide, and the possible need for adding a second drug to counteract the hyperuricemia, why not do just that?

None of the other answer choices have any appreciable desired or untoward effects on serum urate levels, renal handling of urate, or the incidence or severity of gout.

179. The answer is b. (*Craig, pp 114–116, 232–233; Hardman, pp 252, 260, 883–884; Katzung, pp 151–153, 161–162, 170–172.*) β blockers are not only likely to control blood pressure, but also to reduce catecholamine-induced cardiac stimulation (the tachycardia). In addition, β blockers tend to lower intraocular pressure, and so these drugs would probably provide yet another benefit to a patient with glaucoma. (Even though β-blocker therapy for glaucoma usually involves topical ophthalmic preparations, the same desired effect will occur with oral therapy).

Verapamil or diltiazem, calcium channel blockers (CCBs) of the nondihydropyridine class will not only lower blood pressure but also tend to modulate the tachycardia (through direct but β-receptor-independent processes). However, they don't lower intraocular pressure. All other things being equal, then, the β blocker would still be a better choice for the hypertensive, tachycardiac, glaucomatous patient. Thus, we get three potential benefits from β blockade and only two with verapamil or diltiazem.

Why not nifedipine? See the explanation for Question 190.

ACE inhibitors, ARBs, and thiazides, have no actions that would make them particularly suitable for hypertensive patients who are tachycardiac, have glaucoma, or both.

180. The answer is e. (*Craig, pp 201–202, 220–221; Hardman, pp 859–863; Katzung, pp 176, 192–196.*) The vascular calcium channel–blocking actions of verapamil or diltiazem will not only lower systemic blood pressure, but also tend to counter coronary arterial calcium influx that leads to vasospasm. Thus, in this setting we will get both antihypertensive and antianginal effects.

One might argue that nifedipine (answer c) would be a reasonable alternative. However, recall that the dihydropyridines lack cardiac depressant actions. A dihydropyridine is likely to lower blood pressure (the desired antihypertensive effect), but lacking cardiac-depressant actions they may trigger reflex (sympathetic/baroreceptor) cardiac stimulation. The resulting increases of either or both cardiac rate and contractility necessarily may raise myocardial oxygen demand sufficient to cause myocardial ischemia. [The degree to which a dihydropyridine will cause unwanted reflex cardiac stimulation depends on the drug, the dose, and even the dosage form (e.g., immediate-acting vs. extended-acting).] Nonetheless, a member of the nondihydropyridine CCB would have a much better overall profile of cardiac/vascular actions.

ACE inhibitors, an ARB, or a thiazide, might be suitable for a patient with vasospastic angina, but they have no actions other than their antihypertensive effects that would make them a reasonable first choice for the patient with vasospastic angina.

Insofar as β blockers are concerned, see the answers to Questions 176 and 181.

181. The answer is b. (*Craig, pp 114–116, 202–203; Hardman, pp 119, 221–223, 853; Katzung, pp 197–199.*) β *blockers should not be administered (especially by a systemic route) to patients with vasospastic angina* unless for a medical emergency that requires β blockade as a life-saving measure. Recall the dual roles of adrenergic receptors in the coronary vasculature. Activation of β$_2$-adrenergic receptors causes vasorelaxation. Activation of α-adrenergic receptors favors vasoconstriction or—in the setting of variant angina—vasospasm. Normally these receptors are bathed with circulating epinephrine, which causes the opposing vasodilator (β$_2$) and vasoconstrictor (α) effects. Norepinephrine is also activating α-adrenergic receptors. Block only the β (vasodilator) effects in the coronaries and the constrictor (and spasm-producing) effects of the α receptors are left unopposed.

182. The answer is a. (*Craig, pp 212–213; Hardman, pp 828–829; Katzung, p 178.*) ACE inhibitors (and angiotensin receptor blockers) are contraindicated in pregnancy. Normal in utero development of the kidneys and other urogenital structures seems to be angiotensin-dependent. These drugs, given during the second or third trimesters (not the first) have been associated with severe and sometimes fatal developmental anomalies of these structures. Cranial hypoplasia, and neonatal hyperkalemia and hypotension, have also been reported.

Insofar as the other choices are concerned: β blockers are sometimes used during pregnancy, posing no specific or significant risks to the mother or the fetus provided adequate perinatal care is given and blood pressure doesn't fall excessively. None of the calcium channel blockers seem to have any significant benefits or risks during pregnancy, although as parturition draws near they may suppress uterine contractility.

There are some concerns with using thiazides (or other diuretics) during pregnancy: some risk of too great a fall of blood pressure and also volume depletion. If only one effect occurred, and it were mild, there might not be much of an added risk. However, they often occur together and may cause placental hypoperfusion. Nonetheless, thiazides can be used (and are not absolutely contraindicated) during pregnancy without facing the dire risks associated with ACE inhibitors or ARBs.

183. The answer is c. (*Craig, pp 220–221; Hardman, pp 856–859; Katzung, pp 176, 192–196.*) Nifedipine (dihydropyridine CCB) lacks cardiac depressant activity and may reflexly increase cardiac stimulation (via the baroreceptors) in response to its antihypertensive/vasodilator actions. Should this occur, it certainly wouldn't be beneficial for the patient who is already tachycardic. None of the other drugs listed share this problem.

184. The answer is b. (*Craig, pp 115–116; Hardman, pp 252, 257–258; Katzung, pp 151, 157.*) *No β blocker should be administered to patients with asthma,* because of a great risk of severe and potentially fatal bronchoconstriction or bronchospasm (unless the β blocker is being given for a medical emergency that requires β blockade). This applies to all classes of β blockers: nonselective, like propranolol; β_1 "selective," such as atenolol or metoprolol; those with intrinsic sympathomimetic/partial agonist activity, such as pindolol; and those that also have α-blocking activity, i.e., labetalol and carvedilol. The contraindication also applies to all administration routes, including topical (ophthalmic).

The reason? Airways of persons with asthma are exquisitely sensitive to a host of bronchoconstrictor stimuli and exquisitely dependent on the bronchodilator effects of circulating epinephrine (β_2 receptors).

None of the other answer choices given will exacerbate asthma through a bronchoconstrictor mechanism.

185. The answer is d. (*Craig, pp 250, 459; Hardman, pp 772–773.*) You may not have been taught, explicitly, why thiazides (or other) diuretics may pose problems for patients with asthma, but you almost certainly learned the elements you need to think about to arrive at a correct answer.

When we think of asthma we tend to think of two main pathophysiologic elements: chronic airway inflammation and airway hyperreactivity to various bronchoconstrictor stimuli (or, stated differently, a considerable dependence on intact bronchodilator mechanisms). But there's at least one more element to consider. Many asthmatic patients tend to secrete large volumes of mucus. Even though some of those patients may have an impaired ability to remove that mucus (impaired "mucociliary transport"), if the mucus is sufficiently thin the problems may not be that significant.

Now think of what diuretics may do. The thiazides (and, admittedly, to a greater degree the loop agents) cause some additional fluid loss via the kidneys. While you might predict that would cause reduced mucus volume, the predominant effect is an increase of mucus viscosity. This thickened mucus tends to accumulate in the lower respiratory passages and ultimately cause physical impediments to alveolar gas exchange and bronchiolar diameter and air flow.

186. The answer is b. (*Craig, pp 115–116, 232–233, 768; Hardman, pp 258–259, 883–884; Katzung, pp 151–157.*) Unless there are significant overriding factors (e.g., recent MI), a β blocker would be a relatively poor choice for the patient with poorly controlled, insulin-dependent diabetes. First, they prevent sympathetic-mediated cardiac stimulation (e.g., increased heart rate) that is a signal to many diabetics that their blood glucose levels are getting dangerously low. This applies to all β blockers. Moreover, those that also block $β_2$ receptors may (albeit weakly) inhibit glycogenolysis (thereby doing little to raise or maintain blood glucose levels) and inhibit insulin release (thereby impairing a necessary factor to drive glucose into cells that utilize glucose as a metabolic fuel). Finally, there is some evidence that β blockers may delay the recovery of blood glucose levels from hypoglycemic levels. Overall, "cardioselective" β blockers (atenolol, metoprolol) may pose fewer risks than nonselective agents, but if alternative and less problematic antihypertensive drugs from other classes are available (and they certainly are), it's best to avoid a β blocker altogether.

187. The answer is c. (*Craig, pp 170–173; Hardman, pp 869–871; Katzung, pp 226–228.*) Quinidine's main beneficial effect in supraventricular arrhythmias is a suppression of spontaneous depolarization of the S-A node.

Concomitantly, the predominant effect on the A-V node is an increase of nodal electrical impulse conduction velocity (not a slowing, as noted in d). This is a main reason why, when quinidine therapy is to be started and atrial rates are still high, we pretreat the patient with a dose of a drug that "blocks down" the A-V node: often digoxin, sometimes verapamil or diltiazem, and occasionally a β blocker. The main reason why ventricular rates aren't identical (or close to) atrial rates during atrial fibrillation is because the A-V node cannot transmit impulses at such high rates. This protective effect depends on A-V nodal refractoriness and a relative inability to transmit too many impulses per time. If we did not suppress the A-V node before giving quinidine, the A-V nodal effects of the quinidine might increase A-V nodal transmission; ventricular rates might rise to dangerous levels as atrial rate slows in response to the quinidine.

Quinidine is not likely to increase blood pressure, or worsen preexisting hypertension. Quite the contrary: the predominant vascular effect of the drug is dilation, probably due to some α-adrenergic blocking activity. Likewise, quinidine exerts a negative inotropic effect—not a positive one—on ventricular myocardial tissue.

For long-term management of a patient with atrial fibrillation, anticoagulants are important for prophylaxis of thrombosis. The use of quinidine does not preclude or complicate proper oral anticoagulant therapy.

188. The answer is d. (*Craig, pp 235–236; Hardman, pp 787–788; Katzung, p 166.*) A Coombs-positive finding is, among all the antihypertensives, uniquely associated with methyldopa. It occurs in up to about 20% of patients taking this drug long term. Although rare, it may progress to hemolytic anemia. The cause is formation of a hapten on erythrocyte membranes, which induces an immune reaction (IgG antibodies) directed against and potentially lysing the red cell membrane. Many drugs can cause an immunohemolytic anemia. Other drugs with similar actions, and the potential to cause an immunohemolytic anemia, are penicillins, quinidine, procainamide, and sulfonamides.

189. The answer is b. (*Craig, pp 171t, 176–177; Hardman, pp 851–853, 865–867; Katzung, pp 227–228, 230–231, 238.*) All antiarrhythmics have the potential to cause arrhythmias. To a great degree, that occurs because they affect not only cells with abnormal electrophysiologic properties, but also those with relatively normal properties. Although lidocaine certainly can induce some arrhythmias, compared with nearly every other antiarrhythmic (and certainly those listed in the question), it mainly affects abnormal tissues, with minimal effects elsewhere. Lidocaine usually shortens action potential duration and so allows more time for recovery during diastole. It also blocks both activated and inactivated Na channels. Overall, the preferential effects on abnormal tissue makes it suitable for, for example, ventricular arrhythmias arising during acute myocardial ischemia/infarction.

190. The answer is c. *(Craig, pp 219–220, 220t; Hardman, pp 767–773; Katzung, pp 192–196.)* In a nutshell, this question summarizes some of the main and important differences between the dihydropyridine CCBs (e.g., nifedipine, and especially in immediate-release formulations, plus many others) and the nondihydropyridines (diltiazem and verapamil). The dihydropyridines are relatively "selective" for their vascular effects. They cause significant arteriolar dilation, which usually activates the baroreceptor reflex that increases sympathetic influences on the heart: positive inotropy, positive chronotropy (reflex tachycardia can be severe), and increased automaticity and conduction velocity (dromotropic effects).

In contrast, diltiazem and verapamil not only exert arteriolar dilation (via calcium channel blockade there), but also direct cardiac depressant effects (due to calcium channel blockade). These cardiac effects oppose, or blunt, reflex sympathetic cardiac activation: such problems are much less— often nonexistent—with the nondihydropyridines. In fact, when reflex cardiac stimulation caused by other drugs (e.g., nitroglycerin) is problematic and must be controlled, either verapamil or diltiazem may be a reasonable alternative to the traditional agents for blocking the unwanted cardiac responses: the β blockers. Moreover, a nondihydropyridine CCB is the drug of choice for controlling cardiac responses when a β blocker is contraindicated (e.g., in asthma).

191. The answer is d. *(Craig, p 192; Hardman, pp 813–814, 853, 862–864; Katzung, pp 206–208.)* Of the effects listed here, you would expect to find slowed A-V nodal conduction velocity. This is a common and, in many situations useful, effect. For example, when we give the drug as part of the pharmacologic management of atrial fibrillation or flutter, the main desired response is not suppression of the arrhythmia per se, but rather to "block down" the A-V node so that as atrial rates fall (but are still high), the A-V node will be unable to transmit the same frequency of impulses to the ventricles. That is, we "protect" the ventricles from excessive acceleration by inducing a degree of A-V block. In terms of more specific effects on the A-V node, digoxin slows conduction velocity and increases A-V nodal refractory periods.

Other "predominant" effects on the heart—all concentration-dependent—include increases of both atrial and ventricular automaticity and of conduction velocity through those structures and the His-Purkinje system.

192. The answer is d. *(Craig, pp 155, 228–229; Hardman, pp 794–796, 824–825; Katzung, pp 172–174.)* Hydralazine predominately dilates arterioles, with negligible effects on venous capacitance. It typically lowers blood pressure "so well" that it usually triggers the following two unwanted cardiovascular responses that need to be dealt with:

1. Reflex tachycardia is common, and it is typically managed with a β-adrenergic blocker. An alternative approach would be to use either verapamil or diltiazem (but not a dihydropyridine-type calcium channel blocker such as nifedipine, which would not suppress—and, in fact might aggravate—the reflex tachycardia).
2. The renin-angiotensin-aldosterone system is activated. One consequence of this unwanted compensatory response would be increased renal sodium retention that would expand circulating fluid volume and counteract hydralazine's blood pressure–lowering effects. This is typically managed with a diuretic. A thiazide often is sufficient to combat the renal sodium retention, but a more efficacious diuretic (loop diuretic) may be necessary.

Captopril (or another ACE inhibitor, or an angiotensin receptor blocker such as losartan) might be a suitable add-on (it would cause synergistic antihypertensive effects and prevent aldosterone-mediated renal effects). However, combining it with nifedipine (dihydropyridine) is irrational. As noted above, given the "pure" vasodilator actions of nifedipine and no cardiac-depressing activity whatsoever (as we get with verapamil or diltiazem), the net effect on heart rate would be either no suppression of the tachycardia or a worsening of it.

Digoxin, alone or with virtually any other drug, is not rational. There is no indication that there is need for inotropic support in this patient.

Spironolactone, alone or with digoxin, would be of little benefit. One could argue that by virtue of the spironolactone's ability to induce diuresis by blocking aldosterone's renal tubular effects, it would counteract hydralazine's ability to lead to renal sodium retention. That may be true, but spironolactone (with or without digoxin) will do nothing desirable to the unwanted tachycardia.

Nitroglycerin would add to hydralazine's antihypertensive effects, but it would probably aggravate the reflex cardiac stimulation and also increase the unwanted renal response (via a hemodynamic mechanism).

Both triamterene and amiloride are potassium-sparing diuretics. The combination of two diuretics in this class is generally irrational (it can lead to hyperkalemia). Either might beneficially combat a propensity for renal sodium retention in response to hydralazine. But, as with any diuretic alone, either or both would do little if anything to control the cardiac response.

Vitamin K was included as a foil. If you are associating hydralazine with some vitamin-related problem, you should be thinking of vitamin B_6 (pyridoxine): hydralazine can interfere with B_6 metabolism, causing such symptoms as peripheral neuritis, and so prophylactic B_6 supplementation is often used along with long-term hydralazine therapy.

193. The answer is c. (*Craig, pp 269–271; Hardman, pp 884–887; Katzung, pp 568–570.*) Simvastatin (and atorvastatin, fluvastatin, lovastatin, and pravastatin) decreases cholesterol synthesis in the liver by inhibiting HMG-CoA reductase, the rate-limiting enzyme in the synthetic pathway. This results in an increase in LDL receptors in the liver, thus reducing blood levels for cholesterol. These drugs, like other lipid-lowering agents, are best used as adjuncts to exercise and proper diet. They are considered essential components in the primary prevention of coronary heart disease. Some have been shown to lower mortality from cardiovascular causes (MI, stroke, etc.).

194. The answer is b. (*Craig, pp 233–234; Hardman, pp 131, 790–791; Katzung, pp 168–169.*) Guanethidine must be taken up by adrenergic endings in order for it to exert its effects. This involves transport by the same mechanism by which released norepinephrine reenters the neuron, and that process is blocked by tricyclic antidepressants (e.g., amitriptyline, imipramine) and by cocaine. The precise mechanism by which guanethidine exerts its intraneuronal effects isn't known. The initial (but transient) response is rather prompt and significant norepinephrine release (the drug displaces intraneuronal NE, causing a brief sympathomimetic effect). The subsequent and long-lasting effect involves prevention of NE release in response to normal nerve activation (by action potentials). This "sympatholytic" effect accounts for reduced vasoconstriction, reduced blood pressure, and a host of other side effects. Adrenergic uptake is necessary for the hypotensive action of guanethidine.

Amine pump blockers such as the tricyclic antidepressants have no pharmacodynamic effects on the other drugs, as they do not require neuronal uptake to work. Diazoxide and hydralazine act directly on blood vessels (or their endothelia); prazosin and propranolol exert postsynaptic blocking effects on α- and on β-adrenergic receptors, respectively.

195. The answer is d. (*Craig, pp 230–231; Hardman, pp 797–799; Katzung, p 175.*) Cyanide is the ultimate toxic metabolite of nitroprusside sodium. The drug is initially metabolically reduced to nitric oxide, which is responsible for the arteriolar and venular dilation. However, it is another metabolite, CN^-, that is the main cause of or contributor to toxicity.

When CN^- accumulates to sufficiently high levels (as from excessive or excessively prolonged administration of the drug), the vasculature develops what amounts to a tolerance to the drug's vasodilator effects, and so blood pressure usually starts to rise despite the presence of high drug levels. Toxic cyanide accumulation can also lead to severe lactic acidosis: the CN^- reacts with Fe^{3+} in mitochondrial cytochrome oxidase, inhibiting oxidative phosphorylation. Other characteristic signs and symptoms of the toxic syndrome include a cherry red skin (because mitochondrial oxygen consumption is blocked, venous blood remains oxygenated and as "bright red" as normal arterial blood), hypoxia, and, ultimately, hypoxic seizures and ventilatory arrest.

196. The answer is b. (*Craig, pp 230–231; Hardman, pp 797–799; Katzung, p 175.*) Cyanide, whether from nitroprusside metabolism or other sources, normally reacts with endogeous sulfur-containing compounds, mainly thiosulfate; under the influence of mitochondrial rhodanese (a transsulfurase), relatively nontoxic (less toxic than CN^-) thiocyanate is formed and it is readily excreted in the urine. With excessive exposure to nitroprusside (or CN^- from other sources), endogenous sulfur-containing substrate stores are depleted. We manage this, then, by IV infusion of an aqueous sodium thiosulfate solution.

Note: To avoid or at least reduce the risks of nitroprusside-induced cyanide toxicity, some agencies add sodium thiosulfate to the nitroprusside before the drug is administered, thereby providing ample exogenous substrate for the detoxification reaction.

197. The answer is d. (*Craig, p 116; Hardman, pp 235, 240–241; Katzung, pp 153, 156–157, 170–172.*) Propranolol, as well as other nonselective β

blockers, tends to slow the rate of recovery in a hypoglycemic attack caused by insulin. β blockers also mask the symptoms of hypoglycemia and may actually cause hypertension because of the increased plasma epinephrine in the presence of a vascular $β_2$ blockade.

198. The answer is c. (*Craig, pp 202–203, 221; Hardman, p 773; Katzung, pp 196–197.*) Had we referred to variant angina by one of its synonyms, vasospastic angina, perhaps you would have deduced the correct answer (if you didn't already). The etiology involves coronary vasospasm, and that can be blocked well with a calcium channel blocker: diltiazem, verapamil, or dihydropyridines (e.g., nifedipine, for which slow-/extended-acting oral formulations are used). The CCBs block coronary vascular smooth muscle influx of calcium, which is a critical process in triggering spasm.

Nitroglycerin seems to be marginally effective in terms of long-term symptom relief, although it may be the only rapidly acting drug that will be efficacious for acute angina and self-medication.

Aspirin, through its antiplatelet aggregatory effects, would be beneficial, prophylactically, if coronary thrombosis were part of the etiology of variant angina; but it isn't.

Atorvastatin (or other statins) are useful for primary prevention of coronary heart disease, but coronaries that undergo spasm may be remarkably free of atherosclerotic plaque, and the statins have no antispasmodic effects per se.

The β blockers, which are important drugs for many patients with angina due to atherosclerosis (used alone or as adjuncts), can do more harm than good in vasospastic angina. In essence, β-receptor activation in the coronaries tends to cause vasodilation, an effect that to a degree counteracts simultaneous α-mediated constriction. Block only the β receptors and the α-mediated constrictor effects—vasospasm-favoring effects—are left unopposed. Variant angina, then, is likely to be made worse, not better, with β blockers. (You might ask whether a combined α/β blocker like labetalol or carvedilol might be better than a nonselective or cardioselective β blocker. Perhaps in theory, but not in practice. Remember that the α-blocking effects of these drugs are comparatively weak; their β-blocking, spasm-favoring effects will predominate.)

199. The answer is c. (*Craig, pp 210–213; Hardman, pp 743–745, 751–753; Katzung, pp 177–179.*) Losartan, an angiotensin receptor blocker (ARB) has no effect on angiotensin II synthesis (as do the ACE inhibitors).

Its main antihypertensive actions, therefore, include only blockade of angiotensin II–mediated aldosterone release from the adrenal cortex, and of angiotensin II's vasoconstrictor effects.

Captopril and the other ACE inhibitors inhibit angiotensin II synthesis, and that effect accounts (indirectly) for reduced aldosterone release and AII-mediated vasoconstriction. They also inhibit metabolic inactivation of bradykinin, an endogenous vasodilator (bradykininase, angiotensin-converting enzyme, and kininase II are synonyms for essentially the same enzyme).

Neither an ACE inhibitor nor an ARB is associated with an increased incidence of bronchospasm (although some ACE inhibitors may cause cough, presumably from locally increased bradykinin levels, and angioedema, perhaps by the same mechanism). Neither elevates serum urate levels.

There is some evidence that angiotensin II *enhances* (not inhibits) sympathetic-mediated vasoconstriction (by increasing neuronal norepinephrine release and/or blocking neuronal norepinephrine reuptake). Either an ACE inhibitor or an ARB should be equivalent in attenuating that blood pressure–elevating effect.

By reducing aldosterone levels either an ACE inhibitor or an ARB tends to raise serum potassium levels—not cause hypokalemia.

200. The answer is c. (*Craig, pp 172–173, 816–818, 870–871; Hardman, p 919, 966; Katzung, pp 205, 1119.*) Digoxin toxicity is likely to occur within 24 to 48 h unless the digoxin dose is adjusted down. The reason is that quinidine will reduce the renal excretion of digoxin (digoxin's main elimination route).

There is no "reverse interaction"—i.e., an ability of digoxin to cause signs and symptoms of quinidine toxicity. Quinidine has no significant impact on the renal actions of any diuretics, whether these actions are expressed in terms of urine output (volume or concentration) or renal handling of electrolytes or other solutes.

Quinidine-induced digoxin toxicity may suppress cardiac contractility, but that would not be a direct effect of an interaction. Rather, it would be secondary to potential digoxin-induced arrhythmias, and it would not occur "promptly."

[Note: You may have learned that the interaction with quinidine does not apply to digitoxin, another cardiac glycoside that is eliminated mainly by hepatic metabolism. Although that is true, it is likely that you will never encounter any digitalis drug other than digoxin used clinically in the United States. Thus, whether you remember this "noninteraction" with digitoxin is up to you.]

201. The answer is e. *(Craig, pp 169, 180–181; Hardman, pp 844, 851–854, 865, 869; Katzung, pp 231–232.)* Flecainide, propafenone, and to a degree moricizine, the class I-C antiarrhythmics, are associated with a higher incidence of severe proarrhythmic events than virtually any other antiarrhythmics in other classes. This risk partially explains why, when these drugs were first approved, they were indicated only for life-threatening ventricular arrhythmias that failed to respond to all other reasonable (and safer) alternatives. (This risk also contributed to why another I-C agent, encainide, was withdrawn from the market.)

Nowadays, these I-C agents are still used for serious (life-threatening) and refractory ventricular arrhythmias, their efficacy arising from significant sodium channel blockade. However, they also block some potassium channels, which accounts for modestly growing interest in and use of these drugs for some atrial arrhythmias. *Regardless of whether the use is for an atrial or ventricular arrhythmia, the proarrhythmic effects should be of concern.*

You may recall that when these drugs (and others) were evaluated in the Cardiac Arrhythmia Suppression Trial (CAST), the risks of proarrhythmic effects and sudden death were quite prominent in patients with previous myocardial infarction and ventricular ectopic activity. Thus, these drugs are not indicated for arrhythmias during an acute MI. They are poor choices for any patient with low ejection fractions, mainly because they can suppress cardiac contractility (and, overall, cardiac output) further.

Pulmonary fibrosis and alterations of thyroid hormone status (typically, a hypothyroid-like state) are uniquely associated with amiodarone, which is not one of the answer choices given.

Finally, it is probably worth opining that memorizing which antiarrhythmic agents are in which Vaughn-Williams class may not be profitable. Among the reasons why: (1) this classification is based largely on electrophysiologic effects of the drugs in largely normal, isolated cardiac cells, not in diseased intact hearts; (2) some antiarrhythmic drugs have electrophysiologic/ionic mechanisms of action that would place them in more than one class; (3) belonging to a particular Vaughn-Williams class does not necessarily predict clinical use; and (4) side effects profiles of drugs in the same class—both cardiac and extracardiac side effects and toxicities—can differ substantially.

202. The answer is e. (*Craig, pp 273–275; Hardman, pp 892–893; Katzung, pp 571–573.*) Gemfibrozil mainly lowers triglycerides and is used specifically for that purpose. This fibric acid derivative is sometimes classified as a peroxisomal proliferator-receptor activator. It stimulates lipoprotein lipase synthesis and hydrolysis of triglycerides in chylomicrons and VLDL. The net effect is increased clearance of triglycerides. Clofibrate is a related (but lesser used) fibrate. As you should recall, atorvastatin (and other statins) inhibit cholesterol synthesis by inhibiting HMG CoA reductase; cholestyramine and colestyramine are bile acid sequestrants; ezetimibe, a new drug, inhibits uptake of dietary cholesterol from the gut.

203. The answer is b. (*Craig, pp 154, 246; Hardman, pp 703–704; Katzung, pp 208, 212, 254.*) Low K stores due to the effects of potassium-wasting diuretics such as hydrochlorothiazide increase susceptibility to cardiac glycoside toxicity. Note that in this scenario we have listed hydrochlorothiazide as the correct answer choice, but in clinical practice and when we are using a diuretic to manage edema secondary to heart failure, the best choice would be a loop diuretic: also potassium-wasting drugs.

204. The answer is b. (*Craig, pp 272–273; Hardman, pp 889–891; Katzung, pp 570–571.*) Nicotinic acid in large doses stimulates the production of prostaglandins as shown by an increase in blood level. The flush may be prevented by the prior administration of aspirin, which is known to block synthesis of prostaglandins.

205. The answer is a. (*Craig, pp 211, 214, 245–246, 251–252; Hardman, pp 702–703, 743, 750; Katzung, pp 177–178, 179–180.*) Although combined use of an ACE inhibitor [or angiotensin receptor blocker (ARB), e.g., losartan] and a diuretic is quite common, great care must be taken when adding one of the drugs to therapy that has been started with the other. The reason is that some patients develop a sudden fall of blood pressure that may be sufficient to cause syncope or other complications. Volume (and sodium) depletion seem to be among several probable causative factors.

Answer b is incorrect. The effects of ACE inhibitors (or ARBs) and thiazides on renal handling of potassium are the opposite of one another, not synergistic. ACE inhibitors tend to elevate serum potassium levels (in part, by lowering aldosterone levels); the thiazides (and loop diuretics, e.g., furosemide) are potassium-wasting.

There is no evidence that adding one of these drugs to therapy with the other can cause acute (or chronic) heart failure (c); indeed, such a combination is often an essential component in managing chronic heart failure. Blood pressure will fall, not rise, and certainly not cause hypertensive crisis (d); and slowed A-V nodal conduction rates (e) due to this drug combination do not occur.

206. The answer is e. *(Craig, p 191, 222; Hardman, pp 772–773; Katzung, pp 194–197.)* Constipation is a fairly common and sometimes very bothersome response to many calcium channel blockers. If severe and not managed properly, fecal impaction or other significant intestinal problems can occur. The incidence and severity are greatest with the nondihydropyridines, verapamil and diltiazem. The best initial approach—if continued use of an offending drug is needed—is to modify the diet by increasing water and dietary fiber intake.

207. The answer is d. *(Craig, p 212; Hardman, p 750; Katzung, pp 178–179.)* The most consistent of the toxicities of ACE inhibitors is impairment of renal function, as evidenced by proteinuria. Elevations of blood urea nitrogen (BUN) and creatinine occur frequently, especially when stenosis of the renal artery or severe heart failure exists. Hyperkalemia also may occur. These drugs are to be used very cautiously where prior renal failure is present and in the elderly. Other toxicities include persistent dry cough, neutropenia, and angioedema. Hepatic toxicity has not been reported.

208. The answer is d. *(Craig, pp 66t, 260–261; Hardman, p 1346; Katzung, p 548.)* A slow intravenous infusion of protamine sulfate will quickly reverse the bleeding. Protamine binds to heparin, forming a stable complex with no anticoagulant activity. It may also have its own anticoagulant effect by binding with platelets and fibrinogen.

209. The answer is d. *(Craig, p 173; Hardman, pp 868–869; Katzung, pp 228–229.)* Procainamide is uniquely associated with the development of a lupus-like syndrome. The risk is higher in patients who, because of genetically based drug metabolizing capacity, are "slow acetylators"; that is because it appears that the parent drug, not the main metabolite [N-acetylprocainamide (NAPA)], is the culprit. The precise mechanism by which procainamide-associated lupus occurs is not known.

None of the other drugs listed are associated with a lupus-like syndrome, whether administered alone or in combination with one another, or with other drugs not listed here.

Note 1: There is one other drug traditionally discussed in the cardiovascular section of texts and courses that is linked to a lupus-like syndrome: hydralazine. (Such other drugs as quinidine have caused lupus-like responses, but this is quite rare in comparison with the frequency seen with procainamide or hydralazine.)

Note 2: If carvedilol is not familiar to you, learn that it's a β-adrenergic blocker with α-adrenergic blocking activity. In this respect it is similar to labetalol.

210. The answer is e. (*Craig, p 272; Hardman, p 887; Katzung, pp 569–570.*) The findings in Patient 2 are consistent with statin-induced myositis and myopathy, which may progress to rhabdomyolysis and renal failure—both potentially fatal. This syndrome (and hepatotoxicity) is the most serious adverse response to the statins. It is more prevalent in older patients, those with multiple illnesses, and especially chronic renal disease. Coadministration of most other lipid-lowering drugs increases the risk of rhabdomyolysis, hepatotoxicity, or both. As an aside, the risk of rhabdomyolysis (or lesser skeletal muscle changes) is not much different between the currently available statins. However, it was (allegedly) such a problem with one relatively recent drug, cerivastatin, that the drug was pulled from the market.

211. The answer is e. (*Craig, p 165; Katzung, pp 221–222.*) Although you may not consider this question a pharmacology question, being able to answer it correctly is important to the rational and safe use of many drugs.

In general, heart block refers to excessively slowed atrio-ventricular nodal conduction, which you assess by measuring the PR interval on the EKG. Recall that this interval gives information on how long it takes for electrical impulses that originate with SA nodal depolarization to pass through the atrial myocardia and the AV node, ultimately leading to ventricular activation (QRS complex). Impulse conduction through the atria is normally quick; it is the AV node that has the slowest intrinsic impulse conduction rate anywhere in the heart, and it is arguably the structure that is most susceptible to drug- (or disease-) induced changes of supraventricular conduction that lead to the diagnosis of AV block.

In first-degree heart block, the only manifestation is a prolonged PR interval, but each P wave is followed by a normally generated QRS complex. In second-degree heart block, the PR interval is prolonged and some P waves are not conducted through the AV node, and so are not followed by a QRS triggered by the prior atrial activation. In third-degree (complete) heart block, no P waves are conducted normally through the AV node, and ventricular activation is solely dependent on intrinsic automaticity of the ventricles (or conducting tissue therein).

Auscultation of the heart, the presence of blood pressures that are above or below what is generally regarded as normal, or the presence of a slow sinus rhythm, are not reliable indicators of heart block.

212. The answer is f. (*Craig, pp 191–192; Hardman, pp 768–770, 772, 854; Katzung, pp 235–236.*) In essence, we are asking "which drug can suppress AV nodal conduction velocity?" Verapamil (and the very similar nondihydropyridine calcium channel blocker, diltiazem) do that. Recall the profile of verapamil and diltiazem: a vasodilator effect *plus* a direct cardiac "depressant" effect that includes slowing of AV conduction (and potential depression of other cardiac contractile and electrophysiologic phenomena).

[Be sure you can contrast this dual vasodilator/cardiac depressant profile for verapamil and diltiazem with that of the dihydropyridines (e.g., nifedipine; answer c). The dihydropyridines cause vasodilation, but lack any cardiac depressant actions. Indeed, with dihydropyridine dosages sufficient to lower blood pressure enough, and quick enough, there will be reflex (baroreceptor) activation of the sympathetic nervous system. One consequence of increased norepinephrine release at the heart would be increased (faster) AV nodal conduction velocity, which could be construed as an "unblocking" of the AV node—precisely the opposite of what may happen with verapamil or diltiazem.]

Captopril (ACE inhibitor) and losartan (angiotensin receptor blocker) have no significant effects on AV nodal conduction.

Nitroglycerin (nitrovasodilator) and prasosin (vasodilator that acts by competitive α_1 blockade) also have no direct effect on the AV node, but are likely to lead to an indirect quickening of AV conduction via baroreceptor activation.

On a final and important note, be sure you understand that all β-adrenergic blockers (including those with some α-blocking activity, e.g., labetalol and carvedilol) can slow A-V nodal conduction and can cause or worsen heart block.

213. The answer is c. *(Craig, pp 197, 739–740; Katzung, p 189.)* Sildenafil (and the related drugs, tadalafil and vardenafil), a wildly popular and widely prescribed drug for erectile dysfunction (ED), prolongs and enhances erection by a nitric oxide–dependent mechanism. Of course, its effects are systemic—not limited to the penile vasculature. Nitroglycerin causes its vaso- (veno-)dilator effects via a NO/G protein–dependent mechanism also. The ED drug can profoundly intensify nitrate-induced vasodilation and cause life-threatening hypotension and myocardial and cerebral ischemia.

Note the important mechanistic links between vasodilation/hypotension, sexual intercourse, and potentially fatal cardiac responses. Sexual arousal—and, especially orgasm—causes a massive activation of the sympathetic nervous system. One consequence of that, α-mediated vasoconstriction that tends to keep blood pressure up, is too feeble to overcome the hypotensive effects of the sildenafil-nitroglycerin combination. Along with a fall of blood pressure is a fall of coronary perfusion pressure (diastolic blood pressure), i.e., reduced myocardial blood flow/oxygen supply. Yet the sympathetic activation concomitantly causes significant increases of cardiac rate and contractility, i.e., increased myocardial oxygen demand. Oxygen demand rises, supply falls, and the stage is set for acute myocardial ischemia.

214. The answer is d. *(Craig, p 228; Hardman, pp 798, 827–828; Katzung, pp 172–175.)* Hydralazine, minoxidil, diazoxide, and sodium nitroprusside are all directly acting vasodilators used to treat hypertension. Hydralazine, minoxidil, nifedipine, and diazoxide relax arteriolar smooth muscle more than smooth muscle in venules, so the effect on venous capacitance is negligible. Sodium nitroprusside, which affects both arterioles and venules, does not increase cardiac output, a feature that enhances the utility of sodium nitroprusside in the management of hypertensive crisis associated with MI.

215. The answer is a. *(Craig, pp 271–272; Hardman, p 887; Katzung, pp 569–570.)* Lovastatin should not be used in patients with severe liver disease. With routine use of lovastatin, serum transaminase values may rise, and in such patients the drug may be continued only with great caution. Lovastatin has also been associated with lenticular opacities, and slit-lamp studies should be done before and 1 year after the start of therapy. The drug is not toxic to the renal system, and reports of bone marrow depression are very rare. There is a small incidence of myopathy, and levels of creatinine kinase should be measured when unexplained muscle pain occurs. Combination with cyclosporine or clofibrate has led to myopathy. There is no danger in use with bile acid sequestrants.

216. The answer is a. (*Craig, pp 166–169, 192–193; Hardman, p 858; Katzung, pp 227–228, 236.*) Nowadays, IV injection of adenosine is generally regarded as first choice for terminating acute supraventricular tachycardia. Among other reasons, it is preferred over another reasonable alternative, verapamil, because of a faster onset of action.

Digoxin, β blockers, phenylephrine, and edrophonium are older therapies falling into relative disuse. In one way or another their effects revolve around causing or unmasking increased parasympathetic influences on the S-A and/or AV nodes: digoxin via its predominant effects to slow AV nodal conduction; phenylephrine (or other α agonist vasoconstrictors) by increasing blood pressure, which triggers a baroreceptor reflex that reduces sympathetic drive and essentially increases or unmasks parasympathetic tone; propranolol, by blocking β_1-mediated sympathetic influences; and edrophonium, which quickly but briefly inhibits ACh esterase.

217. The answer is b. (*Craig, pp 248–249; Hardman, pp 704–706; Katzung, p 256.*) Amiloride is a K-sparing diuretic with a mild diuretic and natriuretic effect. The parent compound is active, and the drug is excreted unchanged in the urine. Amiloride has a 24-h duration of action and is usually administered with a thiazide or loop diuretic (e.g., furosemide) to prevent hypokalemia. The site of its diuretic action is the late distal tubule and collecting duct, where it interferes with Na reabsorption and allows for K retention.

218. The answer is d. (*Craig, p 246; Hardman, p 702; Katzung, pp 250–251.*) Thiazide diuretics raise serum Ca, possibly through a direct effect on Ca reabsorption in the distal tubule. Although hypercalcemia is seldom caused by the diuretic alone, it is more likely to occur when the patient has a history of carcinoma.

219. The answer is c. *(Craig, p 250; Hardman, p 700; Katzung, pp 247–248.)* Furosemide can cause hypokalemia by blocking Na^+ reabsorption in the loop of Henle, followed by exchange of K^+ with Na^+ in the distal tubules. Hypokalemia is associated with digitalis toxicity. Furosemide also can cause dose-related hearing loss, especially in people with existing hearing loss and/or renal impairment.

220. The answer is c. *(Craig, p 261; Hardman, pp 1347–1348; Katzung, pp 549–551.)* Warfarin is a coumarin derivative that is generally used for chronic anticoagulation. It antagonizes the γ carboxylation of several glutamate residues in prothrombin and the coagulation Factors VII, IX, and X. This process is coupled to the oxidative deactivation of vitamin K. The reduced form of vitamin K is essential for sustained carboxylation and synthesis of the coagulation proteins. It appears that warfarin inhibits the action of the reductase(s) that regenerate the reduced form of vitamin K. The prevention of the inactive vitamin K epoxide from being reduced to the active form of vitamin K results in decreased carboxylation of the proteins involved in the coagulation cascade.

221. The answer is b. *(Craig, p 259; Hardman, pp 1343–1345; Katzung, pp 545–547.)* Heparin binds to antithrombin III (a plasma protease inhibitor), thereby enhancing its activation. The heparin-antithrombin III complex interacts with thrombin. This inactivates thrombin and other coagulation factors such as VIIa, IXa, Xa, and IIa. Heparin accelerates the rate of thrombin-antithrombin binding, resulting in the inhibition of thrombin. The latter effect is not typically seen with low-molecular-weight heparins that are not of sufficient length to catalyze the inhibition of thrombin.

222. The answer is e. *(Craig, pp 263–264; Hardman, p 1351; Katzung, pp 553–554.)* Alteplase is an unmodified tPA. Alteplase activates plasminogen that is bound to fibrin. The plasmin that is formed acts directly on fibrin. This results in dissolving the fibrin into fibrin-split products followed by lysis of the clot.

223. The answer is b. *(Craig, p 263; Hardman, p 1354; Katzung, p 554.)* Clopidogrel inhibits platelet aggregation and the release of platelet granule constituents by inhibiting the binding of ADP to its platelet receptors.

Platelet membrane function is altered irreversibly by inhibition of ADP-induced activation of the platelet glycoprotein GPIIb/IIIa complex, resulting in decreased fibrinogen binding. Decreased platelet aggregation stems from the inability of activated platelets to recruit circulating platelets.

224. The answer is d. *(Craig, pp 187–188; Hardman, p 859; Katzung, pp 233–234.)* Pulmonary fibrosis has been reported with long-term amiodarone therapy, but not in response to other antiarrhythmics. Pulmonary function tests may remain normal for months and then decline quickly and to significant degrees as irreversible fibrosis develops. Changes of thyroid hormone status—sometimes reflecting hypothyroidism and, for other patients, hyperthyroidism—are also uniquely associated with amiodarone: this drug is structurally related to the thyroid hormones. Changes of thyroid hormone status may be subclinical and detectable only with suitable blood tests or may lead to typical signs and symptoms of hyper- or hypothyroidism.

Keep in mind that some adverse responses that are unique to other antiarrhythmic drugs were listed as possible answers. For example, low-grade quinidine toxicity (cinchonism) often includes tinnitus (but that manifestation of ototoxicity cannot be detected with audiometry), and procainamide commonly causes a lupus-like syndrome, for which monitoring of ANA titers is important.

Of course, it's likely that a patient with atrial fibrillation will be placed on warfarin (at least for a while), and so monitoring the prothrombin time [reported as the International Normalized Ratio (INR)] would be essential in that case. And, since this patient may have multiple cardiovascular "risk factors," periodic monitoring of lipid profiles would be essential too. Nonetheless, these do not apply specifically or uniquely to amiodarone.

225. The answer is c. *(Craig, p 263; Hardman, pp 1354, 1356–1357; Katzung, p 554.)* Clopidogrel (and the somewhat older related drug, ticlopidine) decreases platelet aggregation by blocking a proaggregatory interaction between adenosine 5′-diphosphate (ADP) and a population of platelet ADP receptors. There are at least two populations of platelet ADP receptors, and both must be activated to trigger aggregation. Thus, clopidogrel is sufficient to block one of those obligatory pathways. Clopidogrel has no effect on prostaglandin synthesis.

226. The answer is e. (*Craig, pp 198–199; Hardman, pp 762–764; Katzung, pp 186–187.*) Nitric oxide is thought to be enzymatically released from nitroglycerin. It then reacts with and activates guanylyl cyclase to increase GMP, which ultimately causes vasodilation by increasing calcium efflux. It also indirectly causes the dephosphorylation of the light chains of myosin. These actions lead to the vasodilator effect of nitroglycerin. Reaction of nitric oxide occurs with protein sulfhydryl groups. Tolerance may develop in part from a decrease in available sulfhydryl groups. Autonomic receptors are not involved in the primary response of nitroglycerin, but compensatory mechanisms may counter the primary actions.

227. The answer is a. (*Craig, p 212; Hardman, p 750; Katzung, p 178.*) Captopril, and some of the other ACE inhibitors, may cause severe, hacking, and relentless cough in some patients. It is thought to be due to increased levels of bradykinin in smooth muscles in the throat. (Recall that angiotensin-converting enzyme, which forms angiotensin II, is the same enzyme as bradykininase, which metabolically inactivates bradykinin.) Many patients receiving captopril (or other ACE inhibitors) experience no problems of this sort. Still other patients, mainly taking other ACE inhibitors, may develop swelling of the oropharyngeal mucosase, and some may develop life-threatening angioedema.

There are no allergic reactions triggered by digoxin, nor is this ATPase inhibtor displaced from plasma protein or tissue binding sites by captopril or other ACE inhibitors.

Captopril is not a bronchoconstrictor. Hyperkalemia is not a likely explanation. Note that by indirectly lowering aldosterone levels (angiotensin II is the main stimulus for aldosterone release, and we have inhibited angiotensin II synthesis), the main renal effects would be increased sodium excretion and increased potassium retention. However, we are administering bumetanide (a furosemide-like loop diuretic), which causes renal potassium-wasting. Thus, we would not expect hyperkalemia from this combination of drugs (as we would if the diuretic was a potassium-sparing one such as amiloride, triamterene, or sprionolactone).

Cough is not part of the main side effect/toxicity profile of simvastatin or other HMG-CoA reductase inhibitors. Recall that their main toxicities include myositis, myopathy, rhabdomyolysis, renal damage (from the rhabdomyolysis), and hepatotoxicity.

228. The answer is d. (*Craig, p 260; Hardman, p 1346; Katzung, p 545.*) Heparin is a mixture of sulfated mucopolysaccharides and is highly acidic and highly charged. Protamine is a very basic polypeptide that combines with heparin. The complex has no anticoagulant activity. Excess protamine does have anticoagulant activity, so just enough should be given to counteract the heparin effect.

229. The answer is b. (*Hardman, pp 1351–1352; Katzung, pp 547, 552.*) Streptokinase forms a stable complex with plasminogen. The resulting conformational change allows for formation of free plasmin, the active fibrinolytic enzyme.

230. The answer is a. (*Craig, p 193; Hardman, p 953; Katzung, p 236.*) Many patients that receive a therapeutic dose of adenosine experience shortness of breath and fullness or a burning sensation in the chest. These adverse effects are of short duration because of rapid elimination of the drug.

231. The answer is e. (*Craig, pp 105, 108; Hardman, pp 952–953; Katzung, pp 133–135, 209.*) Intravenous infusion of dobutamine may result in an increased heart rate and blood pressure. Patients with a history of hypertension are more likely to have an exaggerated blood pressure response.

232. The answer is b. (*Craig, p 212; Hardman, p 751; Katzung, p 178.*) Angiotensin-converting enzyme inhibitors, especially captopril, can cause alteration or loss of taste sensation.

233. The answer is b. (*Craig, p 237; Hardman, p 789.*) Abrupt discontinuation of clonidine has been associated with a rapidly developing and severe "rebound" phenomenon that includes excessive cardiac stimulation and a spike of blood pressure that may be sufficiently great as to cause stroke or other similar complications. Recall that clonidine is a "centrally acting α-adrenergic agonist." Through its central effects it reduces sympathetic nervous system tone. This, in turn, appears to cause supersensitivity of peripheral adrenergic receptors to direct-acting adrenergic agonists, including endogenous norepinephrine and epinephrine. Once, and soon after, the drug is stopped, endogenous catecholamines trigger hyperresponsiveness of all structures under sympathetic control.

When ACE inhibitors (or angiotensin receptor blockers), hydrochlorothiazide, or nifedipine (long-acting or otherwise) are abruptly stopped, blood pressure will begin to rise from treatment levels, but there will be no sudden "spike" of pressure nor an "overshoot" of it.

Digoxin discontinuation is not associated with the symptoms noted in the question. Besides, the half-life of digoxin (about 36 to 40 h if renal function is normal) is such that stopping the drug abruptly would not lead to any significant events occurring "within a day or two" of discontinuation.

There is no reason to predict that suddenly stopping warfarin would cause tachyarrhythmias, hypertension, or hemorrhagic stroke—and certainly not within 24 to 48 h.

234. The answer is b. (*Craig, p 184; Hardman, p 820; Katzung, p 212.*) This collection of signs and symptoms is characteristic of digoxin toxicity, regardless of the cause (e.g., frank overdose or the development of hypokalemia, which increases the risk of digoxin toxicity). Although a probable cause of the hypokalemia is the furosemide, it is not correct to say that furosemide per se is the cause, because signs and symptoms of furosemide toxicity are not similar at all to those described here. Note, too, that we have administered triamterene. The expected effect of that potassium-sparing diuretic is to counteract renal potassium loss from the furosemide (potassium-wasting).

Do recall that the visual changes described in the question are called chromatopsia.

235. The answer is a. (*Craig, pp 271–272; Hardman, p 887; Katzung, pp 569–570.*) Atorvastatin and other HMG-CoA reductase inhibitors ("statins") occasionally cause myositis and myopathy that can present initially as muscle aches or pains. The onset, severity, and localization of these symptoms is unpredictable, but it is clear that of the drugs listed, the "statins" are the only drugs associated with these symptoms. If the skeletal muscle (and muscle membrane) damage is severe, there are several possible consequences: hyperkalemia from loss of potassium from myocytes; and myoglobin leakage, which can lead to rhabdomyolysis and, eventually, renal failure when the renal tubules are occluded with myoglobin.

236. The answer is b. (*Craig, p 263; Hardman, p 1354; Katzung, p 554.*) Clopidogrel, and the older related drug ticlopidine, selectively block the ADP receptor.

237. The answer is d. (*Craig, pp 262–263; Hardman, p 1353; Katzung, p 554.*) Aspirin (acetylsalicylic acid) inhibits (acetylates) platelet cylooxygenase, thereby inhibiting the conversion of arachidonic acid to thromboxane A_2. This is the antiplatelet effect that occurs with therapeutic blood levels of aspirin. At very high blood levels, aspirin also inhibits prostacyclin synthesis (in the vascular endothelium), but that action tends to be proaggregatory, counteracting the antiaggregatory effects on platelets.

238. The answer is c. (*Craig, p 263; Katzung, p 555.*) Abciximab, and such related drugs as tirofiban and eptifibatide, block the glycoprotein IIb/IIIa receptor on platelets. This is a very important effect, because the formation of fibrinogen bridges between the IIb/IIIa receptors on adjacent platelets is the critical step in causing platelets to attract and aggregate with their neighbors.

It is also noteworthy that activation of the IIb/IIIa receptor can be triggered by thromboxane A_2, thrombin, collagen, ADP, and platelet-activating factor (PAF). Block the activating effects of just one of those factors (e.g., those of ADP with clopidogrel), and the proaggregatory effects of the other activators are left unchecked. Abciximab, in contrast, blocks the "final step" in aggregation, regardless of the presence or absence of influences from the "upstream" activators.

239. The answer is b. (*Hardman, pp 813–814, 862–863; Katzung, pp 206–208.*) Answering this question, of course, requires that you not only know the expected effects of digoxin, but also that you can "translate" those effects into interpretations of findings from a most useful diagnostic tool, the electrocardiogram.

An expected effect of digoxin is slowed atrioventricular nodal conduction velocity, manifest as prolongation of the P-R interval. The effect, which can lead to increasing degrees of heart block, depends on the serum concentration of digoxin and on serum concentrations of several ions, potassium arguably the most important.

Digoxin tends to speed electrical impulse velocity through the atrial myocardium, and so widening of P waves would be the opposite of the expected response. There is no good reason to expect increased P-wave amplitude.

The drug also speeds electrical impulse conduction velocity through the ventricles (e.g., the His-Purkinje system), and so widened QRS complexes, compared with baseline, would be counter to the expected effect.

R-R intervals essentially reflect ventricular rate. Before treatment of heart failure there are varying degrees of compensatory "sympathetic drive" over the heart, leading to tachycardia or, at least, shortened R-R intervals. Once digoxin starts increasing cardiac output, there is a lessening of sympathetic drive (and the physiologic need for it). Thus, compared with baseline heart rate, posttreatment heart rate is slower; this is manifest as a longer R-R interval compared with baseline.

S-T segment elevation is one manifestation of acute coronary syndrome and regional myocardial ischemia. Based on the description of the patient, who appears to be symptom-free and having normal blood profiles, S-T elevation is not a reasonable answer.

240. The answer is d. *(Craig, pp 182–184, 232–233; Hardman, pp 774–775; Katzung, pp 154, 171.)* Labetalol is the best choice. Given its combination of both α- and β-adrenergic (β_1 and β_2) blocking effect, it offers the best approach for managing the hypertension, the tachycardia, the resulting oxygen supply-demand imbalance that leads to both chest discomfort and the ischemic ST-changes; and the ventricular ectopy (which is probably a reflection of excessive catecholamine stimulation of β_1 receptors). If the patient is having an acute myocardial infarction, starting β-blocker therapy early is also decidedly beneficial short term and for the long run. (Most any other β blocker might be a suitable alternative, but only labetalol has the combined α/β-blocking actions that are likely to be of greatest benefit. Carvedilol has the same profile, but it is given orally and in this setting that would not be ideal because of slow onset of action.)

Aspirin will do no harm in this situation, but it will also do no good acutely unless there is ongoing platelet aggregation and coronary occlusion. Even if there were, the aspirin would do little to control heart rate, blood pressure, or the EKG changes.

Nothing in the scenario suggests this patient is volume-overloaded or suffering acute pulmonary edema. Therefore, administering the furosemide in such a situation is not appropriate. Moreover, giving it is likely to cause prompt reductions of blood volume and, along with it, of blood pressure.

The latter effect is likely to lead to further—and unwanted—reflex sympathetic activation that would make matters worse.

Lidocaine might be suitable for the ventricular ectopy. However, we have identified several other important signs and symptoms that would not be relieved by this antiarrhythmic drug. As noted above, the profile of labetalol offers the greatest likelihood of managing multiple problems with one drug.

Increasing the dose of nitroglycerin (and especially giving it as a bolus) is likely to drop blood pressure acutely, triggering reflex (baroreceptor) stimulation of the heart. The usual "anti-ischemic" effects of the drug would be counteracted by such "pro-ischemic" changes as further rises of heart rate and a probable worsening of the premature ventricular beats.

Prazosin would lower blood pressure nicely. However, once again we have to worry about excessive pressure lowering, triggering the baroreceptor reflex, and worsening many of the already worrisome findings (e.g., heart rate, PVCs).

241. The answer is b. (*Craig, p 222; Hardman, pp 767–773; Katzung, pp 176, 192–195.*) A good way to arrive at the answer is to remember the rather narrow cardiovascular profile of nifedipine, the prototype dihydropyridine calcium channel blocker and perhaps to compare it with the two main nondihydropyridines, diltiazem and verapamil.

The dihydropyridines—and diltiazem and verapamil—block vascular smooth-muscle calcium channels, and cause vasodilation. Any of these drugs, therefore, would help lower this patient's blood pressure.

However, nifedipine (and other dihydropyridines) lack any cardiac-depressant effects. The implication is that as the nifedipine drives blood pressure down (and it will, in an uncontrolled fashion with this sometimes-used but wholly inappropriate and unsafe administration method), there will be intense baroreceptor activation. There will be no drug-induced negative inotropic, chronotropic, or dromotropic (conduction velocity) effects to counteract the excessive cardiac stimulation as there would be if we had used either diltiazem or verapamil.

So, under reflex-mediated increases of catecholamines affecting the heart, A-V conduction would increase (not be slowed or blocked); there would be further increases of heart rate (at least, certainly no fall) to accompany lowering of blood pressure (possibly to hypotensive levels); and the current episodes of ventricular ectopy might convert to longer runs, or to ventricular tachycardia or fibrillation.

242. The answer is a. You should know the answer to this from a basic physiology course, so we've added no explicit cross-references to any pharmacology texts. We have mimicked (but not caused) a sudden rise of blood pressure, stretching the baroreceptors and activating the baroreceptor reflex. Consequences of this include a reduction in sympathetic "outflow" from the CNS (and a reduction of catecholamine release), and a simultaneous unmasking and increase of opposing parasympathetic influences. The increased muscarinic receptor activation breaks the tachycardia, mainly by slowing spontaneous (Phase 4) depolarization of S-A nodal cells.

243. The answer is d. (*Craig, pp 165–169, 192–193; Hardman, pp 937–941; Katzung, pp 216–222.*) The origin of the arrhythmia is supraventricular (any structure "above" the A-V node), and in this case both the expected effects of ACh and of carotid massage suggest the origin is the S-A node itself. If you look at the EKG, you should be able to rule out the other (and incorrect) answer choices. The ventricular wave form shows no slurring or "hump" that would suggest preactivation of the ventricles by an accessory pathway (as you might see in Wolff-Parkinson-White syndrome). There is no notching of the QRS that would be consistent with bundle branch block (right or left). And, because ventricular activation follows atrial activation (P waves), we are not dealing with ventricular ectopy.

244. The answer is a. (*Craig, pp 192–193; Hardman, pp 853, 858; Katzung, p 237.*) Adenosine interacts with G protein–coupled receptors, increases maximum diastolic membrane potential. When given as a bolus, which we used here, the main effects are a transient slowing of sinus (nodal) rate, an increase of AV nodal refractoriness, and a slowing of AV nodal conduction velocity. Also, with this administration route, there is no effect on the His-Purkinje system, nor on ventricular myocardial cells per se. Given the lack of ventricular effects, adenosine would not have terminated the arrhythmia if the origin was in the ventricles. Stated otherwise, because the drug does act on the AV node, and it did terminate the original arrhythmia, we must conclude that the arrhythmia originated in the AV node or other supraventricular structures.

Atropine, by blocking the electrophysiologic effects of muscarinic receptor activation (in the S-A node, for example), would have unmasked opposing sympathetic (β_1) influences and probably worsened (but certainly not stopped) the aberrant electrical activity. Isoproterenol or epinephrine would have done the same, albeit by direct activation of β_1-adrenergic receptors.

We can rule-out lidocaine as an acceptable answer in several ways. First, we are dealing with an arrhythmia originating in a supraventricular structure. Lidocaine has no significant effect on SA nodal rate, nor on AV nodal refractory periods. It also has no effects on PR intervals (because it lacks significant effects on AV nodal refractoriness or conduction), QT intervals, or the duration of the QRS. Stated more pragmatically, the drug is not useful for supraventricular arrhythmias (except, perhaps, digoxin-associated atrial arrhythmias). It would not work in the situation described or shown in the EKG.

245. The answer is c. (*Craig, p 229; Hardman, pp 67, 795; Katzung, pp 172–174.*) Hydralazine is probably one of the two "main" cardiovascular drugs (procainamide is the other) associated with a somewhat common incidence of medication-related lupus-like syndrome. As with procainamide, acetylation is the first step in the drug's metabolism, and individuals who metabolize the drug slowly are more susceptible to the arthralgia, fever, and other characteristics of the syndrome. The frequency rises when very high doses of the drug are used long term, as may be done for severe hypertension or (to a lesser degree) heart failure.

246. The answer is b. (*Craig, pp 220–221; Hardman, pp 767–773; Katzung, pp 172–174, 179–180, 209.*) If we must resort to hydralazine for managing hypertension (it can also be indicated for severe heart failure), we must rely on adjunctive drugs too, for several reasons. Hydralazine, which preferentially dilates arterioles (as opposed to venules), usually lowers blood pressure sufficiently that it triggers compensatory renal sodium (and water) retention. That's why a diuretic is necessary, and we have that in this scenario (the furosemide). We also need some drug to control the likely reflex cardiac stimulation that arises from the pressure-lowering effects (arteriolar dilation) of the drug. That's what the carvedilol (α- and β-adrenergic blocker) does. You should note that these adjuncts also contribute antihypertensive effects of their own, and that is important.

Diltiazem (or its related drug, verapamil; both are nondihydropyridine calcium channel blockers) will cause additive pressure-lowering effects and, because of the cardiac/cardiac-depressant effect will reduce the tendency for reflex cardiac stimulation. Diltiazem or verapamil would be the best choice.

Digoxin has no antihypertensive effects per se, nor will it have any appreciable effect on heart rate. At therapeutic blood levels its main net electrophysiologic effect is on A-V nodal conduction velocity.

Nifedipine, a dihydropyridine calcium channel blocker, will help with lowering blood pressure. However, its effects are such that it may add to renal sodium and water retention, and its hypotensive effects may reflexly (via the baroreceptor reflex) add to cardiac stimulation (rate, inotropy), because dihydropyridines lack cardiac-depressant actions. Remember: compared with nondihydropyridines such as verapamil or diltiazem, the dihydropyridines lack any cardiac-depressant actions.

Phentolamine and prazosin are both α-adrenergic blockers. Although they may have synergistic effects to lower blood pressure, they are likely to trigger additional compensatory renal sodium and water retention, and they certainly will worsen reflex cardiac stimulation via the baroreceptor reflex. Because prazosin selectively blocks α-adrenergic receptors, the reflex cardiac stimulation will be less than a nonselective α blocker like phentolamine. Nonetheless, prazosin would not be an ideal choice because our goal is not just to minimize reflex cardiac stimulation that hydralazine might induce, but to have present a drug that actually combats that effect.

247. The answer is c. (*Craig, pp 393–395; Hardman, pp 448–449, 700, 704; Katzung, pp 256, 475–478.*) There is a clinically important relationship between serum sodium concentrations and the concentration-dependent effects of lithium. In essence, Li^+ and Na^+ compete with one another, such that in the presence of hyponatremia the effects of the lithium may be increased to the point of causing toxicity. (Conversely, hypernatremia can counteract lithium's therapeutic effects.) Of the drugs listed, hydrochlorothiazide (and other thiazides and such thiazide-like agents as metolazone) poses the greatest risk of causing hyponatremia. (And you should consider the ultimate renal effects of ACE inhibition to lower serum Na^+ levels further when used with a diuretic. ACE inhibitors used without a diuretic are not at all as likely to cause hyponatremia.)

There are no clinically significant pharmacodynamic or pharmacokinetic interactions between nitroglycerine or HMG CoA reductase inhibitors and the atypical antipsychotics (risperidone, olanzapine, other) or lithium.

248. The answer is e. (*Craig, pp 155–156; Katzung, pp 209–211.*) Vasodilator therapy for CHF has gained prominence in the past 10 years. The ACE inhibitors, such as enalapril, are among the best agents for this purpose, although Ca channel inhibitors and nitroglycerin can also be used. The ACE inhibitors dilate arterioles and veins (reducing preload), as well as inhibit aldosterone production (reducing blood volume), factors considered beneficial in CHF therapy. Both β-adrenergic antagonists and ACE inhibitors have been shown to increase survival in CHF.

249. The answer is e. *(Hardman, pp 110–111, 234–235, 792–793; Katzung, pp 146–147, 151.)* Pheochromocytomas—rare causes of hypertension—involve excessive levels of circulating catecholamines from tumors of the adrenal medulla; other chromaffin cells may be affected, leading to excessive catecholamine production in and release from other sites. The main factor in leading to an increase of blood pressure in this condition is α-mediated vasoconstriction arising from excessive levels of epinephrine, norepinephrine, or both. And, the contributions of epinephrine will involve some β_2 vasodilation. That vasodilator effect, no matter how slight, will be blocked by propranolol or any other β-adrenergic blocker that can block β_2-adrenergic receptors. (So-called cardioselective/β_1 blockers such as atenolol and metoprolol can also block β_2 receptors in the vasculature, and elsewhere, with blood levels that are not too far above the usual "therapeutic" range.) In essence, blockade of β_2 receptors in the vasculature will leave α-mediated constrictor effects unopposed, and blood pressure will rise (concomitant with suppression of cardiac contractility and rate).

250. The answer is d. *(Craig, pp 66t, 261, 781–782; Hardman, pp 1349–1350, 1584–1585; Katzung, pp 552, 556.)* Phytonadione (vitamin K_1) is the antidote. It overcomes (reverses, antagonizes) warfarin's hepatic anticoagulant effects, which involve inhibited synthesis of clotting factors (VII, IX, X, and prothrombin).

Aminocaproic acid is a backup (to whole blood, packed red cells, or fresh-frozen plasma) for managing bleeding in response to excessive effects of thrombolytic drugs [e.g., alteplase (tPA), streptokinase, tenecteplase]. It is not indicated for warfarin-related bleeding. Epoetin alfa is a hematopoietic growth factor that stimulated erythrocyte production in peritubular cells in the proximal tubules of the kidney. Its uses include management of anemias associated with chronic renal failure, chemotherapy (of nonmeleloid malignancies), or zidovudine therapy in patients with acquired immunodeficiency syndrome. It is inappropriate for this patient. Ferrous sulfate (or fumarate or gluconate) is indicated for prevention or treatment of iron-deficiency anemias. It will do nothing to lower the patient's INR or alleviate related symptoms. Protamine sulfate is the antidote for heparin overdoses. It acts electrostatically with heparin, in the blood, to form a complex that lacks anticoagulant activity. It does nothing to the hepatic vitamin K–related problems that are at the root of excessive warfarin effects.

251. The answer is d. *(Hardman, pp 819–820; Katzung, pp 208, 210.)* A potassium-wasting diuretic is usually used as an adjunct to digoxin, or other drugs, for managing heart failure. Almost always the diuretic is a loop agent (e.g., furosemide). These drugs are likely to cause hypokalemia (unless we prescribe another drug to combat that). Recall that for any given serum level of digoxin, reductions of serum K^+ concentrations will enhance binding of digoxin to, and inhibition of, the sodium pump. This "increased" effect of digoxin is often excessive—capable of causing various cardiac and extracardiac signs and symptoms of digoxin intoxication.

Drugs that either inhibit angiotensin II synthesis or block angiotensin receptors have no specific or important effects with respect to the incidence or severity of digoxin intoxication.

Digoxin is eliminated by the kidneys, unchanged. Therefore other drugs that inhibit (or induce) the hepatic drug metabolizing systems will have no appreciable effect on digoxin's levels or effects.

The bile acid–binding resins, cholestyramine and colestipol, can reduce digoxin absorption from the gut (unless the administration of these interactants is separated by several hours). The most likely outcome of this interaction, then, would be reduced digoxin effects.

Quinidine, added to a long-standing digoxin regimen, certainly will raise serum digoxin levels and is likely to induce digoxin toxicity, by reducing digoxin's renal clearance. However, this interaction is so important—and so widely known—that quinidine is not (should not be) used often with digoxin on a long-term basis. It is certainly not "the most common cause" of digoxin toxicity.

252. The answer is d. *(Craig, p 260; Hardman, p 1346; Katzung, p 547.)* This is a fairly typical presentation of heparin-induced thrombocytopenia (HIT) in terms of both physical findings and time-course of onset. If heparin administration lasts for more than about a week, platelet counts should be checked several times a week for the first month or so and then monthly thereafter, because this is a potentially fatal response. It is immune-mediated: antibodies form against a heparin-platelet complex; platelets are activated (thus, the thrombosis and such complications as pulmonary and/or coronary occlusion, as we described); the vascular endothelia are damaged; and ultimately damaged platelets are cleared (hence the thrombocytopenia). The overall incidence is about 10 times higher with unfractionated heparin than with LMW heparins. Should HIT occur, or be suspected, the approach includes stopping the heparin and substituting other anticoagulants. If parenteral therapy is required, that might include using a direct thrombin inhibitor (e.g., bivalrudin). Many oral options are available.

Aspirin, by virtue of its antiplatelet effects, should not induce thrombosis. ACE inhibitors and β blockers (carvedilol, any others) do not interact to cause hemolytic anemias or other blood dyscrasias. Ranitidine (or famotidine or nizatidine, the other two newer H_2 blockers) do not alter the metabolism of other drugs; the prototype H_2 blocker, cimetidine, is a mixed function oxidase inhibitor.

253. The answer is b. (*Hardman, pp 1341–1342, 1350, 1353; Katzung, pp 316, 574.*) Aspirin inhibits cyclooxygenase (I and II). In terms of clotting, the main effect will be inhibition of platelet aggregation by reduced formation of thromboxane A_2. Bleeding time will be prolonged and will remain that way until sufficient numbers of new platelets have been released into the bloodstream, because aggregation of those platelets exposed to the drug will be inhibited for the lifetime of the platelets. The APTT, which should not be affected by aspirin, is used to monitor effects and adjust the dose of heparin. The prothrombin time (and its normalized value, the INR) are used with warfarin. Platelet counts, also not affected by aspirin, are used to assess for the development of thrombocytopenic purpura, which may rarely occur during therapy with (for example), clopidogrel or ticlopidine.

Renal System/Diuretics

Carbonic anhydrase inhibitors
Loop ("high-ceiling") diuretics
Osmotic diuretics

Potassium (K^+)-sparing diuretics
Thiazide diuretics (benzothiadi-
    azides)

Questions

DIRECTIONS: Each item contains a question or incomplete statement that is followed by possible responses. Select the **one best** response to each question.

254. Since diuretic-induced hypokalemia can have clinically significant consequences, it's important to know which diuretics are potassium-wasting and which spare potassium. Which is potassium-sparing?

a. Amiloride
b. Bumetanide
c. Hydrochlorothiazide
d. Metolazone
e. Torsemide

255. Which of the following statements best describes the general mechanism by which potassium-wasting diuretics cause their potassium-wasting effect?

a. Act as aldosterone receptor agonists, thereby favoring K^+ loss (and Na^+ elimination)
b. Block proximal tubular ATP-dependent secretory pumps for K^+
c. Increase delivery of Na^+ to the distal nephron, tubular Na^+ is reabsorbed in exchange with K^+, which is lost into the urine
d. Inhibit a proximal tubular Na,K-ATPase, K^+ is actively pumped into the urine
e. Lower distal tubular urine osmolality, thereby favoring passive diffusion of K^+ into the urine

256. Urinary potassium concentrations are measured before and after several weeks of administering a loop diuretic (typical daily dosages). We find that posttreatment urine K$^+$ *concentrations* are substantially lower than those measured at baseline. This indicates which of the following?

a. An expected response to the drug
b. That loop diuretics cause potassium-wasting only in *in vitro* experimental models
c. That measurements of posttreatment urine K$^+$ concentrations were erroneous
d. The patient has hypoaldosteronism from bilateral adrenalectomy
e. The presence of significantly impaired renal function

257. Which of the following is best avoided, or should be used with extra caution, in a patient with heart failure (or low left ventricular ejection fraction) because it may lower cardiac output further?

a. Amiloride
b. Ethacrynic acid
c. Hydrochlorothiazide
d. Mannitol
e. Spironolactone

258. Furosemide's main mechanism of action involves inhibition of a Na$^+$, K$^+$, 2Cl$^-$ co-transporter located in which of the following?

a. Ascending limb, loop of Henle
b. Collecting duct
c. Descending limb, loop of Henle
d. Distal convoluted tubule
e. Proximal tubule

259. A patient with an infectious disease is being treated with an aminoglycoside antibiotic. Which of the following diuretics should be avoided, if possible, for this patient?

a. Acetazolamide
b. Furosemide
c. Metolazone
d. Spironolactone
e. Triamterene

260. A patient taking a diuretic for several months presents with significantly elevated serum glucose levels and impaired carbohydrate tolerance (i.e., abnormally slow decline of blood glucose levels following a carbohydrate load). You suspect it is diuretic-induced. Which of the following is the most likely cause?

a. Acetazolamide
b. Amiloride
c. Chlorothiazide
d. Spironolactone
e. Triamterene

261. A patient has very high serum uric acid levels and is at imminent risk of developing acute uric acid nephropathy. Which of the following might be used to reduce the risk of this serious response by increasing the solubility of uric acid in the urine?

a. Acetazolamide
b. Antidiuretic hormone (ADH) [vasopressin (VP)]
c. Ethacrynic acid
d. Furosemide
e. Hydrochlorothiazide

262. Which of the following statements correctly describes a property of spironolactone?

a. Contraindicated in heart failure, especially if severe
b. Inhibits Na^+ reabsorption in the proximal renal tubule of the nephron
c. Interferes with aldosterone synthesis
d. Is a rational choice for a patient with an adrenal cortical tumor
e. Is more efficacious than hydrochlorothiazide in all patients who receive the drug

Questions 263–264

Two patients with very different medical conditions present. Which of the following diuretics would be appropriate therapy, whether alone or as an adjunct.

a. Bumetanide
b. Furosemide
c. Hydrochlorothiazide
d. Spironolactone
e. Triamterene

263. Patient 1 has nephrogenic diabetes. Which would reduce (although not normalize) his daily urine output and, indirectly, reduce symptoms such as polydipsia?

264. Patient 2 has idiopathic hypercalciuria: urinary calcium stone formation despite normal serum calcium concentrations and parathyroid function. Which would be your choice?

265. Virtually any diuretic, with the exception of the osmotic agents, can significantly increase the risk of excessive or toxic effects from which of the following?

a. Cholestyramine
b. Lithium
c. Nifedipine
d. Phenylephrine
e. Statin-type cholesterol-lowering drugs

266. A patient with heart failure is treated with digoxin and furosemide. He develops ventricular ectopy, increasing degrees of A-V nodal block, chromatopsia, and other extracardiac signs and symptoms of digoxin intoxication. Blood tests show that serum digoxin levels are well within normal limits. Which of the following mechanisms is involved in the diuretic-induced toxicity?

a. Displacement of digoxin from tissue binding sites
b. Hypocalcemia
c. Hypokalemia
d. Hyponatremia
e. Reductions of digoxin metabolism

267. A patient presents with chronic open angle glaucoma. Which of the following drugs might be prescribed as an adjunct to managing this condition?

a. Acetazolamide
b. Amiloride
c. Furosemide
d. Sprionolactone
e. Triamterene

268. A patient with heart failure has been managed with digoxin and furosemide and is doing well by all measures, for 3 years. He develops acute rheumatoid arthritis and is placed on rather large doses of a very efficacious nonsteroidal antiinflammatory drug—one that inhibits both cyclooxygenase pathways (COX-1 and -2). Which of the following is the most likely outcome of adding the NSAID?

a. Hyperchloremic acidosis indicative of acute diuretic toxicity
b. Dramatic increase of furosemide's potassium-sparing effects
c. Edema, weight gain, and other signs/symptoms indicative of reduced diuresis
d. Rapid onset of digoxin toxicity due to reduced digoxin excretion
e. Reduced digoxin effects because the NSAID competes with digoxin for myocyte receptor-binding sites

269. An edematous patient is taking therapeutic doses of a loop diuretic. Which of the following would you expect to occur along with the increased urine volume?

a. Dilute (hypotonic) urine because normal urine concentrating mechanisms are impaired
b. Hypercalcemia due to impaired renal Ca^{2+} excretion
c. Reduced net excretion of Cl^-
d. Metabolic acidosis due to increased renal bicarbonate excretion
e. Reduced serum uric acid (urate) concentrations because of increased urate excretion

270. Triamterene and amiloride cause their potassium-sparing effects mainly by which of the following?

a. Blocking distal tubular sodium channels and, ultimately, Na^+-K^+ exchange
b. Enhancing the affinity of aldosterone for its renal tubular receptors
c. Hastening metabolic inactivation of aldosterone
d. Inhibiting a proximal tubular Na,K-ATPase
e. Suppressing cortisol and aldosterone release from the adrenal cortex

271. A hypertensive patient has been on long-term therapy with lisinopril, a long-acting angiotensin-converting enzyme inhibitor, for hypertension. The drug isn't controlling pressure as well as wanted, so the physician decides to add triamterene as the (only) second drug. What is the most likely outcome of adding this diuretic to the ACE inhibitor regimen?

a. Blood pressure would rise abruptly
b. Better BP control, but with a risk of hyperkalemia
c. Cardiac depression, because both drugs directly depress the heart
d. Cough that may be severe, even though there was no cough with lisinopril alone
e. Hypernatremia, because ACE inhibitors counteract triamterene's natriuretic effect

Questions 272–273

Your patient, who lives at the bottom of Death Valley, California, (altitude 240 feet below sea level) is planning a vacation that includes a short hike to the top of Mount Everest (alt. approx. 29,000 feet above sea level). You're concerned about "altitude sickness."

272. Which of the following drugs would you recommend that this adventurer take before, and probably during, his trek?

a. Acetazolamide
b. Amiloride
c. Bumetanide
d. Furosemide
e. Sprionolactone
f. Triamterene

273. Assume this patient is also taking digoxin and torsemide; serum digoxin levels are therapeutic, and all electrolyte profiles are normal. Now your patient starts taking the altitude sickness medication you recommended. Which of the following is the most likely outcome?

a. Acute pulmonary edema
b. Antagonism of torsemide's expected and desired actions
c. Hyperkalemia
d. Increased and possibly excessive effects of the digoxin
e. Metabolic alkalosis

274. A patient with edema fails to respond adequately to maximum recommended dosages of chlorthalidone. Which of the following is the most appropriate and most fruitful next step?

a. Add hydrochlorothiazide
b. Add metolazone
c. Replace chlorthalidone with furosemide
d. Replace chlorthalidone with hydrochlorothiazide
e. Try increasing the chlorthalidone dose anyway

275. Five patients are placed on long-term diuretic therapy, each getting a different drug (below). Assuming the dose of each drug is "correct" and each patient is like the other in just about every respect that could affect drug action (overall health, diet, taking no other drugs, etc.), the patient who is most likely to develop hyponatremia is the one taking which of the following drugs?

a. Bumetanide
b. Ethacrynic acid
c. Furosemide
d. Hydrochlorothiazide
e. Torsemide

Questions 276–280

The table below shows the urinary electrolyte excretion patterns typical of various diuretics. These are *qualitative* changes and do not reflect the magnitude of the changes. They reflect whether excretion of an electrolyte (net amount) is increased or decreased; they do not reflect changes in urine *concentrations* of these substances.

Drug	Na⁺	K⁺	Ca²⁺	Mg²⁺	Cl⁻	HCO₃⁻
a.	↑	↑	↓	↑	↑	0/↑
b.	↑	↑	↑	↑	↑	0
c.	↑	↓	0	0	↑	↑
d.	↑	↑	0	0	↓	↑

↑, increased net loss into urine; ↓, decreased loss into urine (i.e., reduced elimination); 0, no change; ↑↓, increase or decrease, largely dependent on dose.

For each numbered diuretic listed below, choose the letter representing the urine electrolyte profile it is most likely to cause. A letter may be used once, more than once, or not at all.

276. Triamterene

277. Furosemide

278. Hydrochlorothiazide

279. Acetazolamide

280. Amiloride

Renal System/Diuretics

Answers

254. The answer is a. (*Craig, pp 247–249; Hardman, pp 692, 704–706; Katzung, pp 256–257.*) Amiloride is potassium-sparing. Its mechanism of action is largely similar to triamterene (see Question 270). The other available potassium-sparing diuretic, sprionolactone, causes natriuresis and potassium loss by blocking aldosterone receptors.

255. The answer is c. (*Craig, pp 241, 243–244; Hardman, pp 690, 692, 697–699, 701–702; Katzung, p 244.*) Thiazides (and thiazide-like agents such as metolazone) and loop diuretics (furosemide, bumetanide, torsemide, ethacrynic acid) increase delivery of Na^+ to the distal nephron because they inhibit reabsorption of Na^+ at more proximal sites. This extra Na^+ reaches the distal tubules, and some of it is taken from the tubular fluid and returned to the blood by a process that involves sodium channels. This reclamation of Na^+ leads to exchange of K^+, which is lost into the urine (i.e., potassium "wasting"). In essence, the more Na^+ delivered (and recovered) distally, the more K^+ that is eliminated in exchange.

256. The answer is a. (*Craig, pp 249–250; Hardman, pp 699–700; Katzung, p 247.*) One expected response to therapeutic doses of loop diuretics, which are clearly and correctly classified as potassium-wasting, is a reduction of urinary potassium *concentrations*. How can this be? Note that the term concentration reflects the amount of a substance (here, potassium) per unit volume. The loop diuretics do increase K^+ excretion in exchange for an added load of Na^+ delivered to the distal nephron. They also impair the ability of the kidneys to form a concentrated urine—i.e., they promote formation of a larger volume of more dilute urine. The net loss of K^+ (say, on a 24-h basis) is increased, but it's accompanied by a disproportionate increase in free water loss such that urine K^+ concentration (but not total amount) is decreased. (Be sure to see the explanation to Question 275 for a different look at this important amount vs. concentration issue.)

257. The answer is d. (*Craig, pp 250–251; Hardman, pp 695–696; Katzung, pp 252–253.*) Mannitol is an osmotic diuretic, the prototype of that small class of drugs (glycerin/glycerol is another somewhat noteworthy member of the group) with indications and potential side effects that are quite different from those of "typical" diuretics like the thiazides or loop agents. What happens when you inject (intravenously) this nonmetabolizable sugar (its structure is similar to that of glucose, and its molecular weight is the same)? Initially, and until it is excreted by glomerular filtration, mannitol increases plasma osmolality. That, in turn, osmotically withdraws water from the extracellular space and, ultimately, from the parenchymal cells, and into the blood. If the patient has good renal function, renal blood flow and GFR rise, and the drug is eventually excreted. If he or she has adequate cardiac function, circulating that extra volume (up to a limit) is not a problem.

However, if the patient has a sufficiently low ejection fraction or contractility to begin with, the increased blood volume and pressure may be such that the heart simply cannot handle the added work load. Indeed, in a futile attempt to circulate that additional volume and eject it against a higher afterload, the heart may fail acutely.

258. The answer is b. (*Craig, p 249; Hardman, pp 697–698; Katzung, p 247.*) As soon as you realize (it should be instantaneous) that furosemide (and bumetanide, torsemide, and ethacrynic acid) is a loop diuretic, you're half-way toward picking the right answer. These agents inhibit a Na^+, K^+, $2Cl^-$ co-transporter in the ascending limb. You should recall that unimpaired Na^+ and Cl^- reabsorption in the ascending limb is what is responsible and necessary for making the medullary milieu hypertonic, thereby providing the osmotic force necessary for withdrawing water (i.e., concentrating the urine) as urine passes through the collecting ducts. Note, too, that the ability of loop agents to increase Ca^{2+} and Mg^{2+} excretion involves actions in the ascending limb.

259. The answer is b. (*Craig, p 250; Hardman, p 700; Katzung, pp 248, 767–768.*) Both the loop diuretics and the aminoglycosides (tobramycin, streptomycin, gentamicin, others) are potentially ototoxic—capable of causing vestibular damage (e.g., balance problems) or cochlear damage (tinnitus or, in some cases, sensorineural hearing loss). The ototoxic effects of each drug is enhanced (often significantly) by the other's. The loop diuretic furosemide is an example of a drug that can cause several drug-drug interactions.

260. The answer is c. (*Craig, p 246; Hardman, pp 702–704; Katzung, p 250.*) Thiazides and thiazide-like diuretics (e.g., chlorthalidone, metolazone) may elevate blood glucose levels and cause frank hyperglycemia. The loop diuretics may do the same.

Several mechanisms have been proposed to explain the effect: decreased release of insulin from the pancreas, increased glycogenolysis and decreased glucogenesis, and a reduction in the conversion of proinsulin to insulin.

[You might want to recall that diazoxide (mainly used as a parenteral drug for prompt lowering of elevated blood pressure) can be used, orally, to raise blood glucose levels in some hypoglycemic states. It is, chemically, a thiazide but is not a diuretic.]

261. The answer is a. (*Craig, pp 244–245, 442, 445; Hardman, pp 725–726, 766–767; Katzung, pp 248, 250, 596, 599.*) Here we asked about reducing the risk of urate nephropathy acutely by increasing uric acid solubility. One key to answering this question correctly is to realize that uric acid becomes *more* soluble (less likely to precipitate or crystallize) as local pH rises. Recall that normal urine is acidic. By alkalinizing the urine, which is precisely what acetazolamide does, we can reduce the risk of stone formation. Note that acetazolamide is only an adjunct, and in addition to (or instead of) using it, we might also administer sodium bicarbonate, which will alkalinize the urine. Maintaining adequate hydration to help form relatively large volumes of a dilute urine is important.

Allopurinol, the xanthine oxidase inhibitor that blocks urate synthesis, can be (often is) used for prophylaxis. However, it takes some time to lower serum urate levels and so would be of little immediate value when urate stone formation is imminent or has occurred. Moreover, allopurinol does not change urine pH. Note that furosemide forms a dilute urine. Although that might lower urate concentrations in the urine and reduce the risk of crystallization there, it concomitantly increases serum urate levels, thereby increasing the risk of such other problems as acute gout. Thiazides are problematic too and should be avoided. They cause formation of a concentrated urine (increasing the likelihood of concentration-dependent urate crystallization) and also elevate serum urate levels.

262. The answer is d. (*Craig, pp 247–248; Hardman, pp 706–708; Katzung, pp 250–252.*) Spironolactone is a potassium-sparing diuretic. Its active metabolite displaces aldosterone from aldosterone receptors in the collecting ducts. The drug is ineffective in the absence of aldosterone. (Recall that aldosterone normally causes renal Na^+ retention and K^+ loss. The effects of aldosterone are, qualitatively the opposite: Na^+ loss, K^+ retention.)

Owing to the ability of sprionolactone to counteract the effects of aldosterone, it is particularly suited for patients with primary or secondary hyperaldosteronism (e.g., adrenal cortical tumor or hepatic dysfunction, as might occur with long-term/high-dose alcohol consumption, respectively). There is abundant data that the drug is beneficial in heart failure and probably reduces morbidity in severe heart failure.

In addition to the potential for causing hyperkalemia (especially if combined with oral potassium supplements, which should not be done) and hyponatremia (overall risk is low), spironolactone may cause several other side effects. CNS side effects include lethargy, headache, drowsiness, and mental confusion. Other side effects that are fairly common arise from the drug's androgen receptor–blocking actions: gynecomastia (in men and women) and erectile dysfunction. It may also cause seborrhea, acne, and coarsening of body hair. (Paradoxically, the drug can cause hirsutism in some patients, but it is also used to manage hirsutism in others.)

263. The answer is c. (*Hardman, p 704; Katzung, pp 244, 249–250.*) Recall that thiazides form a concentrated urine. That is, they interfere with physiologic mechanisms by which the kidneys form a normally (more) dilute urine. They are, therefore, useful adjuncts for nephrogenic diabetes insipidus.

264. The answer is c. (*Craig, p 246; Hardman, p 704; Katzung, p 249.*) Thiazides reduce renal Ca^{2+} excretion. Although these drugs tend to form a concentrated urine (which would favor calcium stone formation), the desired reduction of Ca^{2+} excretion predominates. The risk of Ca^{2+} stone formation can be reduced further by keeping the patient well hydrated. The loop diuretics increase renal Ca^{2+} excretion. Even though they help form a dilute urine, that effect occurs late in the nephron, and so these drugs would not "dilute" Ca^{2+} in sites proximal to the ascending limb of the loop of Henle. Thus, the risk of calciuria and stone formation is not at all reduced and probably is increased.

265. The answer is b. (*Craig, pp 393–395; Hardman, pp 448–449; Katzung, p 478.*) In essence, the intensity of effects from any given serum level of lithium are inversely related to serum sodium concentrations. When serum sodium concentration falls, the effects of lithium can be intensified to the point of causing toxicity. Via their actions to increase renal sodium loss, virtually all the common diuretics also reduce renal lithium excretion.

266. The answer is c. (*Craig, pp 154, 246; Hardman, p 700; Katzung, pp 208, 211–212.*) Significant digoxin toxicity can occur even when lab test results indicate that serum digoxin levels are "therapeutic." The most likely cause is hypokalemia, and the most common cause of that is coadministration of *any* potassium-wasting diuretic and inattention to falling serum potassium concentrations. The problem is due to the hypokalemia. Digoxin's binding to and inhibition of sarcolemmal Na^+,K^+-ATPase is significantly affected by $[K^+]_o$. When $[K^+]_o$ falls, as it can do in response to these diuretics, digoxin's binding and enzyme-inhibitory effects are intensified—often undesirably so. Conversely, hyperkalemia counteracts digoxin's effects. Note that digoxin is eliminated mainly by renal excretion, not by metabolism, and that none of the diuretics have significant stimulatory or inhibitory effects on the metabolism of any drugs.

267. The answer is a. (*Craig, p 245; Hardman, pp 694–695, 1623, 1633–1636, 1642; Katzung, pp 245–246.*) Aqueous humor formation (as well as that of cerebrospinal fluid) involves carbonic anhydrase activity. Acetazolamide is, of course, "the" carbonic anhydrase-inhibiting diuretic; lower aqueous humor synthesis and, all other factors being equal, pressure goes down. Note that when a carbonic anhydrase inhibitor is used to manage glaucoma, the drug's renal/diuretic effects, which certainly occur if the drug is given systemically, have nothing to do with the beneficial effects that are due to an ocular (ciliary body) site of action. If fact, those extraocular effects aren't needed for glaucoma control. That is why when a carbonic anhydrase inhibitor is used for glaucoma, we choose a topical ophthalmic agent (e.g., dorzolamide drops—don't memorize the name!), not a systemic agent like acetazolamide itself.

268. The answer is c. (*Hardman, p 700; Katzung, p 247.*) An important element in the renal responses to furosemide is maintenance of adequate renal blood flow. That is, to a degree, prostaglandin-mediated. The NSAIDs, such as the hypothetical one described here, inhibit prostaglandin synthesis. That, in turn, antagonizes the desired effects of the loop diuretic, leading to less fluid and salt elimination: edema, weight gain, and other markers of heart failure are likely to develop as a result. Hyperchloremic alkalosis is incorrect, in part, because chronic or acute excessive effects of loop diuretics are characterized by *hypo*chloremic metabolic *alkalosis*. Regardless, NSAIDs are not likely to potentiate the effects of these diuretics. "Dramatic increases of furosemide's K-sparing effects" is incorrect. Recall that loop diuretics are K-wasting. The NSAIDs do not reduce digoxin excretion appreciably, nor do they bind to and inhibit the myocyte Na^+,K^+-ATPase, which is digoxin's cellular receptor.

269. The correct answer is a. (*Craig, pp 249–250; Hardman, pp 697–700; Katzung, pp 247–248.*) Recall one of the main mechanisms by which a concentrated urine is formed: a hypertonic milieu in the renal medulla—and a medullary-to-cortical osmotic gradient—osmotically withdraws water (but not solute) from the tubular fluid as it passes through the collecting ducts. What creates that hypertonic medullary-to-cortical gradient? Reabsorption of Na^+ and Cl^- as tubular fluid ascends the loop of Henle, which ultimately increases interstitial osmolality. However, that process of ion resorption is impaired by loop diuretics. That reduces osmolality in the medullary interstitium, thereby dramatically reducing the osmotic gradient that enables the tubular fluid to become hypertonic as water is lost in the distal nephron. Thus, in the presence of a loop diuretic the urine remains dilute and hypotonic.

Metabolic acidosis from increased bicarbonate excretion doesn't occur. Recall that the main anion excreted (along with Na^+, K^+, etc.) is chloride. Bicarbonate tends to be reabsorbed. So, if there is any change of blood pH, it's one that can be characterized as alkalosis. Indeed, hypochloremic alkalosis is one potential adverse response of loop diuretics.

Loop diuretics do not lower serum urate concentrations. Rather, urate levels tend to rise, in part, because of reduced urate excretion combined with a "concentration" of urate in the blood owing to increased free water loss via the urine.

Hypercalcemia is not an expected accompaniment. Loop diuretics (in contrast with thiazides) increase renal Ca^{2+} elimination.

Serum uric acid concentration tends to rise. The loop diuretics reduce urate excretion. In addition, the proportionally large extra free water loss shrinks blood volume and tends to increase solute concentration, independent of any renal tubular effects on urate elimination.

270. The answer is a. (*Craig, p 248; Hardman, pp 704–706; Katzung, p 251.*) Triamterene and amiloride block distal tubular Na^+ channels that provide for Na^+ reabsorption in exchange for K^+, which is lost into the urine. The actions of these drugs have nothing to do with effects on aldosterone metabolism or aldosterone receptors (the latter being blocked by sprionolactone, which is the third potassium-sparing diuretic). None of these agents should be administered to patients who are hyperkalemic, and to avoid causing hyperkalemia, they should not be administered with oral potassium supplements or other drugs that increase circulating potassium levels.

271. The answer is b. (*Craig, p 249; Hardman, pp 706, 750–751; Katzung, pp 178–180, 252–256.*) The combined use of an ACE inhibitor and a diuretic is quite common, because the combination often provides better blood pressure control than can either agent alone. However, this combination usually involves a thiazide, not triamterene or another K-sparing diuretic because of the risk of hyperkalemia. Recall that one ultimate effect of any ACE inhibitor is potassium retention (and, of course, renal Na$^+$ loss); add to this the K-sparing effects of triamterene, amiloride, or sprionolactone, and there's a definite risk of causing hyperkalemia that can be more of a problem than the prior issues with blood pressure control.

You should also recall that although it is common to use both an ACE inhibitor and a thiazide, adding the thiazide is often associated with an excessive (but, fortunately, transient) fall of blood pressure that may lead to symptoms of hypotension. So, caution is required.

There is no known interaction involving a rise of blood pressure when adding a diuretic (triamterene or other) to an ACE inhibitor regimen. Neither drug has cardiac-depressant activity. Cough from an ACE inhibitor— not uncommon, and often severe—apparently involves inhibition of bradykinin metabolism by bradykininase, an enzyme that is, for all practical purposes, identical to angiotensin-converting enzyme. Diuretics do not potentiate that particular effect.

Hypernatremia is not a reasonable answer. Note that through different mechanisms both ACE inhibitors and diuretics (all) increase renal sodium loss. If anything, there would be a risk of hyponatremia.

272. The answer is a. (*Craig, pp 244–245; Hardman, pp 694–695; Katzung, p 246.*) The signs and symptoms of altitude sickness are related to the development of respiratory alkalosis: ventilatory rate is increased in response to breathing the rarefied air, which increases net ventilatory loss of CO_2. Blood pH rises. Acetazolamide increases bicarbonate loss, inducing a metabolic acidosis that counteracts the ventilatory-induced rise of blood pH.

273. The answer is d. (*Craig, p 245; Hardman, pp 694–695, 699–700; Katzung, p 246.*) Among other things, acetazolamide is potassium-wasting. Although serum potassium concentrations *might* be normal while taking the torsemide (loop diuretic) alone, adding acetazolamide might be sufficient to induce hypokalemia, which as we've said, is an important and common cause of digoxin toxicity. Pulmonary edema is not likely to occur merely by adding the acetazolamide. This drug addition will potentiate, rather than counteract, the effects of torsemide on renal sodium and potassium loss. As noted elsewhere, acetazolamide increases urinary bicarbonate loss and causes metabolic acidosis.

274. The answer is c. (*Craig, p 253; Hardman, pp 710–711; Katzung, pp 249–250, 254–256.*) Chlorthalidone is a thiazide-like diuretic. If maximum dosages don't yield the desired effects, there's little likelihood that switching to another thiazide or thiazide-like agent (e.g., hydrochlorothiazide, metolazone, many others) will do better. Likewise, and given the relatively "flat" dose-response relationship for these drugs, nothing good is likely to be gained by adding "yet another" agent that works in precisely the same way as the drug that has already proven inadequate. If a maximum recommended dose isn't adequate, giving more of the same or a similar drug won't be better. So, in situations such as this, it's time to switch to a drug that is intrinsically more efficacious and works via a different mechanism: a loop diuretic.

275. The answer is d. (*Hardman, pp 702–703; Katzung, p 250.*) Diuretic-induced hyponatremia is almost always due to a thiazide or thiazide-like agent.

This may seem like a picky question, but don't jump to that conclusion. Although you probably know that furosemide is a loop diuretic, you may not remember (probably you should) that bumetanide, ethacrynic acid, and torsemide are loop diuretics, too. So then you may begin splitting hairs, wondering which of those loop diuretics is more likely than another to cause hyponatremia. But that's irrelevant for this question. Would you have arrived at the correct answer if your only choices were hydrochlorothiazide and furosemide? Would you have realized (correctly) that loop diuretics are more efficacious (in many respects, including the natriuretic effect) than a thiazide, and then (*incorrectly*) concluded that the risk of hyponatremia was, therefore, higher with the loop agent?

The essential point here lies in the "definition" of hyponatremia. It does not mean an abnormally low *amount* of sodium, whether in the body overall or in just one compartment, such as the blood. It reflects an abnormally low *concentration* of blood sodium—mEq/mL.

Loop diuretics are more efficacious than thiazides in terms of the amount of extra Na^+ that appears in the urine, but also that increased urinary Na^+ loss is accompanied by a comparatively great loss of free water in the urine. That is because, in essence, loop diuretics impair the normal urine concentrating mechanisms in the nephron. (See the answer to Question 256, which focuses on the same concept, but in the context of urine potassium concentration after a loop diuretic.) Compared with a thiazide, there is less of a mismatch between the amounts of Na^+ and water lost.

In contrast, although thiazides may cause only a modest amount of Na^+ being lost into the urine, the amount of extra water that is lost is comparatively low: the urine is more concentrated with respect to many solutes, Na included. Arginine vasopressin "kicks in" and helps promote renal water retention. Rather than focusing on the urine, look instead at the blood, which is what we test to decide whether a patient is hyponatremic. What we have said is that, in relative terms, with a thiazide, we have depleted a larger amount of Na^+ than of water. Serum Na^+ concentration goes down, often to the point that the patient becomes clinically hyponatremic.

This fundamental difference is clinically important in a way you may not have thought about, nor thought was logical: a loop diuretic (by definition, a drug that increases renal Na^+ excretion) can be used to *treat* hyponatremia, such as that caused by a thiazide, precisely because it will increase water loss more than Na^+ loss, thereby helping to raise serum Na^+ concentration.

276–280. *(Craig, p 244; Hardman, p 692; Katzung, p 254; and pages nearby each.)* Rather than rehashing the sites and mechanisms by which the "main" diuretics cause their effects—that's largely all been addressed above—what follows provides some tips for arriving at the correct answer easily. We'll add some additional comments if they haven't been emphasized before.

Note that all the profiles show an increased (qualitative) renal excretion of Na. The essence of this is that it reflects the fact that all the common diuretics do that. Indeed, this natriuretic effect is at the root of the "definition" of "diuretic."

The next step is to identify which agents increase renal K excretion and which do the opposite, because the main diuretics are either K-sparing or K-wasting. That will narrow your choices nicely. You should be able to place a drug in the proper K-related class instantaneously (with the possible exception of acetazolamide, a K-wasting drug, because we tend to emphasize its carbonic acid–inhibitory effects and overload other important properties).

Finally, once you see that a drug's profile involves increased K^+ elimination, you have narrowed your choices to a thiazide or thiazide-like agent (hydrochlorothiazide, chlorthalidone, metolazone, many others), a loop agent, or a carbonic anhydrase inhibitor.

Look now at what happens to urinary Ca^{2+} excretion. If it's reduced, it's a thiazide or a related agent (recall we can use these drugs for idiopathic hypercalciuria, an effect that capitalizes on reduced presence of Ca^{2+} in the urine). If Ca^{2+} excretion is increased, it's a loop diuretic.

Now how do you identify which agent is a carbonic anhydrase inhibitor (i.e., acetazolamide)? In addition to looking at Na^+ and K^+, note what happens to HCO_3^- and Cl^-. Acetazolamide causes profound urinary alkalinization from the HCO_3^- loss; so much so that the blood's other major anion, Cl^-, is retained. Just looking at the table you would probably rule out a thiazide (a) as being acetazolamide because we indicate that the effect on that anion is variable ($0/\uparrow$).

How could you rule out triamterene, because we showed increased HCO_3^- loss with it? (It's a slight effect, by the way, and carbonic anhydrase inhibition is not its main nor an important mechanism or outcome, but you can't tell from the table.) Look at the Cl^- profile and you will see that acetazolamide is the *only* diuretic that lowers Cl^- excretion. That's because one of the blood's major anions, HCO_3^-, is lost to such a great degree that the other main anion, Cl^-, is conserved.

276. Answer c shows the profile for triamterene.

277. Answer b shows the profile for furosemide or other loop diuretics.

278. Answer a shows the profile for hydrochlorothiazide (and related drugs).

279. Answer d represents what occurs with acetazolamide.

280. Answer c is amiloride's profile (same as for triamterene, which is largely identical in most pharmacodynamic respects).

Respiratory System: Asthma/COPD

Adrenergic agonists
Antimuscarinics
Methylxanthines
Leukotriene synthesis inhibitors
and receptor blockers

Mast cell "stabilizers"
Mucolytics
Antitussives
Histamine receptor (H_1) blockers

Questions

DIRECTIONS: Each item contains a question or incomplete statement that is followed by possible responses. Select the **one best** response to each question.

281. The most important goal to achieve, pharmacologically, in optimal management of asthma is which of the following?

a. Ensure that serum levels of adrenergic bronchodilators are therapeutic around the clock (24 h/day)
b. Limit use of rescue inhalers to a maximum of 3 times per week
c. Provide prompt reversal of bronchospasm
d. Suppress airway inflammatory processes
e. Use inhaled drugs only; avoid use of oral agents

282. Which of the following adrenergic agonists lacks bronchodilator activity, and so has no role in managing asthma long term or acutely?

a. Albuterol
b. Epinephrine
c. Norepinephrine
d. Salmeterol
e. Terbutaline
f. Theophylline

283. A patient with asthma is taking an oral methylxanthine. Which of the following is an accurate characterization of this drug class?

a. Eliminated almost exclusively by renal excretion, unchanged
b. Excellent anti-inflammatory actions
c. Frequently causes drowsiness, lethargy
d. Remarkably free of significant interactions with other drugs
e. Unusually high (large) margin of safety/therapeutic index
f. Useful only for symptom prophylaxis

284. A patient with asthma has moderate bronchospasm and wheezing about twice a week. Current medications are inhaled albuterol, used for both prophylaxis and to abort ongoing attacks (rescue therapy), and inhaled beclomethasone, because the physician deems the steroid beneficial. If the physician chooses to use salmeterol, it should be used as which of the following?

a. A replacement for the albuterol
b. A replacement for the corticosteroid
c. An add-on to current medications for additional prophylactic benefits
d. Primary (sole) therapy, replacing both albuterol and the steroid
e. The preferred agent for acute symptom control (rescue therapy)

285. A patient took a lethal dose of theophylline. Which of the following was the most likely cause of death?

a. Bradycardia and heart block
b. Hepatotoxicity (liver failure)
c. Hypertensive crisis
d. Paradoxical bronchospasm leading to apnea
e. Seizures and, consequently, hypoxia from inability to breathe during the seizures

286. A 16-year-old boy with breathing difficulty is seen in the emergency department. He is diagnosed with asthma and given urgent care. The next day he visits his primary physician, who starts him on therapy with albuterol, to be inhaled "as needed" (for acute symptom control—rescue therapy). After several weeks the patient says he needs to use the inhaler several times a day, nearly every day, because "breathing just gets real hard; I can't get much air in." The physician's assessment is that symptom severity and frequency are getting progressively and quickly worse.

Which *initial* therapeutic modification for outpatient management would be most reasonable, with the greatest likelihood of controlling the asthma?

a. Add an inhaled corticosteroid
b. Add cromolyn
c. Add oral prednisone
d. Add theophylline
e. Double the albuterol dose to be taken with each episode
f. Replace the albuterol with salmeterol

287. A 16-year-old girl treated for asthma develops skeletal muscle tremors that is drug-induced. Which of the following is the most likely cause?

a. Albuterol
b. Beclomethasone
c. Cromolyn
d. Ipratropium
e. Zileuton

288. A 23-year-old with asthma has what is described as "aspirin sensitivity" and experiences severe bronchospasm in response to even small doses of the drug. The most likely explanation for this is that the aspirin

a. Blocks synthesis of endogenous prostaglandins that have bronchodilator activity
b. Induces formation of antibodies directed against the salicylate on airway mast cells
c. Induces hypersensitivity of H_1 receptors on airway smooth muscles
d. Induces hypersensitivity of muscarinic receptors on airway smooth muscles
e. Prevents or reduces epinephrine binding to β_2-adrenergic receptors (airways and elsewhere)

289. An asthma patient has been receiving oral anhydrous theophylline (theophylline base) for some time, and now we plan to switch to the sodium glycinate salt—one of several theophylline salts available—for continued oral therapy. How does the sodium glycinate salt, or any theophylline salt for that matter, differ from anhydrous theophylline?

a. Eliminated renally; no dependence on metabolism
b. Have much greater margins of safety
c. Less potent on a mg-for-mg basis
d. Radically different side effects profiles
e. Unquestionably more efficacious as bronchodilators than anhydrous theophylline

290. An elderly man with COPD is being managed with several drugs, one of which is inhaled ipratropium. Which of the following is the main effect that accounts for the beneficial effects of this drug?

a. Blockade of an endogenous bronchoconstrictor mediator
b. Enhanced release of epinephrine from the adrenal medulla
c. Inhibition of cAMP breakdown via phosphodiesterase inhibition
d. Prevention of antigen-antibody reactions that lead to mast cell mediator release
e. Stimulation of ventilatory rates (CNS effect in brain's medulla)
f. Suppression of inflammatory processes

291. A 26-year-old patient with asthma is receiving montelukast. Which of the following is the main mechanism by which this drug works?

a. Enhanced release of epinephrine from the adrenal medulla
b. Increased airway adrenergic receptor responsiveness to catecholamines
c. Inhibition of cAMP breakdown via phosphodiesterase inhibition
d. Prevention of antigen-antibody reactions that lead to mast cell mediator release
e. Stimulation of ventilatory rates (CNS effect in brain's medulla)
f. Suppression of inflammatory processes

292. A young boy, in obvious respiratory distress from a severe asthma attack, presents in the emergency department. One drug ordered by the physician, to be administered by the respiratory therapist, is *N*-acetylcysteine. Which of the following is the purpose of this drug?

a. Block receptors for the cysteinyl leukotrienes
b. Inhibit metabolic inactivation of epinephrine or β_2 agonists that were administered
c. Inhibit leukotriene synthesis
d. Promptly suppress airway inflammation
e. Reverse ACh-mediated bronchoconstriction
f. Thin airway mucus secretions for easier removal by suctioning

293. A young boy is diagnosed with asthma. His primary symptom is frequent cough, not bronchospasm or wheezing. Other asthma medications are started, but until their effects develop fully we wish to suppress the cough without running a risk of suppressing ventilatory drive or causing sedation or other unwanted effects. Which of the following would best meet these needs?

a. Codeine
b. Dextromethorphan
c. Diphenhydramine
d. Hydrocodone
e. Promethazine

294. An adult patient with asthma begins taking furosemide for another indication. After several weeks on the diuretic he complains of more breathing difficulty than he had before. Pulmonary function tests confirm his perceptions. Which of the following is the most likely mechanism by which the furosemide worsened the clinical picture?

a. Blocking the endogenous bronchodilator effects of circulating epinephrine
b. Causing greater bronchoconstriction by releasing more ACh in the airways
c. Directly causing bronchoconstriction
d. Drying the airways, increasing mucus viscosity
e. Enhancing metabolic clearance of other asthma medications (lowering their serum levels)
f. Releasing histamine

295. An asthma patient has symptom flare-ups during hay fever season. He visits the local superstore and purchases an over-the-counter antihistamine/allergy remedy containing diphenhydramine. After a few days of using it, his breathing becomes worse. You evaluate him and conclude that what the patient viewed as the allergy cure was actually the cause of the problems. Which of the following is the most likely mechanism by which the diphenhydramine worsened this patient's condition?

a. Blocking the endogenous bronchodilator effects of circulating epinephrine
b. Causing greater bronchoconstriction by releasing more ACh in the airways
c. Directly causing bronchoconstriction
d. Drying the airways, increasing mucus viscosity
e. Enhancing metabolic clearance of other asthma medications (lowering their serum levels)
f. Releasing histamine

296. A patient suffering status asthmaticus presents in the emergency department. Blood gases reveal severe respiratory acidosis and hypoxia. Even large parenteral doses of a β_2 agonist fail to dilate the airways adequately; rather, they cause dangerous degrees of tachycardia. Which of the following should be done, pharmacologically, to manage the pulmonary problems and restore the efficacy of the adrenergic drug.

a. Add inhaled cromolyn
b. Give a parenteral corticosteroid
c. Give parenteral diphenhydramine
d. Switch to epinephrine
e. Switch to isoproterenol (β_1/β_2 agonist)

297. In the context of asthma, what property is shared by acetylcholinesterase inhibitors, muscarinic agonists such as pilocarpine, and β blockers?

a. Are preferred topical antiglaucoma drugs for patients with asthma
b. Contraindicated, or pose great risks, for people with asthma
c. Degranulate mast cells, cause bronchoconstriction
d. Trigger bronchoconstriction by directly activating H_1 histamine receptors on airway smooth muscle cells
e. Useful for acute asthma, not for ambulatory patients

Respiratory System: Asthma/COPD

Answers

281. The answer is d. (*Craig, p 460; Hardman, pp 659–660, 678–679; Katzung, pp 319–322, 328–329, 332.*) Control of airway inflammation is the single most important factor in optimal asthma control. Although one often focuses on bronchoconstriction (which is no doubt important to control), that is almost always a *consequence* of ongoing inflammatory responses. Controlling inflammation satisfactorily may (and hopefully) eliminate the need for bronchodilators altogether or may enable marked reductions in adrenergic bronchodilator doses or the frequency with which they might be needed. Treating asthma with bronchodilators only, especially if episodes are severe and/or frequent, is almost certainly doomed to fail.

282. The answer is c. (*Craig, pp 93, 101; Hardman, pp 110–111, 209–210; Katzung, p 86.*) By way of a brief but essential review of autonomic pharmacology, recall that "adrenergic bronchodilation" requires activation of β_2-adrenergic receptors on airway smooth-muscle cells. Norepinephrine is an α and β_1 agonist, with no ability to activate β_2s, and so it has no bronchodilator activity. Final note: theophylline is not an adrenergic drug in any respect.

283. The answer is f. (*Craig, p 463; Hardman, pp 672–675; Katzung, pp 325–327.*) First, you should remember that the methylxanthines are anhydrous theophylline and its various salts. They are bronchodilators that are indicated only for prophylaxis. (The EDTA salt, aminophylline, is sometimes used for acute control, but it is given intravenously, and we asked about oral therapy.) We do not know the precise mechanism of action in vivo: postulated ones are inhibition of phosphodiesterase and blockade of receptors for adenosine, which has bronchoconstrictor activity.

Methylxanthines have no anti-inflammatory activity; they cause dose- (concentration-) dependent CNS stimulation; their elimination (inactivation) is heavily dependent on hepatic metabolism, and, as such, the drug's half-life and effects are clinically significantly affected by a variety of drugs that induce or inhibit the liver's mixed function oxidase system; and they have an extremely low margin of safety/therapeutic index. All these can be considered major limitations, therapeutically, and they account for the declining use of these largely outmoded drugs (except in some very selected patient populations).

Note: Although it may be picky (but someone may ask you), a related drug, dyphylline, differs from the typical methylxanthines in one important way: this theophylline derivative (not a theophylline salt) is eliminated by renal excretion, not by hepatic metabolism. The implication is that dyphylline might be a "preferred" choice for patients who could benefit from a methylxanthine but have impaired liver function or are taking other drugs that interact by altering hepatic drug metabolism. Nonetheless, as with the methylxanthines in general, given the other limitations of this drug class and the availability of other drug classes that are arguably more effective or safer for asthma control, there's little good reason to use dyphylline either.

284. The answer is c. (*Craig, p 462; Hardman, pp 215, 665; Katzung, pp 324–325, 332.*) If we were to decide to use salmeterol, in this case it would be best to consider it as an add-on. It can be administered separately, or the physician might prescribe one of the proprietary fixed-dose combination products containing both salmeterol and a steroid (inhaled). Recall that salmeterol, like albuterol, is mainly a β_2 agonist, but salmeterol's onset of action is much slower, its duration longer. The slow onset makes it a useful prophylactic agent for some patients, but renders it completely inappropriate for rescue therapy. One could reasonably argue that salmeterol is also dangerous if used as the sole intervention for rescue, because serious ventilatory compromise can develop before its bronchodilator effects develop. The patient described needs a corticosteroid (and probably should be put on an oral steroid for a while, given symptom frequency and severity with the current regimen). Replacing either just the current steroid with salmeterol, or (worse) replacing both the albuterol and the steroid with it, would be unconscionable.

285. The answer is e. (*Craig, p 463; Hardman, p 675; Katzung, pp 326, 924.*) Increasing serum levels of theophylline, the prototype methylxanthine bronchodilator, cause increasing degrees of CNS stimulation (e.g., of the cerebral cortex, medulla). Ultimately, seizures develop, and during the resulting tonic-clonic convulsions the patient cannot breathe adequately. Cerebral hypoxia and death ensue.

Through a variety of mechanisms—inhibition of phosphodiesterase probably an important one—theophylline and other methylxanthines increase cardiac contractility, heart rate, and electrical impulse conduction. Tachycardia and potential arrhythmias are likely, not bradycardia and/or heart block. For some patients, lethal cardiac responses might occur before status epilepticus and brain hypoxia cause death.

Blood pressure would probably rise, but it would be a response to cardiac stimulation (increased contractility and stroke volume), not due to any peripheral vasoconstriction, and the blood pressure rise is not likely to be so great as to qualify it as a hypertensive crisis.

Hepatotoxicity is not a common concern with methylxanthines, whether acutely or chronically.

286. The answer is c. (*Craig, pp 464–465; Hardman, pp 666, 670; Katzung, pp 328–329, 332.*) Given the severity of symptoms and the speed with which they are worsening, the only appropriate approach is to start the patient on an daily oral steroid until symptom control is deemed adequate and sufficiently long-lasting. At that time, carefully tapering the oral steroid and starting the inhaled agent (beclomethasone, triamcinolone, others) might be appropriate.

Although corticosteroid therapy, per se, is the correct approach, beginning the therapy change by adding an inhaled steroid (rather than starting oral treatment) would not be suitable. Inhaled steroids are efficacious, but it takes roughly 2 or more weeks of continued use until meaningful control of airway inflammation and symptoms develops. Given the nature of the patient's rapidly worsening symptoms, we do not have the luxury of time. (As noted in the paragraph above, however, it would be very reasonable to add an inhaled steroid to the sympathomimetic regimen after we have good control with an oral drug such as prednisone.)

Cromolyn would not be a good choice. The onset of this inhaled drug is slow, too, and it will be of little benefit with the quickly worsening asthma attacks. It might be considered as a prophylactic measure sometime later (after the current situation is well under control), and it would probably be suitable as an add-on only if we can determine that the asthma attacks are largely due to atopy (allergic responses).

Theophylline is not a good choice. Although it may have some prophylactic value, it will be of little benefit should acute attacks continue, as they are likely to do for a while. Other reasons why theophylline is not a good choice are its low therapeutic index (or margin of safety), the prevalence of side effects (CNS and cardiovascular stimulation), and the need for frequent blood testing to help guide dosing adjustments. Overall, theophylline and other methylxanthines are becoming passé.

Doubling the albuterol dose is a poor approach. The continuation of asthma attacks—indeed, the apparent worsening—may be due to at least two issues: (1) continued and perhaps worsening airway inflammation, which will not be suppressed with any sympathomimetic; and (2) potential airway tolerance to the actions of the adrenergic agent. Doubling the dose may briefly overcome the tolerance, but tolerance to the increased dose eventually would develop too. Moreover, increasing the dose of this "selective" β_2 agonist would likely be associated with adverse cardiovascular stimulation, because preferential β_2 activation is lost with increased dosages; the lost selectivity implies increased β_1 stimulation.

Switching from albuterol to salmeterol would be a poor choice. This slow- and long-acting adrenergic agonist is useful for prophylaxis (for some patients), but it will be of little help for this boy, given his frequent and worsening attacks. The salmeterol would be largely useless should an acute attack occur again. Even if we started therapy with salmeterol and instructed the patient to keep his albuterol inhaler and use it to abort attacks, we would be doing nothing beneficial for the underlying pathophysiologic problem: the airway inflammation.

287. The answer is a. (*Craig, p 462; Hardman, p 215; Katzung, p 325.*) Skeletal muscle tremor is a side effect associated with β_2-adrenergic agonists—albuterol and others. It is almost always a dose-dependent phenomenon. None of the other drugs listed are associated with skeletal muscle tremor. (Note: Some physicians titrate the dose of adrenergic bronchodilators upward, stopping when tremors develop and equating the blood level associated with that dose as being therapeutic with respect to controlling the pulmonary disease. That is poor management; proper dosage adjustments or other therapy changes should be based on pulmonary symptom relief in general and pulmonary function tests ideally.)

288. The answer is a. (*Craig, pp 313, 426–427; Hardman, pp 606, 610, 622–624; Katzung, pp 319–321, 581.*) Aspirin, a nonsteroidal antiinflammatory drug (NSAID), inhibits cyclooxygenases and the "arachidonic acid cascade." One outcome of that is inhibited synthesis of PGE_2. The PGE_2 (along with circulating epinephrine) is a physiologically important endogenous bronchodilator, particularly for most asthmatics. Inhibit this synthesis, with aspirin or another nonselective cyclooxygenase inhibitor/NSAID, and bronchoconstriction or bronchospasm is likely to ensue in that population of asthmatics who often are exquisitely sensitive to these drugs. Virtually all other NSAIDs may cross-react, although the incidence of severe pulmonary reactions seems to be among the highest with aspirin itself. Selective COX-2 inhibitors (celecoxib, rofecoxib, others) pose less of a problem, but they are not absolutely free from the potential problem. If one needs a drug to manage fever or mild pain in an asthmatic, acetaminophen is preferred: it does not cross-react (owing to negligible effects on prostaglandin synthesis: it is not classified as an NSAID).

289. The answer is c. *(Hardman, p 673; Katzung, pp 325–327.)* Do not get misled by a question that addresses knowledge of a very simple concept. The various theophylline salts (sodium glycinate, monohydrate, others, made mainly to increase solubility compared with anhydrous theophylline) are less potent on a mg-for-mg basis than the "gold standard," anhydrous theophylline (theophylline base). Once absorbed, the salts dissociate and form theophylline in the blood. Because we are giving theophylline itself, albeit in salt form, everything you should have learned about the pharmacokinetics and actions of anhydrous theophylline (theophylline base) still applies: see Question 283 for an overview. The salts are no more efficacious, don't have other important unique properties, and so on.

(Here's one way to look at it. Imagine, hypothetically, that we had a pill that contained 100 mg of anhydrous theophylline—100% by weight is the active drug; if the pill were 100 mg of a salt, only a portion of that total weight would be due to the active drug; the rest would be the inactive salt. Some of the salts are large, weight-wise, in comparison with the weight of theophylline itself. For example, 100 mg of the sodium glycinate salt contains only about 50 mg of theophylline. If the correct dose of anhydrous theophylline was x mg, we'd have to give $2x$ mg of this salt in order to get effects of equivalent intensity.)

290. The answer is a. *(Craig, pp 137–138, 463–464; Hardman, pp 152, 154–155, 665; Katzung, pp 327–328, 332.)* You should be able to deduce quickly (if not simply know outright) that ipratropium is an atropine-like drug—an antimuscarinic that blocks the bronchoconstrictor effect of ACh on airway smooth muscle. It is a quaternary, inhaled antimuscarinic: that is, it acts locally in the airways, and very little of the "always charged" molecule diffuses into the circulation to cause systemic effects. Ipratropium has no effects on the adrenal medulla, on mast cells or other elements of the inflammatory response, or in the CNS. Ipratropium is approved for managing COPD, but is often used for some asthma patients. The drug has a rapid onset of action. However, some studies indicate that it is not as efficacious a bronchodilator as β_2 agonists, and so it is not a suitable agent for rescue therapy. Finally, the bronchodilator effects of ipratropium and β agonists are synergistic (same effect, different mechanisms), and so there's some logic to using them both.

291. The answer is f. (*Craig, pp 465–466; Hardman, p 644; Katzung, pp 330–331.*) Montelukast (and a related drug, zafirlukast) block receptors for leukotrienes (LTs). (When you see "leuk" or "luk" as part of these drugs' generic names, think leukotrienes or leukotriene modifiers.)

Recall that the LTs, which are pro-inflammatory and bronchoconstrictor mediators, are formed as part of normal arachidonic acid metabolism via the 5'-lipoxygenase pathway. (Recall that the other main part of arachidonic acid metabolism, involving cyclooxygenases, forms various prostaglandins and thromboxane A_2.) A somewhat related drug, zileuton, inhibits 5'-lipoxygenase directly, thereby mainly blocking LT synthesis rather than mainly blocking LT receptors.

These are oral agents, indicated for prophylaxis only. They will do virtually no good in a short enough time if they were administered to suppress ongoing bronchoconstriction, mainly because they are too slow-acting. And, although this class of drugs is the newest one to be approved for asthma in many years, they are not panaceas for all asthma patients, and for some patients their efficacy is not all that great.

Note: One probable advantage of montelukast or zafirlukast over zileuton is that they don't appear to participate in well-documented, clinically significant drug-drug interactions.

In contrast, zileuton inhibits theophylline's metabolism to a degree that is likely to be clinically significant for some patients (e.g., envisage a scenario in which these two asthma drugs are prescribed for the same patient) and also inhibits hepatic clearance of warfarin. It can also cause liver damage (as evidenced by increased transaminase levels in the blood). It is contraindicated for patients with acute liver disease and probably also should be avoided in chronic liver disease.

292. The answer is f. (*Hardman, p 632; Katzung, p 333.*) N-acetylcysteine is a mucolytic (mucus-thinning) drug, given to reduce the viscosity of airway mucus. It has no effects, in the context of pulmonary disease, other than that. It is given by inhalation, usually with a nebulizer in hypertonic saline, mainly to facilitate mucus removal (whether by airway suctioning or by postural changes that allow better drainage from the airways). This is an important emergency adjunct for asthma—one that you should know better in its other main role, as an antidote for acetaminophen poisoning.

293. The answer is b. (*Craig, p 327; Hardman, pp 551–552; Katzung, p 512.*) Dextromethorphan is a centrally acting antitussive drug that is about as efficacious a cough-suppressant as codeine. However, unlike codeine and hydrocodone (another useful antitussive in some cases), dextromethorphan is not an opioid and so lacks the potential for ventilatory suppression (and generalized CNS depression, analgesia, dependence risks, and other typical traits of the opioids). Diphenhydramine and promethazine also have antitussive action. However, they, too, can cause generalized CNS (and ventilatory) depression. Moreover, they have significant antimuscarinic effects. Although that may be good in terms of inhibiting ACh-mediated bronchoconstriction, they may also cause thickening of airway mucus, leading to some mechanical plugging of the airways with viscous mucus deposits.

294. The answer is d. Although you may not have learned this explicitly, nor are there any explicit comments in the texts we have cross-referenced, you should be able to integrate your knowledge of drugs and pathophysiology to arrive at the answer. Dehydration (whether caused by an efficacious diuretic such as furosemide, excessive exercise, or failure to consume adequate amounts of water) renders the airways more reactive to a variety of bronchoconstrictor stimuli and can also favor formation of viscous mucus that can cause physical obstruction to gas transfer or movement. Maintaining adequate hydration—and avoiding dehydration—are important elements in asthma management.

Look at the other possible (and wrong) answers listed and refresh your memory: you did *not* learn that furosemide, or any other diuretics, block epinephrine receptors, release ACh, cause bronchoconstriction directly, alter metabolism of other drugs, or release histamine. That is because furosemide does not cause those effects.

295. The answer is d. (*Craig, pp 136–137, 459, 464; Hardman, pp 588–590; Katzung, pp 115, 266, 319–321.*) Diphenhydramine, and most of the other older antihistamines (H_1 histamine-receptor blockers) have varying degrees of antimuscarinic (atropine-like) activity. With diphenhydramine and several others, that effect is quite intense. These antihistamines do block the bronchoconstrictor effects of both histamine (via H_1 receptors) and ACh (muscarinic), and so in those regards they can be beneficial. However, the muscarinic blocking activity also thickens airway mucus, and as was the case with the patient described in Question 294 (but by a different mechanism), this increased mucus viscosity and the tendency for mucus plugs to form can do more harm than the good provided by the other effects. If the patient chooses to take an antihistamine, they might be better off taking one of the second-generation agents (e.g., fexofenadine, loratadine, others), which lack the antimuscarinic/mucus-thickening effects caused by the older agents. If an antihistamine that can cause mucus thickening must be used, then ensuring that the patient is well hydrated is paramount.

Notes: Diphenhydramine and a very similar antihistamine, doxylamine, are also common ingredients in OTC sleep aids. Airway problems from mucus thickening may also arise, therefore, with these products.

Paradoxically (you may think), atropine is an important element in managing status asthmaticus. Why use it in this life-threatening situation, but avoid it or other antimuscarinics in ambulatory patients? When used for severe asthma, the atropine is given by inhalation. It is nebulized and given with a mucus-thinning drug plus ample "moisture"—e.g., saline— along with steroids and adrenergic bronchodilators. It is this use of drug and other adjuncts that will maximize atropine's bronchodilator actions while simultaneously and virtually eliminating all the potential problems related to mucus thickening and airway obstruction.

296. The answer is b. (*Craig, p 467; Hardman, pp 669–670; Katzung, pp 127, 325, 332.*) When pulmonary function deteriorates so much that respiratory acidosis ensues (because sufficient amounts of CO_2 aren't being eliminated by ventilation) and severe hypoxia develops (because of inadequate oxygen transfer), acute tolerance (in essence, desensitization) develops to the bronchodilator effects of drugs with β_2 agonist activity—all of them. If this is ignored, repeated administration of a β_2 agonist will lead to increasing degrees of cardiac stimulation (rate, contractility, automaticity, conduction) because under these conditions they lose their selectivity for β_2 receptors and also begin activating β_1s very effectively. (They become isoproterenol-like in their profiles.)

Even epinephrine won't work as a good bronchodilator under these conditions, and repeated injections of it will do little more than cause further cardiac stimulation plus vasoconstriction via α activation. Through mechanisms that are not quite clear, administering suitable doses of a parenteral steroid under these conditions of acidosis and hypoxia "restores" a substantial degree of airway responsiveness to β agonists. Giving a steroid (plus oxygen, which helps correct the underlying blood gas and pH changes) is essential.

Giving diphenhydramine, even though it blocks the bronchoconstrictor effects of both ACh and histamine, will not do much good for the acute and life-threatening signs and symptoms. Giving cromolyn will prove largely worthless and certainly not life-saving.

297. The answer is b. (*Craig, pp 87, 93, 115–116, 124–125, 130; Hardman, pp 119, 158, 183–184, 252–258; Katzung, p 297.*) By now you should be able to recall the classifications and actions of the drugs listed in this question. Acetylcholinesterase inhibitors and such muscarinic agonists as pilocarpine are sometimes used as topical miotics for managing glaucoma (mainly angle-closure/narrow angle forms of the disease). Certain topical β blockers are used for open-angle glaucoma, probably working by inhibiting aqueous humor production. However, all these drugs (and others in the class, used systemically for a host of other common medical conditions) are contraindicated for asthma patients—even if or when they are used topically on the eye(s). An important element in the pathophysiology of asthma is airway smooth-muscle hyperresponsiveness to various bronchoconstrictor stimuli, ACh clearly among them.

You may recall that the choline ester, methacholine, is used to help diagnose asthma when the diagnosis is otherwise questionable. The basis of this "methacholine challenge" centers on the concept that airway smooth muscles of people with asthma are much more sensitive (hyperreactive) to choline esters (and several other drugs) than those of people who do not have asthma. Small doses of methacholine are given, by inhalation, while pulmonary function tests are recorded. Asthmatics experience significant (sometimes damgerous) bronchoconstrictor responses to methacholine doses that are far lower than those that would provoke even slight changes in nonasthmatics.

Recall that ACh esterase inhibitors cause what amounts to a "build-up" of ACh at the neuroeffector junction. These drugs, whether used for glaucoma or such other conditions as myasthenia gravis, can have lethal effects for some asthma patients. (Note, too, that ACh esterase inhibitors are found in some insecticides, so there is a risk to the asthma patient in agricultural or gardening/lawn care activities.) Muscarinic agonists, whether those used for glaucoma or for stimulating the gut or urinary tract (e.g., bethanechol for functional urinary retention) may prove lethal too. Finally, asthmatics tend to be extremely dependent on the bronchodilator actions of circulating epinephrine. Block the β_2 receptors that mediate that effect and the outcome can be disastrous. Even the so-called "cardioselective" β blockers (atenolol, metoprolol) can cause serious problems for asthmatics. That is because their ability to block β_1 receptors is relative, not absolute: they may pose no pulmonary problems for persons without asthma, but may be deadly in those who do.

Local Control Substances: Autacoids, Drugs for Inflammatory Processes

Histamine-receptor antagonists
Serotonin agonists
Serotonin antagonists
Hyperuricemia, gout
Ergot alkaloids

Prostaglandins and related
   eicosanoids
NSAIDs (eicosanoid synthesis
   inhibitors)

Questions

DIRECTIONS: Each item contains a question or incomplete statement that is followed by possible responses. Select the **one best** response to each question.

298. Arachidonic acid is metabolized by two main pathways: cyclooxygenase and lipoxygenase. The latter, initially involving 5′-lipoxygenase (LP), is responsible for synthesizing which of the following?

a.   Leukotrienes
b.   Platelet-activating factor (PAF)
c.   Prostacyclin (PGI$_2$)
d.   Prostaglandins
e.   Thromboxanes

299. Which of the following drugs interrupts/inhibits the cyclooxygenase pathway of eicosanoid formation by nonselectively inhibiting both cyclooxygenase-1 and -2 (COX-1 and -2)?

a.   Allopurinol
b.   Aspirin
c.   Acetaminophen
d.   Misoprostol
e.   Celecoxib
f.   Zileuton

300. In terms of inflammatory responses and underlying metabolic reactions, which of the following is inhibited by pharmacologic doses of glucocorticoids?

a. Cyclooxygenases (COX-1 and -2)
b. Histidine decarboxylase
c. 5′-lipoxygenase
d. Phospholipase A_2 (PLA_2)
e. Xanthine oxidase

301. A patient has mild cutaneous and systemic manifestations of an allergic response. Before you prescribe a short course of diphenhydramine for symptom relief, you should realize that this drug has one mechanism of action resembling, causes many side effects similar to, and shares many contraindications that apply to which of the following prototypic "autonomic" drugs?

a. Atropine
b. Bethanechol
c. Norepinephrine
d. Phentolamine
e. Physostigmine
f. Propranolol

302. Bradykinin plays important roles in local responses to tissue damage and a variety of inflammatory processes. It also has vasodilator activity. Which of the following statements is correct about this endogenous peptide?

a. Captopril inhibits its metabolic inactivation
b. Drugs that are metabolized to, or generate, nitric oxide, counteract bradykinin's vascular effects
c. Increased blood pressure is the predominant cardiovascular response
d. Newer H_1 blockers (e.g., fexofenadine; "second-generation" antihistamine) also competitively block bradykinin receptors
e. The main renal responses are arteriolar constriction and reduced GFR

303. A patient with an allergic disorder experiences significant broncho-constriction and urticaria. Histamine, released from mast cells, is incriminated as an important contributor to these responses. Which of the following drugs may pose extra risks for this patient—not because it has any bron-choconstrictor effects in its own right, but because it quite effectively releases histamine from mast cells?

a. Atropine
b. Isoproterenol
c. Neostigmine
d. Pancuronium
e. Propranolol
f. *d*-tubocurarine

304. A patient presents with a history of frequent and severe migraine headaches. When we give one of the more commonly used drugs for abortive therapy, we capitalize on its ability to modify or mimic the actions of which "local control" substance?

a. Histamine
b. $PGF_{2\alpha}$
c. Prostacyclin
d. Serotonin
e. Thromboxane A_2

305. A newborn has blood gas and hemodynamic problems because of a patent (open) ductus arteriosus. Which of the following drugs would be administered in an attempt to close the ductus?

a. Cimetidine
b. Diphenhydramine
c. Indomethacin
d. Prostaglandin E_1 (PGE_1; alprostadil)
e. Zileuton

306. The second-messenger pathway that mediates the responses to H_1 histamine receptor activation involves which of the following?

a. Activation of cellular Na^+ influx
b. Activation of tyrosine kinases
c. Elevation of intracellular cyclic AMP (cAMP) levels
d. Increased formation of inositol trisphosphates (IP_3)
e. Inhibition of adenylate cyclase activity

307. A patient with severe arthritis will be placed on long-term therapy with indomethacin. All other factors being equal, which of the following drugs is the most likely choice to administer as an add-on (adjunct) to prevent gastric ulcers caused by this NSAID?

a. Celecoxib
b. Cimetidine
c. Diphenhydramine
d. Misoprostol
e. Sumatriptan

Questions 308–314

The next 7 questions apply to a patient for whom you have prescribed aspirin (acetylsalicylic acid).

308. At usual therapeutic doses (blood levels), expected effects of aspirin include which of the following?

a. Efficacy greater than acetaminophen as an anti-inflammatory agent
b. Efficacy less than acetaminophen for relieving simple headache pain
c. Inhibited growth, or killing, of bacteria that cause fever as a symptom of infection
d. Inhibition of leukotriene synthesis, protection against bronchospasm in asthmatics
e. Inhibition of uric acid synthesis

309. Aspirin's desired (and sometimes unwanted) effects on blood clotting involve which of the following?

a. Activating antithrombin III, inhibiting thrombin
b. Blocking platelet aggregation by preventing bridging between glycoprotein IIb/IIIa receptors on neighboring platelets
c. Blocking platelet receptors for ADP
d. Inhibiting hepatic vitamin K–dependent clotting factor synthesis
e. Preventing platelet aggregation by inhibiting thromboxane A_2 synthesis
f. Simulating fibrinogen synthesis, enhancing thrombolysis

310. Aspirin causes significant bronchoconstriction and bronchospasm in a patient who was subsequently described as being "aspirin-sensitive." The mechanism involves which of the following?

a. Drug-mediated hypersensitivity of H_1 receptors on airway smooth muscles
b. Drug-mediated hypersensitivity of muscarinic receptors on airway smooth muscles
c. Enhanced formation of antibodies directed against the salicylate on airway mast cells
d. Inhibited synthesis of endogenous prostaglandins that have bronchodilator activity
e. Reduced (blocked) epinephrine binding to β_2-adrenergic receptors on airway smooth-muscle cells

311. Which of the following signs or symptoms would be suggestive that serum levels of aspirin are getting too high—supratherapeutic, although not necessarily toxic? Assume the patient does not have asthma.

a. Constipation
b. Cough
c. Hypertension
d. Myopia
e. Tinnitus

312. At high (but not necessarily toxic) blood levels, another drug with which you should be familiar causes many signs and symptoms that resemble what you see with "low-grade" aspirin toxicity (salicylism). Which is it?

a. Atropine
b. Captopril
c. Diphenhydramine
d. Morphine
e. Propranolol
f. Quinine or quinidine

313. A patient takes an acute, massive overdose of aspirin that, without proper intervention, will be fatal. Which of the following would you expect in the advanced (late) stages of aspirin (salicylate) poisoning?

a. Hypothermia
b. Metabolic alkalosis
c. Respiratory alkalosis
d. Respiratory plus metabolic acidosis
e. Ventilatory stimulation

314. In addition to providing symptomatic, supportive care, which of the following would be a helpful adjunct to manage severe aspirin poisoning.

a. Acetaminophen
b. N-acetylcysteine
c. Amphetamines (e.g., dextroamphetamine)
d. Phenobarbital
e. Sodium bicarbonate

315. Which of the following is an H_2-receptor antagonist?

a. Sumatriptan
b. Cyproheptadine
c. Ondansetron
d. Cimetidine
e. Fluoxetine

Questions 316–317

A 29-year-old woman presents with frequent, debilitating migraine headaches. Sumatriptan is prescribed for abortive therapy.

316. Which of the following conditions should be ruled-out before pre-scribing the triptan for this woman?

a. Arthritis (rheumatoid, osteo-, or gouty)
b. Coronary artery disease/vasospastic angina
c. Glaucoma
d. Hearing loss
e. Hypotension

317. Not long after using the drug she is rushed to the hospital. Her vital signs are unstable, and she has muscle rigidity, myoclonus, generalized CNS irritability and altered consciousness, and shivering. You learn that for several months she had been taking another drug with which the triptan interacted. Which of the following was the most likely drug?

a. Acetaminophen
b. Codeine
c. Diazepam
d. Fluoxetine
e. Phenytoin

318. Which of the following is the primary cause of death from massive acetaminophen overdoses?

a. Acute nephropathy
b. A-V conduction disturbances, heart block
c. Liver failure
d. Status asthmaticus
e. Status epilepticus

319. The antidote that may be of great benefit in early management of acetaminophen's organ-specific toxicity is which of the following?

a. N-acetylcysteine
b. Atropine
c. Physostigmine
d. Pralidoxime
e. Warfarin

320. Which of the following is a highly selective inhibitor of cyclooxygenase 2 (COX-2)?

a. Acetaminophen
b. Aspirin
c. Celecoxib
d. Ibuprofen
e. Ketoprofen

321. How do methotrexate, gold salts, hydroxychloroquine, or penicillamine differ from "traditional" NSAIDs such as aspirin or indomethacin in the context of managing arthritic/inflammatory disease?

a. Activate the immune system/inflammatory responses
b. Are primary therapies for hyperuricemia, gout, gouty arthritis
c. Are remarkably free from serious toxicities
d. Provide much quicker relief of arthritis signs, symptoms
e. Slow, stop, possibly reverse joint pathology in rheumatoid arthritis

322. A 29-year-old woman has recently developed migraine headaches. For various reasons you cannot prescribe a triptan for abortive therapy, so you prescribe ergotamine. Which of the following is the main mechanism of action of this drug in terms of the migraine?

a. Activates serotonin receptors
b. Inhibits thromboxane synthesis/improves cerebral blood flow
c. Propranolol-like blockade of β-adrenergic receptors
d. Reduces cerebral metabolic rate (reduced oxygen demand)
e. Strong antimuscarinic activity

323. The main reason for using a "coxib" (selective COX-2 inhibitor) rather than a nonselective COX-inhibitor (aspirin, others) is that the coxibs

a. Are associated with a lower risk of gastric or duodenal ulceration
b. Cure arthritis, rather than just give symptom relief
c. Effectively inhibit uric acid synthesis
d. Have a lower risk of cardiotoxicity
e. Have significantly faster onsets of action

324. Which of the following enzymes is responsible for ultimate formation of uric acid, which contributes to hyperuricemia and the pathophysiology of chronic and acute gout?

a. 5′-Lipoxygenase
b. Cyclooxygenase 1
c. Cyclooxygenase 2
d. Phospholipase
e. Xanthine oxidase

325. A patient develops acute gout. Which of the following is an accurate description of how uric acid causes the arthritic response?

a. Activates microtubular formation in leukocytes
b. Directly activates leukotriene B_4 receptors
c. Has intrinsic tumor necrosis factor (TNF) activity
d. Mechanically damages articulating surfaces of the joints
e. Uncouples oxidative phosphorylation leading to tissue damage

326. Which of the following drugs specifically inhibits uric acid synthesis?

a. Allopurinol
b. Aspirin
c. Celecoxib
d. Corticosteroids (glucocorticoids)
e. Probenecid
f. Zileuton

327. Aspirin generally should be avoided as an anti-inflammatory or analgesic drug by patients with hyperuricemia or gout. That is because it *counteracts* the effects of one important drug the hyperuricemic patient may be taking. Identify the drug.

a. Acetaminophen
b. Allopurinol
c. Colchicine
d. Indomethacin
e. Naproxen
f. Probenecid

328. A hyperuricemic patient who is asymptomatic (no gouty arthritis or other expected signs or symptoms; merely elevated serum uric acid concentrations) is started on probenecid. In a couple of days he develops acute gout. Which of the following is the most likely explanation for this patient's symptoms?

a. Accelerated synthesis of uric acid by the probenecid
b. Co-precipitation of probenecid and urate in the joints
c. Idiosyncratic response
d. Probenecid-induced systemic acidosis, favoring uric acid crystallization
e. Reduced renal excretion of uric acid

329. A patient with hyperuricemia is placed on an "antigout" drug. Before starting the drug you measure the total uric acid (amount, not concentration) in a 24-h urine sample and then do the same several weeks after continued drug therapy at therapeutic doses. The posttreatment sample shows a significant reduction in urate content. There were no new pathologies developing during therapy, and the patient's daily purine intake did not change at all. Which of the following drugs was given?

a. Acetaminophen
b. Allopurinol
c. Colchicine
d. Indomethacin
e. Probenecid

330. A patient has acute gout. The physician initially thinks about prescribing just one or two oral doses of colchicine, 12 h apart, but then decides otherwise. The main reason for avoiding colchicine, even with a very short oral course, is the development of which of the following?

a. Bone marrow suppression
b. Bronchospasm
c. GI distress that is almost as bad as the acute gout discomfort
d. Hepatotoxicity
e. One or two oral doses seldom relieve gout pain
f. Refractoriness/tolerance with just a dose or two

Local Control Substances: Autacoids, Drugs for Inflammatory Processes

Answers

298. The answer is a. (*Craig, p 425; Hardman, pp 602–605; Katzung, pp 298–301, 581.*) The arachidonic acid (AA) "cascade" begins with AA synthesis from membrane phospholipids by phospholipase A_2. Once arachidonic acid is formed, the metabolic pathways diverge into the lipoxygenase pathway (that forms cysteinyl leukotrienes (LTs) and the cyclooxygenase pathways). One important intermediate early on in the LP pathway is LTA_4. From that we get LTB_4, which mainly regulates chemotaxis (cytokine activity) and activates phagocytosis in white blood cells. Also derived from LTB_4 are, sequentially, LTC_4, LTD_4, and LTE_4 (cysteinyl leukotrienes, historically and collectively called SRS-A, for slow-reacting substance of/in anaphylaxis), which individually and collectively cause mainly bronchoconstriction. 5'-lipoxygenase can be inhibited therapeutically by zileuton. The leukotriene receptors can be blocked by montelukast and zafirlukast. These three drugs are used prophylactically to suppress airway inflammation and bronchoconstriction in asthma.

299. The answer is b. (*Craig, p 427; Hardman, pp 620–622; Katzung, pp 299, 577–582.*) Aspirin (and indomethacin and many other NSAIDs) inhibits both COX-1 and COX-2. This differs from the "coxibs" (celecoxib, rofecoxib, a couple of others), which are relatively selective for inhibiting COX-2.

Acetaminophen has no appreciable effects on the arachidonic acid cascade, whether through inhibition of the COX or the lipoxygenase pathways. Misoprostol is a synthetic analog of PGE_1, and has no synthesis-inhibitory actions. Zileuton, as explained in Question 291, inhibits 5'-lipoxygenase but not the COXs. Allopurinol inhibits xanthine oxidase, which is not part of the arachidonic acid metabolic pathways but rather of purine metabolism and the ultimate formation of uric acid.

300. The answer is d. (*Craig, p 425; Hardman, pp 603–605, 1470–1472; Katzung, pp 577, 580, 643–646.*) Glucocorticoids ultimately inhibit phospholipase A_2 activity. In doing so, they inhibit arachidonic acid synthesis and, therefore, synthesis of all products of the cyclooxygenase and lipoxygenase pathways, because both originate with arachidonic acid. This action of glucocorticoids is indirect because their initial or direct effect is induced synthesis of annexins (previously called lipocortins); the annexins are the molecules that directly inhibit PLA_2 activity. Glucocorticoids have no intrinsic or direct inhibitory effects on later steps in AA metabolism, i.e., no effects on cyclooxygenase or lipoxygenase activity.

As noted in Questions 291 and 299, zileuton inhibits 5'-lipoxygenase. We have no clinically useful inhibitors of histamine synthesis (which involves histidine decarboxylase activity).

Cyclooxygenases are inhibited by NSAIDs such as aspirin (nonselective COX-1 and -2 inhibitors) or the "coxibs" (celecoxib, rofecoxib, a few others) that relatively selectively inhibit COX-2.

301. The answer is a. (*Craig, p 454; Hardman, p 588; Katzung, pp 266, 319–321.*) Diphenhydramine, an older or "first-generation" antihistamine, is a competitive antagonist of histamine's effects on H_1 receptors, and also strongly blocks muscarinic cholinergic receptors. Other older H_1 blockers (but none of the second-generation H_1 blockers, such as fexofenadine) possess this atropine-like effect, often to a lesser degree than diphenhydramine. (If you wished to argue that because diphenhydramine was more like scopolamine, because it causes not only anticholinergic effects but also a considerable degree of sedation, you would be correct.) Thus, common side effects related to antimuscarinic activity include sedation, dry mouth, photophobia, and cycloplegia (paralysis of accommodation). Key contraindications include prostatic hypertrophy, bowel or bladder obstruction or hypomotility, tachycardia, and narrow-angle (angle-closure) glaucoma.

To refresh your memory about the other drugs listed, bethanechol is a muscarinic agonist, norepinephrine is an effective agonist for β_1- and α-adrenergic receptors, phentolamine is a nonselective α blocker, physostigmine is an acetylcholinesterase inhibitor, and propranolol is, of course, the prototypic nonselective β-adrenergic blocker.

302. The answer is a. (*Craig, pp 212–215; Hardman, pp 590–591, 594, 743–745; Katzung, pp 177, 285–288.*) Bradykinin is metabolized to biologically inactive peptides by an enzyme that has three names: angiotensin-converting enzyme (ACE; recall that the prototype ACE inhibitor is captopril), bradykininase, and kininase II.

Bradykinin, whether injected experimentally or derived from endogenous sources (kininogens cleaved by specific proteases called kallikreins), exerts significant vasodilator effects that can lower systolic and diastolic blood pressures. Although this may not be an important pressure-regulating mechanism in normotensive individuals, it probably is in many (most?) patients with essential hypertension.

Recall that ACE inhibitors lower blood pressure in many hypertensive patients. One mechanism involves "preserving" bradykinin by inhibiting its enzymatic inactivation. Bradykinin also causes prerenal arteriolar vasodilation and increases GFR, leading to diuretic effects.

The peptide's vascular effects are mediated by endothelial cell–derived nitric oxide, and they are enhanced by other drugs that cause vasodilation by a nitric oxide–related mechanism.

Bradykinin receptor blockers prevent the peptide's vasodilator effects. However, no currently approved drugs exert that effect.

303. The answer is f. (*Craig, p 451; Hardman, p 648; Katzung, pp 260, 438.*) Tubocurarine, arguably the prototypic nondepolarizing skeletal neuromuscular blocker (competitive antagonist of the effects of ACh on skeletal muscle nicotinic receptors), differs from most of the other nondepolarizing neuromuscular blockers (including pancuronium) because it quite effectively triggers histamine release. It is a "direct" effect on mast cells, not one involving activation of antibodies on the mast cells. This effect is not clinically significant for patients who do not have asthma, but for many who do, the bronchoconstriction can be problematic (even though the patient is intubated while they are receiving the blocker). In the absence of (released) histamine, curare and the other neuromuscular blockers would have no effect on airway smooth-muscle activity.

(Note: In addition to tubocurarine, morphine and several intravascular contrast media used in diagnostic radiology—particularly some of the iodinated compounds—also have a reputation as "histamine-releasers." Some venoms and other animal toxins also cause mast cell degranulation, a component of which is histamine release.)

Atropine causes bronchodilation by blocking muscarinic receptors on airway smooth muscle cells. Isoproterenol, the β_1/β_2 agonist, is a bronchodilator. Propranolol triggers airway smooth-muscle contraction in asthmatics, but that is due to blockade of epinephrine's agonist (bronchodilator) actions on β_2 receptors. Histamine is not involved in the responses to any of these drugs.

304. The answer is d. (*Craig, pp 283–284; Hardman, pp 248, 278–281; Katzung, pp 268–272.*) Acute migraine therapy often involves giving a drug that mimics the effects of endogenous serotonin, thereby reversing the cerebrovasodilation that contributes significantly to migraine signs and symptoms. A good example is sumatriptan (member of a small group of drugs called triptans). These are 5-HT$_{1B/2D}$ receptor agonists. Histamine [and, to a lesser extent, prostacyclin (PGI$_2$)] are vasodilators, too, but they don't seem to have appreciable roles in migraine, nor are they targets of antimigraine drug activity. Activation of β_2-adrenergic receptors in the cerebral vasculature also leads to vasodilation and migraine symptoms. The β-adrenergic blockers (particularly the nonselective ones, i.e., atenolol and metoprolol, which are called "cardioselective") are useful for some migraineurs, but only for prophylaxis, not for abortive therapy.

305. The answer is c. (*Craig, p 721; Hardman, p 706; Katzung, p 585.*) The ductus arteriosus in the fetus, and sometimes in the neonate, remains patent largely because of the vasodilator effects of endogenous PGE$_1$, formed via the cyclooxygenase pathway. When the goal is to close a ductus that remains open after birth, we generally use the very efficacious prostaglandin synthesis inhibitor, indomethacin. [Conversely, there are times when surgical procedures are required on a congenitally anomalous heart in newborns, and we want to keep the ductus open until surgery. In that case, alprostadil (PGE$_1$) may be administered.] Administration of H$_1$ or H$_2$ histamine receptor blockers (diphenhydramine, cimetidine, respectively) will be of no benefit. Zileuton, as you know by now, inhibits leukotriene synthesis and so will have no impact on prostaglandin synthesis or the anomaly we wish to treat.

306. The answer is d. (*Craig, p 452; Hardman, p 647; Katzung, pp 260–261.*) Activation of H$_1$ receptors appears to be linked to phospholipase C and increased intracellular formation of inositol-1,4,5-trisphosphate (IP$_3$) and 1,2-diacylglycerol. IP$_3$ binds to an endoplasmic reticulum receptor, triggering release of Ca^{2+} into the cytosol, where it activates Ca-dependent protein kinases. Diacylglycerol activates protein kinase C. Additionally, stimulation of H_1 receptors may activate phospholipase A_2 and trigger the arachidonic acid cascade, leading to prostaglandin production.

The H_2 receptors are the ones associated with adenylate cyclase; activating them increases cytosolic cAMP levels and activates cAMP-dependent protein kinase.

307. The answer is d. (*Craig, p 481; Hardman, pp 694, 709, 1011–1012, 1018; Katzung, pp 299, 309, 1043.*) Misoprostol is a long-acting synthetic analog of PGE_1, and its only use (outside of reproductive medicine) is prophylaxis of NSAID-induced gastric ulcers. Its main effects are suppression of gastric acid secretion and enhanced gastric mucus production (a so-called mucotropic or cytoprotective effect). The need for the drug arises, of course, because such drugs as indomethacin (and most other COX-nonselective inhibitors) inhibit PGE_1 synthesis (as well as that of other prostaglandins, prostacyclin, and thromboxane A_2).

Although cimetidine might help reduce gastric acid secretion (via H_2 blockade) and diphenhydramine may too (via antimuscarinic effects), their antisecretory effects are weak and nonspecific in this situation, and they don't increase formation of the stomach's protective mucus.

Celecoxib (and other coxibs) are associated with a lower risk or incidence of peptic ulcers than more traditional NSAIDs, mainly because the former are relatively selective COX-2 inhibitors: it is the COX-1 pathway that, when inhibited, mainly allows gastric HCl secretion to rise and mucus production to fall. However, we asked about which drug would be an add-on to indomethacin therapy, and adding a COX-2 inhibitor would be of little benefit. Sumatriptan, a serotonin receptor agonist, also would be of little benefit in this situation and would not be prescribed for this purpose.

308. The answer is a. (*Craig, pp 426–429; Hardman, pp 696–701; Katzung, pp 578–581.*) Aspirin inhibits synthesis of prostaglandins that are important in the pathophysiology, signs, and symptoms of a host of inflammatory or arthritic states. It does so, of course, by inhibiting both COX-1 and -2. Acetaminophen lacks this property, and so acetaminophen is much less efficacious for managing inflammation. Aspirin and acetaminophen are equally efficacious (and, for all practical purposes, equipotent) for relieving simple headache pain for most patients. (Note, however, when pain

involves a component of inflammation, aspirin is clearly superior to acetaminophen because it suppresses both the inflammation and the pain
caused by it.)

Aspirin usually helps normalize or lower body temperature in febrile
states, but this, too, involves inhibited synthesis of prostaglandins (peripherally perhaps, leading to increased heat loss through diaphoresis, but also in
such central structures as the hypothalamus, which is a prime temperature-
regulating structure). Aspirin does not exert bacteriostatic or bactericidal
effects (at any level encountered *in vivo*), and so antibiotic effects do not contribute to its antipyretic actions.

Although aspirin is an effective cyclooxygenase inhibitor, it has no
effects on the lipoxygenase pathway that leads to leukotriene synthesis. It
does not affect uric acid synthesis (xanthine oxidase) at all.

309. The answer is e. (*Craig, pp 262–263, 427; Hardman, pp 694–695,
699, 1534; Katzung, p 601.*) Aspirin exerts its antiplatelet effects by inhibiting synthesis of one (of several) platelet aggregatory agent, TXA_2. It does
not activate antithrombin III or inhibit thrombin (heparin does that), block
glycoprotein IIb/IIIa receptors (abciximab), block ADP receptors (clopidogrel), cause thrombolysis (tPA/alteplase; streptokinase, others), or inhibit
clotting factor synthesis in the liver (warfarin).

310. The answer is d. (*Craig, pp 425–426; Hardman, pp 695, 703;
Katzung, p 581.*) Inhibited synthesis of prostaglandins that are bronchodilators (mainly PGE_2) are thought to be responsible for severe or fatal
responses to aspirin in some asthmatics. Note that aspirin inhibits the synthesis of $PGF_{2\alpha}$ and of TXA_2, both of which are bronchoconstrictors. As a
result, one would predict reduced bronchoconstriction with aspirin. However, in those patients with aspirin-sensitive asthma (indeed, in many asthmatics overall), the adverse effects arising from inhibited PGE_2 synthesis
tend to predominate, and so aspirin and other efficacious NSAIDs are generally contraindicated.

311. The answer is e. (*Craig, p 429; Hardman, pp 702–703; Katzung, pp
581–582.*) Tinnitus, along with a feeling of dizziness or lightheadedness, GI
upset (including nausea and some pain or other discomfort, and diarrhea
more so than constipation), and such visual changes as blurred or double-
vision, all or collectively are part of a low-grade aspirin "toxicity" called sal-

icylism. It is not necessarily worrisome (to the physician, provided he/she prescribed the drug and the patient is compliant with dosing), dangerous, or indicative of imminent and severe toxicity. Indeed, some patients experience one or more signs or symptoms of salicylism in response to high (antiarthritic) doses of aspirin.

312. The answer is f. (*Craig, pp 172, 429; Hardman, pp 702, 966, 1088–1089; Katzung, pp 227, 581–582.*) Many of the signs and symptoms of salicylism are similar to those caused by high blood levels of quinine (antimalarial) or quinidine (antiarrhythmic, mainly). These drugs are called cinchona alkaloids, and the syndrome is called cinchonism. Aspirin and the cinchona alkaloids are chemically similar in some important ways. [It is up to you to decide whether this question is important, just interesting (or not), or outright trivial.]

313. The answer is d. (*Craig, p 429; Hardman, pp 702–703; Katzung, pp 581–582, 991.*) Late, severe aspirin poisoning is characterized by a combination of respiratory and metabolic acidosis. In early stages of aspirin poisoning (or even with high "therapeutic" doses of the drug), ventilatory stimulation occurs. That induces a respiratory alkalosis (net CO_2 loss, relative HCO_3 retention). The kidneys compensate for this by increasing HCO_3 excretion to help normalize blood pH. As serum levels of aspirin rise, however, blood pH falls precipitously. Part of that is due to the accumulation of acidic salicylic acid in the blood, and part is due to inhibited oxidative phosphorylation that shifts metabolism from oxidative to glycolytic (with lactic acid being the key end product). No longer synthesizing ATP effectively, the mitochondria generate metabolic heat, which contributes to fever (not hypothermia!). Ventilatory failure ensues, adding respiratory acidosis (from CO_2 retention) to the metabolic acidosis. Cardiovascular collapse and seizures eventually cause death. Note that hepatotoxicity is not a component of this: that is the main cause of morbidity and mortality with acetaminophen poisoning.

314. The answer is e. (*Hardman, pp 702–703; Katzung, pp 581–582, 991.*) Adjunctive use of sodium bicarbonate (IV) can be an important adjunct to managing severe salicylate poisoning for two main reasons: (1) it helps raise blood pH, which as stated earlier is profoundly reduced from metabolic plus respiratory acidosis; (2) it alkalinizes the urine, which (via a pH-dependent mechanism) converts more aspirin molecules into the ionized form in the tubules, thereby reducing tubular reabsorption of a toxin we want to eliminate from the body as quickly as possible.

Acetaminophen, even though it is usually an effective antipyretic, is not ideal in managing fever of severe aspirin poisoning. It would add yet another drug that might complicate the clinical picture, and ordinary (ordinarily safe) doses aren't likely to do much to lower temperature quickly or sufficiently. (Thus, we use physical means to lower body temperature.) N-acetylcysteine, the antidote for acetaminophen poisoning, does nothing for salicylate poisoning. Amphetamines might seem rational for managing ventilatory depression that characterizes late stages of severe aspirin poisoning. The more likely outcome is simply to hasten the onset of seizures. Phenobarbital, or other CNS depressants, would aggravate an already bad state of CNS/ventilatory depression. (However, if seizures develop they must be managed—e.g., with IV lorazepam and phenytoin, even though they cause CNS depression. Without them, the patient may quickly die from status epilepticus.)

315. The answer is d. (*Craig, pp 455, 479; Hardman, pp 1009–1011; Katzung, pp 268, 1035–1038.*) Cimetidine is an H_2 antagonist that decreases gastric acid secretion. Sumatriptan is a $5\text{-}HT_{1D}$ serotonin agonist. Cyproheptadine is a histamine and serotonin antagonist. Ondansetron is a serotonin antagonist. Fluoxetine is an antidepressant agent that selectively inhibits serotonin reuptake (SSRI).

316. The answer is b. (*Hardman, p 281; Katzung, pp 272, 276–278.*) Triptans can cause significant coronary vasoconstriction, particularly if administered to patients with variant (vasospastic or Prinzmetal's) angina. However, any coronary artery disease or other conditions that put the patient at extra risk of myocardial ischemia will also weigh strongly against using a triptan.

317. The answer is d. (*Hardman, p 468; Katzung, pp 271, 483, 492–494, 991.*) This patient has what is almost certainly the serotonin syndrome. The triptan "adds" serotonin to the circulation, and its neuronal reuptake will be blocked by fluoxetine (or sertraline, others), which is classified as a selective serotonin reuptake inhibitor (SSRI) antidepressant. When sumatriptan (or other triptans used for migraine) is added, rapid accumulation of serotonin and/or the triptan in the brain can occur. The other drugs listed are not likely to interact—at least not in the way described here.

318. The answer is c. *(Craig, pp 66, 314; Hardman, pp 704–705; Katzung, pp 595–596.)* The primary cause of death from acetaminophen overdoses is hepatic necrosis. One of the drug's main (and most toxic) metabolite binds to sulfhydryl groups that are constituents of key macromolecules in the liver. If acetaminophen doses are low, glutathione conjugates the metabolite. With toxic doses, however, glutathione is depleted and other –SH groups on hepatocyte proteins are attacked and irreversibly altered. Concomitant with overall hepatic damage we find, eventually, profound hypoglycemia (as the liver's stores of glycogen are depleted) and coagulopathies (as hepatic clotting factor synthesis stops and the patient begins bleeding spontaneously).

319. The answer is a. *(Craig, pp 66, 314; Hardman, pp 704–705; Katzung, pp 595–596, 988–999.)* N-acetylcysteine is a –SH-rich drug. It provides the extra –SH groups that acetaminophen's toxic metabolite can react with instead of attacking sulfhydryl groups on/in hepatocyte proteins. To be effective, acetylcysteine must be given early on (it prevents or delays, but does not reverse acetaminophen-induced hepatotoxicity) and in repeated doses.

Atropine is an antidote for muscarinic agonist poisoning and plays an adjunctive role in managing muscarinic responses in acetylcholinesterase (AChE) poisoning. Pralidoxime (2-PAM), a cholinesterase reactivator, may be a life-saving adjunct for poisoning with "irreversible" AChE inhibitors (e.g., organophosphate insecticides, nerve gases such as soman and sarin). Physostigmine (an AChE inhibitor) is used to manage severe poisoning with atropine or other drugs with appreciable antimuscarinic actions (e.g., diphenhydramine, tricyclic antidepressants, phenothiazine antipsychotics). Warfarin will be of no benefit in protecting the liver or reversing its damage.

320. The answer is c. *(Craig, p 431; Katzung, pp 582–584.)* Celecoxib is the selective COX-2 inhibitor. Acetaminophen has no effect on cyclooxygenases and negligible (and not clinically useful) anti-inflammatory activity. All the others (and many more, not named) are classified as nonselective (COX-1 and -2) inhibitor NSAIDs.

321. The answer is e. (*Craig, pp 432–437; Hardman, pp 716–718; Katzung, pp 588–594.*) Methotrexate, gold salts, and penicillamine are members of a diverse group of drugs called DMARDs (disease-modifying antirheumatic drugs) or SAARDs (slow-acting antirheumatic drugs). The former term derives from the ability of these drugs to slow, stop, or in some cases reverse joint damage associated with rheumatoid arthritis (RA). They do more than merely mask or relieve RA symptoms, which is mainly what the traditional NSAIDs do. The second acronym derives from the fact that it may take a month (or a couple more) for meaningful symptom relief to develop; they are not at all quick-acting drugs. Their actions probably are due to suppression of immune responses that often contribute to the etiology of RA.

Their toxicities can be serious, which is one reason why, until not long ago, these agents were considered third-line or even last resort treatment for refractory disease. (Methotrexate is now being used much earlier, and safely, for RA, now that we know better how to use it and monitor for serious toxicities; see the chapter, "Cancer Chemotherapy and Immunosuppressants.") Most of these drugs can cause serious blood dyscrasias; in addition, penicillamine can cause renal and pulmonary toxicity; hydroxychloroquine is associated with vision impairments/retinopathy.

322. The answer is a. (*Hardman, pp 248, 283–284; Katzung, pp 273–278.*) Ergotamine has several pharmacologic properties. The one that seems to be responsible for its efficacy in migraines is activation (as a typical agonist) of serotonin receptors ($5\text{-}HT_{D1}$) in the cerebral vasculature, thus causing a triptan-like effect (but the drug should not be used *with* a triptan). The drug works best in prodromal phases (classical signs and symptoms the migraineur should learn to recognize before a full-blown migraine attack develops). It's less effective once the full onslaught of migraine has developed. It lacks intrinsic sedative or analgesic activity.

In addition to the effects just mentioned, toxic doses of ergotamine cause peripheral vasoconstriction intense enough to cause hypertension and tissue ischemia (including gangrene of such structures as the fingers and toes). The syndrome of poisoning is called ergotism.

The ergot alkaloids, as a group, also cause intense, prolonged uterine-contracting effects. This contraindicates their use during pregnancy, but explains the use of the related drugs ergonovine and methylergonovine postpartum to control uterine bleeding (bleeding is reduced by the strong uterine contractions).

323. The answer is a. (*Craig, p 431; Katzung, pp 582–584.*) Celecoxib and related drugs, by virtue of their selective COX-2 inhibition, do not interfere as much with synthesis of PGE_2, which normally suppresses a component of gastric acid secretion and mucus production. Overall, then, the risks of gastric and duodenal ulcers are reduced. The selectivity also means that the COX-2 inhibitors do not interfere with the production of other eicosaniods, such as TXA_2. That is both good and bad, clinically. On the good side, this means that COX-2 inhibitors don't cause antiplatelet effects and increase the risk of excessive or spontaneous bleeding. On the other hand, this lack of effect renders them unsuitable for causing antiplatelet-aggregatory effects, as might be wanted when we administer aspirin.

COX-2 inhibitors, like the nonselective alternatives, aren't cures for arthritis; they just alleviate symptoms. Compared with (and like) aspirin and other older NSAIDs, they have no effect on uric acid metabolism or excretion and cause no cardiotoxicity, and their onsets of action are, overall, no faster.

324. The answer is e. (*Craig, pp 445–446; Hardman, p 721; Katzung, p 599.*) Xanthine oxidase catalyzes the last two steps in (human) purine degradation: the conversion of hypoxanthine to xanthine and the conversion of xanthine to uric acid. This pathway is not part of the arachidonic acid-cyclooxygenase-lipoxygenase pathways.

325. The answer is d. (*Craig, p 442; Hardman, p 719.*) The clinical problems that arise with uric acid relate to its poor solubility in body fluids—solubility that gets less as local pH falls. When a part of the body (e.g., a joint in the great toe, which is a common site of a gout attack) is damaged or otherwise insulted, uric acid crystals concentrate and precipitate in the area. These crystals cause mechanical damage to the joint surfaces and also evoke a typical inflammatory response. Leukocytes are attracted to the area, and in an attempt to phagocytize the crystals release acidic metabolites that lower local pH, favoring precipitation of even more uric acid and amplifying the entire unwanted series of pathologic reactions.

326. The answer is a. (*Craig, pp 445–446; Hardman, p 721; Katzung, pp 598–599.*) Allopurinol (through its active metabolite, oxypurinol, which is a xanthine oxidase substrate) inhibits xanthine oxidase and so blocks synthesis of xanthine and its metabolite, uric acid. Purine degradation stops at the production of hypoxanthine, which is more soluble in body fluids than the two subsequent products of xanthine oxidase activity, xanthine, and uric acid.

Allopurinol has no effect on other inflammatory pathways or arthritides other than those related to hyperuricemia, nor does it directly affect renal function to enhance or inhibit urate excretion.

327. The answer is f. (*Craig, p 445; Hardman, pp 699, 725–726; Katzung, pp 597–598.*) Probenecid (and the related drug, sulfinpyrazone) are classified as uricosurics: at sufficiently high (therapeutic) doses they enhance the renal elimination of uric acid by inhibiting tubular reabsorption of filtered urate. Aspirin significantly impairs the uricosurics' actions.

Important note: Aspirin (given alone) has blood level–dependent effects on urate elimination by the kidneys. At "low doses" perhaps up to about 1 gram/day, it selectively inhibits tubular secretion of urate and so elevates serum urate levels. At doses much higher than that (including doses sometimes prescribed for arthritis other than gout), the predominant effect (and the net, or overall, effect) is uricosuria due to blockade of tubular reabsorption of urate (this effect is greater than the drug's inhibitory effect on tubular secretion of urate). Nonetheless, aspirin is not used as a uricosuric drug because the doses/serum levels needed to cause that are sufficiently high to cause significant side effects (e.g., salicylism; see Question 312) that don't arise with the traditional uriciosurics such as probenecid.

328. The answer is e. (*Craig, pp 444–445; Hardman, p 723; Katzung, pp 597–598.*) It has been said that the initial phase of uricosuric therapy is the most worrisome period. Probenecid is a uricosuric drug, but that effect depends on having high (therapeutic) blood levels that are sufficient to inhibit active *tubular reabsorption* of urate. At subtherapeutic blood levels the main effect is inhibition of *tubular secretion* of urate, which reduces net urate excretion and raises serum urate levels (sometimes to the point of causing clinical gout). It is only once drug levels are therapeutic that the desired effects to inhibit tubular reabsorption of urate predominate. Thus, and intuitively, once a patient starts probenecid therapy drug levels must pass through that stage in which urate excretion will actually go down.

Some texts suggest using a short course of colchicine or another (nonaspirin) NSAID that is indicated for gout when probenecid therapy is started. That is for prophylaxis of acute gout that might occur. Although that may be acceptable, other rules are perhaps more important: (1) do not administer a uricosuric during a gout attack; (2) if the patient has had a gout attack recently, suppress the inflammation for 2 to 3 months with a suitable anti-inflammatory and consider starting a uricosuric only after that 2- to 3-month symptom-free interval; and (3) do not use uricosurics for patients with "severe hyperuricemia" and/or poor renal function. Doing otherwise is associated with a great risk of potentially severe renal tubular damage as the uricosuric shifts large amounts of uric acid from the blood (with its large volume, that keeps urate relatively "dilute") into a small volume of acidic urine, which concentrates urate and lowers its solubility via pH-dependent mechanisms.

(The patient who skips doses of probenecid also becomes very vulnerable to the "paradoxical" extra risk, because doing this may allow drug levels to fall into that subtherapeutic range in which more urate is retained than eliminated.)

329. The answer is b. (*Craig, pp 445–446; Hardman, pp 721–722; Katzung, pp 598–599.*) You may think that reductions in urate content in a 24-h urine sample would be bad for the hyperuricemic patient, but that is because you probably automatically (and incorrectly) equate less urine urate with increased serum urate. Not necessarily so. Allopurinol inhibits uric acid synthesis: less uric acid made, less to be excreted in the urine, and less to be detected there. This is one manifestation of allopurinol "at work."

330. The answer is c. (*Craig, pp 443–444; Hardman, p 720; Katzung, pp 596–597.*) The main reason why many physicians are shunning oral colchicine for acute gout is that many patients develop horrible GI discomfort, vomiting, diarrhea, and the like. For some, the "cure" is almost as bad as the disorder for which the drug is given. This GI distress can be alleviated somewhat by giving colchicine IV, but more serious systemic responses can develop if the IV dose is too great or too many IV doses are given in a short period of time. Indomethacin seems to have become one of the preferred alternatives for anti-inflammatory therapy of acute gout or prophylaxis of recurrences. (And clearly indomethacin is not without side effects or toxicities; the risks are simply more acceptable, for some patients, with it.)

But when colchicine does work in acute gout, relief may be dramatic and occur literally "overnight" with just a dose or two. The likely mechanism of action involves impaired microtubular assembly or function in leukocytes, which limits their migration to the area of crystal deposition and so limits their ability to amplify the inflammatory reaction.

Bone marrow suppression can occur, but that is mainly with long-term, high-dose oral or parenteral colchicine administration (the latter of which must be avoided). The same applies to frank gastric damage (with the possibility of gastric bleeding or hemorrhage) and to blood dyscrasias (bone marrow toxicity).

Gastrointestinal System and Nutrition (Vitamins)

Acid secretion inhibitors
  (H$_2$ blockers, proton pump
  inhibitors, others)
Antacids
Antidiarrheals
Emetics, antiemetics
Gallstone-dissolving drugs

Inflammatory bowel disease drugs
Laxatives, cathartics
Mucosal protective drugs
Pancreatic enzyme replacement
Prokinetic agents
Vitamins

Questions

DIRECTIONS: Each item contains a question or incomplete statement that is followed by possible responses. Select the **one best** response to each question.

331. The most complete (greatest) suppression of gastric acid suppression, whether baseline or stimulated (e.g., by meals, gastrin) is afforded by therapeutic doses of:

a. Atropine
b. Bismuth subsalicylate
c. Calcium salts
d. Cimetidine
e. Misoprostol
f. Omeprazole (or esomeprazole)

332. On your first day on a general medicine clerkship you encounter a patient who is taking a proton pump inhibitor, bismuth, metronidazole, and tetracycline. The most likely purpose for this drug combination is to treat or manage which of the following?

a. Antibiotic-associated pseudomembranous colitis
b. Irritable bowel syndrome (IBS)
c. Refractory or recurrent, and severe, gastric or duodenal ulcers
d. "Traveler's diarrhea," severe, *Escherichia coli*–induced, from drinking contaminated water
e. Ulcers that occur in response to long-term, high-dose NSAID therapy for arthritis

333. In the context of gastrointestinal disorders, misoprostol is specifically indicated for which of the following?

a. Routine management of gastroesophageal reflux disease (GERD)
b. Prophylaxis of ulcers during long-term therapy with some nonsteroidal anti-inflammatory drugs
c. Eradicating *Heliobacter pylori* in patients with acute duodenal ulcers
d. Prevention of acute stress ulcers (e.g., in the postoperative setting)
e. Managing ulcers that tend to develop during pregnancy

334. We prescribe bismuth subsalicylate for a patient with a disorder affecting the GI tract. This drug:

a. Powerfully inhibits the parietal cell "proton pump"
b. Is a rational, safe, and effective drug to give to children suffering GI upset that accompanies influenza
c. Is a powerful histamine (H_2) receptor blocker
d. Tends to cause a host of side effects due to its strong antimuscarinic activity
e. Exerts antibiotic activity against *H. pylori*
f. Tends to cause diarrhea

335. A patient with multiple medical problems is taking several drugs, including theophylline, warfarin, quinidine, and phenytoin. Despite the likelihood of interactions, dosages of each are adjusted carefully so their serum concentrations and effects are acceptable. However, the patient suffers some GI distress and purchases and begins consuming an over-the-counter "heartburn" remedy. He presents with excessive or toxic effects from all his other medications. He almost certainly took which OTC drug?

a. Cimetidine
b. Famotidine
c. Nizatidine
d. Omeprazole
e. Ranitidine

336. A patient with renal failure is undergoing periodic hemodialysis while awaiting a transplant. Between dialysis sessions we want to reduce the body's phosphate load by reducing dietary phosphate absorption and removing some phosphate already in the blood. Which would we administer (orally)?

a. Aluminum hydroxide
b. Magnesium hydroxide/oxide
c. Omeprazole (or another drug in its class)
d. Sodium bicarbonate
e. Sucralfate

337. We have two patients. One requires suppression of emesis caused by an anticancer drug that causes a high incidence and severity of vomiting (highly emetogenic drug). Another patient has severe diabetic gastroparesis and gastroesophageal reflux, which requires relief. Which one drug would be suitable for both indications (assuming no specific contraindications)?

a. Diphenoxylate
b. Dronabinol
c. Loperamide
d. Metoclopramide
e. Ondansetron

338. A patient is being treated with sulfasalazine. The most likely purpose for giving it is for which of the following?

a. Antibiotic-associated pseudomembranous colitis
b. *E. coli*–induced diarrhea
c. Gastric *H. pylori* infections
d. Inflammatory bowel disease
e. NSAID-induced gastric ulcer prophylaxis

339. A woman has severe, irritable bowel syndrome characterized by frequent, profuse, and symptomatic diarrhea. She has not responded to first-line therapies and is started on alosetron. The most worrisome adverse effect of this drug is which of the following?

a. Cardiac arrhythmias (serious, e.g., ventricular fibrillation)
b. Constipation, bowel impaction, ischemic colitis
c. Parkinsonian extrapyramidal reactions
d. Pulmonary fibrosis
e. Renal failure

340. A patient has steatorrhea due to pancreatic insufficiency secondary to cystic fibrosis. The most reasonable and usually effective drug for managing the symptoms and consequences is which of the following?

a. Atorvastatin (statin-type cholesterol-lowering drug)
b. Cimetidine (or an alternative, e.g., famotidine)
c. Bile salts
d. Metoclopramide
e. Pancrelipase

341. Bismuth salts are thought to be effective adjuncts in managing, if not healing, refractory or recurrent gastric ulcers because they have bactericidal properties against:

a. *Bacteriodes fragilis*
b. *Clostridium difficile*
c. *E. coli*
d. *H. pylori*
e. *Staph. aureus*

342. A patient presents with severe abdominal pain and a "burning" sensation. Endoscopy reveals several benign ulcers in the antral mucosa of the stomach. When therapy is started, which will provide the fastest—albeit probably the briefest—relief of the discomfort with just a single dose?

a. Antacids
b. Cimetidine or another H_2 blocker
c. Misoprostol
d. Omeprazole
e. Propantheline

343. A patient is receiving chenodeoxycholic acid (chenodiol). The most likely reason for administering this drug is to:

a. Dissolve cholesterol stones in the bile ducts
b. Enhance intestinal digestion and absorption of dietary fats
c. Help treat dietary deficiencies of fat-soluble vitamins
d. Lower gastric pH in patients with achlorhydria
e. Suppress steatorrhea and its consequences

344. Which would we administer for adjunctive management of a patient with hepatic portal-systemic encephalopathy?

a. Diphenoxylate
b. Lactulose
c. Loperamide
d. Omeprazole
e. Ondansetron

345. A patient has multiple gastric ulcers but has done nothing about them. Shortly after consuming a large meal and large amounts of alcohol, he experiences significant GI distress. He takes an over-the-counter heartburn remedy. Within a minute or two he develops what he will later describe as a "bad bloated feeling." Several of the ulcers have begun to bleed and he experiences searing pain.

The patient becomes profoundly hypotensive from upper GI blood loss and is transported to the hospital. Endoscopy confirms multiple bleeds; the endoscopist remarks that it appears as if the lesions had been literally stretched apart, causing additional tissue damage that led to the hemorrhage. The drug or product the patient most likely took was:

a. An aluminum salt
b. An aluminum-magnesium combination antacid product
c. Magnesium hydroxide
d. Ranitidine
e. Sodium bicarbonate

346. The two most common ingredients in over-the-counter antacid combination products are a magnesium salt and an aluminum salt. The rationale for this particular combination is that:

a. Al salts counteract the gastric mucosal-irritating effects of Mg salts
b. Al salts require activation by an Mg-dependent enzyme
c. Mg salts cause a diuresis that helps reduce systemic accumulation of the Al salt by increasing renal Al excretion
d. Mg salts potentiate the ability of Al salts to inhibit gastric acid secretion
e. Mg salts tend to cause a laxative effect (increased motility) that counteracts the tendency of an Al salt to cause constipation

347. An opioid abuser, seeking something to self-administer for subjective responses, gets a large amount of diphenoxylate and consumes it all at once. He is not likely to do this again because he has consumed a combination product that contains not only the opioid but also another drug that causes a host of unpleasant systemic responses. That other ingredient is:

a. Apomorphine
b. Atropine
c. Ipecac
d. Magnesium sulfate
e. Naltrexone

348. Over-the-counter medications containing bismuth are quite popular for managing diarrhea and several other common GI maladies. However, the bismuth salt they contain is the (sub)salicylate. Given the presence of salicylate, these should not be administered to children:

a. Under 14 years old
b. With diarrhea lasting more than 18 h
c. With flatus
d. With flu, common cold, chickenpox
e. With otitis media

349. Which vitamin or nutrient, also an ingredient in some prescription medications for severe, refractory acne vulgaris, is "highly" teratogenic and should not be administered to pregnant women?

a. A
b. B_{12}
c. C
d. E
e. Folic acid

350. Fat-soluble vitamins, compared with their water-soluble counterparts, generally have a greater potential toxicity. They are:

a. Administered in larger doses
b. Avidly stored by the body
c. Capable of dissolving membrane phospholipids
d. Involved in more essential metabolic pathways
e. Metabolized much more slowly

351. Which is *not* a fat-soluble vitamin?

a. Vitamin A
b. Vitamin C
c. Vitamin D
d. Vitamin E
e. Vitamin K

352. A patient with tuberculosis is being treated with isoniazid. She develops paresthesias, muscle aches, and unsteadiness. Which vitamin needs to be given in supplemental doses in order to reverse these symptoms—or used from the outset to prevent them in high-risk patients?

a. Vitamin A
b. Vitamin B_1 (thiamine)
c. Vitamin B_6 (pyridoxine)
d. Vitamin C
e. Vitamin K

353. A patient presents with malaise, and skin and mucous membranes appear pale. Among the key findings from blood work are hypochromic, microcytic red cells and reduced red cell count; reduced hematocrit; reduced reticulocyte count; and reduced total hemoglobin content. Assuming the most likely diagnosis is correct, the proper approach would be to administer supplemental:

a. Cyanocobalamin (B_{12})
b. Folic acid
c. Iron
d. Vitamin C
e. Vitamin D

354. The patient should be told to avoid taking supplemental vitamin B_6 (pyridoxine) if he/she is being treated with which of the following?

a. Digoxin for heart failure
b. Haloperidol for Tourette's syndrome
c. Levodopa/carbidopa for Parkinson's disease
d. Niacin for hypertriglyceridemia
e. Phenytoin for epilepsy

355. You have a patient who has been consuming extraordinarily large amounts of alcohol for several years. He goes into acute withdrawal and manifests nystagmus and bizarre ocular movements and confusion (Wernicke's encephalopathy). Although this patient's alcohol consumption pattern has been accompanied by poor nutrient intake overall, you specifically manage the encephalopathy by administering which of the following?

a. α-tocopherol (vitamin E)
b. Cyanocobalamin (vitamin B_{12})
c. Folic acid
d. Phytonadione (vitamin K)
e. Thiamine (vitamin B_1)

Gastrointestinal System and Nutrition (Vitamins)

Answers

331. The answer is f. (*Craig, pp 477–480; Hardman, pp 1006–1007; Katzung, pp 1035–1038.*) Omeprazole (actually a prodrug that requires metabolic activation) and related drugs (esomeprazole, lansoprazole, rabeprazole, pantoprazole) inhibit the parietal cell $H^+,K^+ATPase$—the "proton pump"—that is the "final common pathway" for acid secretion triggered by all the major stimuli of gastric acid secretion.

Recall that the main agonists that provoke acid secretion include gastrin; histamine [arises from enterochromaffin-like (ECL) cells], which activates H_2 receptors that can be blocked by cimetidine and famotidine (and ranitidine and nizatidine); and ACh, which activates muscarinic receptors on both ECL cells and parietal cells and which can be blocked by atropine, propantheline, pirenzipine, and other drugs with antimuscarinic activity.

Misoprostol is unique in several ways. One way is that this prostaglandin analog mimics the effects of endogenous prostaglandins (mainly PGE_2) on parietal cell PG receptors. Unlike the agonists noted above, one result of activating parietal cell PG receptors is *inhibition* of acid secretion. Overall, the anti-acid-secretory effects are relatively weak. (It inhibits a G protein/adenylate cyclase–mediated pathway that is activated when histamine causes acid secretion.)

Ultimately, however, regardless of whether gastrin, ACh, or histamine is present, parietal cell acid secretion ultimately "funnels through" the proton pump. Block the receptors for any of the mediators noted above and you will suppress acid secretion caused only by that mediator—but that is only a fraction of total acid secretion. Block the proton pump and acid secretion will be inhibited nearly fully, no matter which one or more agonists are present.

332. The answer is c. (*Craig, pp 473, 483; Hardman, pp 1016–1018; Katzung, pp 1035–1038.*) Several professional organizations, including the

American College of Gastroenterology, have guidelines for managing severe, refractory, or recurrent duodenal and/or gastric ulcers, for which *H. pylori* clearly plays an important pathophysiologic role. Although several regimens have been suggested, all of them include an anti-acid-secretory drug (usually a proton pump inhibitor, sometimes an H_2 blocker), two or three antibiotics (e.g., amoxicillin, clarithromycin, or tetracycline, usually with metronidazole), and bismuth. In many cases, this so-called eradicative therapy can cause a clinical cure and prevent recurrences after about 8 weeks of treatment. (The treatment is expensive, but pales in comparison with the cost of treating recurrent episodes or potentially serious complications such as GI bleeding or hemorrhage, either pharmacologically or surgically.)

333. The answer is b. (*Craig, p 481; Hardman, pp 1011–1012; Katzung, p 1043.*) Misoprostol is sometimes used as an adjunct to prevent ulcers in the GI tract caused by NSAIDs used for managing such chronic inflammatory disorders as rheumatoid arthritis. [The NSAIDs to which we are specifically referring includes the nonselective COX-1 and -2 inhibitors—i.e., all but the "coxibs" (celecoxib, others) that are selective COX-2 inhibitors.] Misoprostol is not at all used for "routine" management of acid-peptic disorders such as gastric or duodenal ulcers or gastroesophageal reflux disease (GERD).

The NSAIDs can cause mucosal damage by inhibiting prostaglandin synthesis, one consequence of which is reduced formation of mucus that protects the mucosal cells. Misoprostol, a prostaglandin-like agonist, stimulates mucus formation (mucotropic effect), has some weak acid-antisecretory activity, stimulates HCO_3 secretion, and may protect mucosal cells in other ways (cytoprotective effect).

Just as it is important to know this use, it's equally important to know that pregnancy contraindicates using misoprostol for its GI actions. The drug's prostaglandin-like properties can trigger uterine contractions (oxytocic effect) that may lead to premature labor or abortion.

Note that misoprostol is sometimes used in conjunction with either mifepristone (RU 486) or methotrexate as alternatives to surgical termination of early pregnancy. The prostaglandins related to misoprostol, carboprost tromethamine and dinoprostone, are sometimes used instead of the misoprostol for pharmacologic induction of abortion (mainly in the second trimester).

334. The answer is e. (*Craig, pp 473, 483; Hardman, pp 1014, 1018; Katzung, p 1044.*) Bismuth salts such as the subsalicylate (best known, perhaps, as the brand-name product Pepto-Bismol®) exert antibiotic activity against *H. pylori*. However, for the eradicative treatment of this organism—a common cause of severe or refractory PUD—it is usually part of a multidrug regimen that includes an antibiotic and metronidazole.

Bismuth salts lack significant effects on acid secretion (whether triggered by histamine, ACh, gastrin, etc.), and clearly have no "powerful" inhibitory effect on the proton pump.

The salicylate in this particular formulation contraindicates its use in children with influenza or any other viral illness, owing to the risk of Reye's syndrome. The salicylate component also poses risks in other situations for which a salicylate should be avoided. Aspirin-sensitive asthma is a prime example. Other bismuth "subsalts" besides the salicylate are available.

The drug has no H_2-blocking or muscarinic receptor–blocking activity. In the absence of any contraindications, bismuth subsalicylate may be useful for managing some cases of diarrhea, such as "traveler's diarrhea" that often is caused by *E. coli*.

335. The answer is a. (*Craig, p 479; Hardman, pp 55, 1010–1011; Katzung, pp 1086–1087, 1128–1129, 1119.*) Cimetidine differs (significantly) from the other H_2 blockers, famotidine, nizatidine, and ranitidine, in that it is a very effective inhibitor of the hepatic mixed function oxidase (P450) drug-metabolizing enzyme systems. The alternatives have no significant P450-inhibiting activity, nor do they cause side effects as frequent or as problematic as those caused by cimetidine, especially at high doses. The outcome of P450 inhibition, of course, is reduced hepatic clearance of the interactants, leading to excessive serum concentrations and effects if their dosages are not reduced properly. The examples cited in the question—phenytoin, warfarin, quinidine, and theophylline—are among the most important interactants with cimetidine. They, and other interactants such as lidocaine, have rather low margins of safety, so even slight increases in serum levels may be enough to cause toxicity. Given the fact that the alternative H_2 blockers don't inhibit the P450 system, there's no rational reason or excuse for prescribing cimetidine to patients on multiple drug therapy (and in this case, the patient should have been warned about self-medicating with it).

Omeprazole and the related proton pump inhibitors participate in no clinically significant interactions with the drugs noted here, or others.

336. The answer is a. *(Hardman, pp 1012–1013, 1721; Katzung, pp 1035.)* Aluminum hydroxide has a high affinity for phosphate. In the gut it binds phosphate and prevents its absorption quite well. It also induces a blood-to-gut gradient that favors elimination of circulating phosphate. (Used inappropriately, it may cause hypophosphatemia: sustained, high-dose use of aluminum-containing antacids is one of the most common causes of hypophosphatemia.) None of the other drugs listed are effective in or used for reducing phosphate absorption or lowering serum levels.

The main limitation to using an aluminum salt by itself is its tendency to cause constipation. This is usually dealt with, when aluminum salts are used as typical "antacids," by coadministering a magnesium salt, which alone tends to cause laxation. (Giving Mg would be inadvisable for patients with renal failure, who are often unable to excrete Mg at rates sufficient to avoid hypermagnesemia.)

337. The answer is d. *(Craig, pp 472, 477; Hardman, pp 1026, 1032; Katzung, pp 1044–1046.)* Metoclopramide has clinically useful antiemetic and prokinetic actions and would be suitable for either of the patients described in the question. The antiemetic effect arises from blockade of dopamine (and, probably, serotonin) receptors in the brain's chemoreceptor trigger zone (CTZ). The drug is indicated for not only chemotherapy-induced nausea and vomiting, but also that which may occur with radiation therapy, postoperatively, or in response to opioid analgesics or emetogenic toxins.

The enhanced gastric and upper intestinal motility probably reflects an enhancement of the expected effects of ACh on muscarinic receptors found on longitudinal smooth muscle in the GI tract. Metoclopramide raises the lower esophageal sphincter tone and relaxes the pyloric sphincter, which hastens gastric emptying. This helps explain its beneficial effects in both gastroparesis and GERD.

Diphenoxylate is an oral opioid indicated only for managing diarrhea. Typical antidiarrheal doses inhibit bowel motility well but cause no central opioid-like effects (ventilatory depression, analgesia, euphoria, etc.). Loperamide, a meperidine analog, also lacks opioid- or meperidine-like systemic or central effects at usual doses. It probably works not only by suppressing bowel motility, but also fluid secretion into the intestines. Dronabinol is a cannabiniod, and the principal psychoactive chemical in marijuana. It is used to suppress chemotherapy-induced nausea and vomiting. The drug has no role in managing gastroparesis or GERD. Ondansetron, also used exclusively to manage emetogenic drug-induced symptoms, is a serotonin receptor (5-HT$_3$) blocker that acts mainly in the CTZ and on vagal efferents to parts of the upper GI tract.

338. The answer is d. (*Craig, pp 480–481; Hardman, pp 1174–1175; Katzung, pp 1053–1055.*) Sulfasalazine, which is a combination of sulfapryidine and 5-aminosalicylic acid (5-ASA) linked covalently (azo bond), is quite effective for managing inflammatory bowel disease (e.g., ulcerative colitis and Crohn's disease). Some of the sulfasalazine is absorbed, and a portion of that is excreted unchanged back into the colon. Colonic bacteria split the azo linkage, releasing the two drugs. The 5-ASA is responsible for local anti-inflammatory activity (suppression of inflammatory mediators, but how, which, is not well understood) and symptom relief. The other metabolite, sulfapyridine, is primarily responsible for side effects associated with this "two drugs in one" combination: nausea, vomiting, and headaches (dose-dependent); sulfonamide allergic reactions in "sulfa-sensitive" patients; and rare but potentially fatal blood reactions including immune-mediated hemolysis and aplastic anemia.

A related drug, mesalamine, contains only the active 5-ASA. Lacking any sulfapyridine, the side effects and adverse responses are very low compared with sulfasalazine. An even neater strategy is used by olsalazine: the drug is comprised of two azo-linked 5-ASA molecules; the bond is cleaved by gut bacteria, releasing two 5-ASA molecules for every molecule of olsalazine administered.

339. The answer is b. (*Craig, p 473; Hardman, pp 1033–1034, 1041; Katzung, pp 1049–1050.*) Constipation is the most common and most worrisome adverse response to alosetron. This drug's mechanism of desired action involves selective blockade of serotonin receptors (5-HT$_3$) in the gut; the main outcomes include slowing of colonic transport time, increased sodium and water reabsorption from the colon, and reduced secretion of water and electrolytes into the colon.

Although constipation might be viewed as "trivial" or a minor complaint with most drugs, with alosetron it is the most worrisome one. Constipation may (and has) progressed to fecal impaction, bowel perforation or obstruction, and ischemic colitis. Fatalities have occurred.

The risks are such that the drug was pulled from the market in early 2000 and reapproved 2 years later with a limited indication (prolonged, severe diarrhea-predominant IBS in women); abundant warnings in the package insert; and a comprehensive risk-management/-avoidance program that includes a requirement for (among other things) a special "sign-off" by both the prescriber and the patient that they understand and acknowledge and can identify the risks and agree to treatment anyway.

340. The answer is e. *(Hardman, pp 1055–1056; Katzung, p 1058.)* Pancrelipase is an alcoholic extract of hog pancreas that contains lipase, trypsin, and amylase. (The related drug, pancreatin, is similar.) The goal here is not so much to control the diarrhea, but do so by attacking the cause, which is endogenous pancreatic enzyme deficiency (lipases, amylase, chymotrypsin, and trypsin) that leads to impaired fat digestion and absorption. None of the other drugs mentioned have actions that would be as effective or specific as pancrelipase. "Traditional" antidiarrheals, for example, would only treat the symptoms, not the underlying cause.

Note: You may find pancrelipase administered with antacids, or an acid secretion inhibitor (H_2 blocker or proton pump inhibitor). The purpose of combined therapy is not related to preventing adverse effects of acid on the gastric mucosa, but rather to raise gastric pH and prevent the pancrelipase from being hydrolyzed and inactivated by acid.

341. The answer is d. *(Craig, p 473; Hardman, pp 1017–1018; Katzung, p 1044.)* Most of us have *H. pylori* colonies in our gut and probably don't suffer much from it. However, this acid-stable organism appears to be a major factor in the etiology of refractory, recurrent, severe, or multiple gastric ulcers. Bismuth salts are bactericidal for many organisms, but especially for spirochetes. Colloidal bismuth salts (subsalts, such as subsalicylate) also have a lesion-coating or cytoprotective action. Antimicrobials and GI antisecretory drugs are also used in combination with bismuth compounds.

342. The answer is a. *(Craig, p 478; Hardman, pp 1012–1013; Katzung, pp 1034–1035.)* The typical symptoms of acid-peptic disease are caused by acid. (You might want to remember the "no acid, no pain" concept, but also

258   Pharmacology

recognize that the phrase "no pain, no ulcer" is clearly *incorrect* because ulcers may be present in the absence of symptoms.)

Although antacids seem to have no ability to accelerate ulcer healing, they act almost instantaneously to neutralize acid (provided adequate dosages are given), thereby relieving pain and other discomforts that are due to the acid in a matter of a minute or so.

All the other drugs can, to varying degrees, suppress gastric acid secretion and ultimately get the patient near or to a "no acid, no pain" state. However, it takes some time (variable, but clearly longer than it takes for an antacid to work) for those medications to be absorbed and reach blood levels sufficient to suppress acid production and then reduce symptoms.

Note: You should be familiar with propantheline, but in case you're not: it's an antimuscarinic drug, but with "preferential" effects on the gut. Nonetheless, it shares virtually all the potential systemic side effects, adverse reactions, contraindications, and precautions, that apply to atropine.

343. The answer is a. *(Hardman, pp 1053–1055; Katzung, p 1058.)* Chenodeoxycholic acid (chenodiol), one of several naturally occurring bile acids, is effective in some patients with cholesterol gallstones. Its main initial action is reduced hepatic cholesterol synthesis. That, in turn, lowers the cholesterol content in the bile, which favors the spontaneous dissolution of cholesterol stones that have formed already and reduces the incidence of new stone formation. Related drugs are ursodiol (ursodeoxycholic acid) and monooctanoin; the former is given orally, the latter by direct infusion into the common bile duct.

344. The answer is b. *(Hardman, pp 1043–1045.)* Lactulose is a synthetic, nonabsorbable disaccharide (galactose-fructose). In moderate doses it acts as a laxative. In higher doses it binds intestinal ammonia and other toxins that accumulate in the intestine in severe liver dysfunction. These toxins, and perhaps more so the ammonia, contribute to the signs and symptoms of encephalopathy. None of the other drugs listed provide this benefit.

345. The answer is e. *(Katzung, pp 1034–1036.)* You've all done the experiment: mix vinegar and baking soda (sodium bicarbonate) and one product is CO_2. This gas is formed when sodium bicarbonate—still used as a lay remedy for heartburn and other acid-related GI disturbances—reacts with HCl.

Normally intragastric pressure is kept in check when the gastro-esophageal sphincter opens. However, when pressure can't be relieved quickly enough, or adequately, the stomach will distend. In the presence of ulcers the lesions can be stretched mechanically, favoring further damage that can lead to acute bleeding. Even in the absence of ulcers, any weakness of the gastric wall can lead to gastric rupture. (This ostensibly bizarre outcome, leading to bleeding or rupture, has been documented.)

None of the other antacids listed, whether alone or in combination, lead to production of CO_2 or any other gas that might lead to the outcome described in the scenario.

346. The answer is e. (*Craig, p 479; Hardman, pp 1012–1013; Katzung, p 1046.*) Magnesium salts used alone tend to cause a laxative effect. (Indeed, at dosages higher than those used for acid neutralization, magnesium salts are used for their laxative or cathartic effects.) Aluminum (and calcium) antacids, given alone, tend to cause constipation. Combining a magnesium salt with an aluminum (and/or calcium antacid) is an often successful approach to minimizing antacid-induced changes of net gut motility.

Magnesium salts do not potentiate the antisecretory actions of Al or any other antacid. Indeed, none of the antacids inhibit gastric acid secretion (i.e., they don't have an antisecretory effect to begin with). They merely neutralize acid that has already been secreted (Mg, Ca, sodium bicarbonate) or adsorb acid and pepsins (most of the aluminum compounds).

Although high concentrations of Mg salts may cause gastric irritation, the amounts and concentrations found in antacid products are not sufficient to do that. Regardless, Al salts don't protect against any such potential effect.

Magnesium salts do contribute to a diuresis, but it is not a significant effect. Regardless, Al salts are "nonsystemic" antacids: they are not absorbed to any appreciable degree, and therefore they don't depend on renal processes for their elimination.

Al salts are effective in the form in which they are administered and don't require any enzymatic (or other type of) "activation" to exert their effects (which involves adsorption of acid, pepsins, etc.).

347. The answer is b. (*Craig, p 473; Hardman, pp 594, 1040; Katzung, pp 511, 1047.*) Diphenoxylate is an opioid that has predominant antidiarrheal activity, and that is its sole use. It inhibits peristalsis and, hence, increases the passage time of the intestinal bolus. Typical antidiarrheal doses do not cause ventilatory depression, analgesia, or the euphoria for which opioids are mainly abused. However, should one attempt to take high doses to become euphoric, unpleasant effects will appear. That is because the product contains a small amount of atropine—usually not enough to cause side effects when the proper dose of the product is consumed, but clearly able to cause all the typical antimuscarinic side effects of which you should be aware (see the chapter, "Autonomic Nervous System") when excessive doses are taken. This pharmaceutical manufacturing "trick" discourages diphenoxylate abuse.

Apomorphine and ipecac are dopaminergic emetics (for parenteral and oral administration, respectively) that are used in some poisonings where inducing emesis is desired. Magnesium sulfate (clearly a foul-tasting salt) is used as a laxative or cathartic. Naltrexone, of course, is an opioid antagonist (μ and κ receptors, naloxone-like, but given orally.)

348. The answer is d. (*Craig, p 429; Hardman, p 696.*) Viral illnesses such as the common cold or flu, or chickenpox, contraindicate bismuth subsalicylate use in children (regardless of age). The reason is a risk of Reye's syndrome from the salicylate: precisely the same reason that aspirin or other salicylates should be avoided. No other common analgesics or antipyretics that might be used for a child needing symptom relief, e.g., ibuprofen or acetaminophen, pose this risk.

349. The answer is a. (*Craig, pp 487–488, 778; Hardman, pp 1778–1779; Katzung, pp 919, 1023–1024.*) Pregnant women should not take more than a 25% increase in the normal (recommended) daily dietary intake of vitamin A, because it is definitely teratogenic, especially in the first trimester of pregnancy. Note that the vitamin A-like drugs tretinoin and isotretinoin, which are mainly used for treating refractory or severe acne vulgaris, or to relieve wrinkled facial skin, are contraindicated too.

350. The answer is b. (*Hardman, pp 1751–1752.*) Fat-soluble vitamins, especially A and D, can be stored in massive amounts and, hence, have a potential for serious toxicities. (On the bright side, this abundant storage means that relatively brief periods of inadequate intake are not likely to cause clinical signs and symptoms of deficiency.) Water-soluble vitamins are easily excreted by the kidneys and accumulation to toxic levels is much less common. Conversely, inadequate dietary intake will lead to manifestations of deficiency relatively faster.

351. The answer is b. *(Craig, pp 779–781; Hardman, pp 1753, 1773.)* Vitamin C is water-soluble. The easy way for you to remember the fat-soluble vitamins—to avoid getting "faked-out" on an exam? F(at) soluble: A, K, E, D

352. The answer is c. *(Craig, pp 558–559, 780, 782; Hardman, pp 1276, 1760–1761; Katzung, p 784.)* Pyridoxine deficiencies arise often during isoniazid therapy because the antimycobacterial drug interferes with metabolic activation of the vitamin. The treatment or prophylaxis for at-risk patients is to administer relatively large doses of B_6 (pyridoxine).

353. The answer is c. *(Craig, pp 782–783; Hardman, pp 1497–1500; Katzung, pp 531–532.)* The description contains many of the characteristics of "iron-deficiency anemia." Oral iron salts (e.g., ferrous sulfate, gluconate, or fumarate) are usually the first choice for management (after ruling out such causes as blood loss). Diarrhea (or constipation), nausea, and heartburn are common complaints with oral iron salts, but using these drugs is often preferable to (and safer than) using parenteral iron products such as iron-dextran (risk of anaphylaxis) or other iron complexes, which typically involve erythropoietin administration adjunctively.

Megaloblastic anemia (in contrast with the microcytic anemia we described here) would be treated differently. If it is caused by vitamin B_{12} deficiency (vitamin malabsorption due to deficiency of intrinsic factor), we would treat with cyanocobalamin. The other cause, folate deficiency (inadequate dietary intake) is managed with oral folic acid. Deficiencies of vitamin C or D don't typically cause anemias.

354. The answer is c. *(Craig, p 782; Hardman, pp 555–557, 1761; Katzung, pp 448–449.)* Recall that DOPA decarboxylase, an enzyme whose activity is dependent on pyridoxine, is responsible for metabolizing orally administered levodopa to dopamine in the gut and that only unmetabolized levodopa crosses the blood-brain barrier to be efficacious in relieving parkinsonian signs and symptoms. Recall, too, that levodopa is often administered with carbidopa, a drug that inhibits the peripheral decarboxylase, sparing levodopa for entry into the brain and whose actions are antagonized by pyridoxine. Administering supplemental B_6 will reduce the bioavailability of levodopa, thereby counteracting its antiparkinson effectiveness.

355. The answer is e. (*Craig, pp 415–416, 780; Hardman, pp 430–431, 434–435, 1755–1756; Katzung, pp 368–372.*) Thiamine, administered parenterally with glucose, is the specific intervention for Wernicke's encephalopathy. It dramatically ameliorates the signs and symptoms as well as the underlying causes. Thiamine deficiency is also responsible for Korsakoff's psychosis, another accompaniment of severe, long-term alcohol consumption (especially without adequately nutritional diets). Unfortunately, the signs and symptoms of Korsakoff's (short-term memory problems, a tendency to fabricate, polyneuropathies) are not reversible.

Endocrine System

Anabolic steroids, testosterone, related drugs

Calcium-regulating drugs, including parathyroid hormone and vitamin D

Corticosteroids

Diabetes mellitus and hypoglycemia

Diagnosis, management, of adrenal dysfunction

Erectile dysfunction

Estrogens, progestins, contraceptives, fertility agents

Thyroid disorders

Uterine stimulants and relaxants (oxytocics, tocolytics)

Questions

DIRECTIONS: Each item contains a question or incomplete statement that is followed by possible responses. Select the **one best** response to each question.

356. A patient with a previously undiagnosed thyroid cancer presents with thyrotoxicosis (thyroid storm). One drug that is administered as part of early management is propranolol. The main goal of giving it is to promptly:

a. Block parenchymal cell receptors for thyroid hormones
b. Block thyroid hormone release by a direct effect on the gland
c. Inhibit thyroid hormone synthesis
d. Lessen dangerous secondary signs and symptoms of thyroid hormone excess
e. Lower TSH levels

357. A 44-year-old traveling salesman was recently diagnosed with type 2 diabetes mellitus. The physician prescribed an exercise and diet plan, but this gentleman wouldn't be compliant. He habitually has a morning cup of coffee, gets in his car in the morning, and drives until he gets to his next appointment late afternoon. He says he rarely stops and eats in between.

The next approach is to use a single oral antidiabetic drug, but you are concerned about the drug causing or worsening hypoglycemia in this "meal-skipper." Which of the following drugs poses the greatest relative risk of causing or exacerbating hypoglycemia?

a. Acarbose
b. Glyburide
c. Metformin
d. Pioglitazone
e. Repaglinide

Questions 358–359

A woman deemed at high risk of postmenopausal osteoporosis is started on alendronate.

358. Which of the following is this representative bisphosphonate's main mechanism of action?

a. Activate vitamin D
b. Directly form hydroxyapatite crystals in the bone
c. Provide supplemental calcium in the diet
d. Provide supplemental phosphate, which indirectly elevates serum Ca^{2+}
e. Reduce the number and activity of osteoclasts in bone

359. Which of the following is the most serious adverse response to administration of low doses of alendronate or another bisphosphonate, such as those generally used for osteoporosis?

a. Cholelithiasis
b. Esophagitis
c. Fluid/electrolyte loss from profuse diarrhea
d. Hepatic necrosis
e. Renal damage from calcium stone formation
f. Tetany

360. Some patients who are taking high doses of a bisphosphonate for Paget's disease of the bone develop an endocrine-metabolic disorder. Which of the following is the most likely disorder?

a. Cushing's disease (cushingoid symptoms)
b. Diabetes insipidus
c. Diabetes mellitus
d. Hyperparathyroidism
e. Hyperthyroidism

361. A 75-year-old man had surgery for prostate carcinoma, and local metastases were found intraoperatively. Which of the following is the most appropriate follow-up drug aimed at treating the metastases?

a. Aminoglutethimide
b. Fludrocortisone
c. Leuprolide
d. Mifepristone
e. Spironolactone

362. Which of the following is a naturally occurring substance that is useful in treating Paget's disease of the bone?

a. Etidronate
b. Cortisol
c. Calcitonin
d. Parathyroid hormone (PTH)
e. Thyroxine (T_4)

363. A 75-year-old woman with diabetes is taking an oral antidiabetic drug. One day she goes without eating for 18 h. Her serum glucose concentration is 48 mg/dL (hypoglycemic) upon arrival at the emergency department, where she is deemed to be in critical condition. Which of the following drugs most likely aggravated this fasting hypoglycemia?

a. Acarbose
b. Glyburide
c. Metformin
d. Pioglitazone
e. Rosiglitazone

364. Metyrapone is useful in testing endocrine function of which of the following?

a. α cells of pancreatic islets
b. β cells of pancreatic islets
c. Leydig's cells of the testes
d. Pituitary-adrenal axis
e. Thyroid gland's response to TSH

365. A man with type 2 diabetes is receiving a combination of oral drugs used to maintain glycemic control. If he becomes hypoglycemic, ingesting some sugar (sucrose) will work less well, and certainly less quickly, to restore blood glucose levels if he is taking which of the following drugs?

a. Acarbose
b. Glyburide
c. Metformin
d. Repanglinide
e. Rosiglitazone

366. A woman with a cardiac arrhythmia is being treated long-term with amiodarone. This drug can cause biochemical changes and clinical signs and symptoms that resemble those associated with which of the following endocrine diseases/disorders?

a. Addisonian crisis
b. Cushing's syndrome
c. Diabetes insipidus
d. Diabetes mellitus
e. Hypothyroidism
f. Ovarian hyperstimulation syndrome

367. A 35-year-old woman has Graves' disease, a small goiter, and symptoms that are deemed "mild-to-moderate." Propylthiouracil is prescribed. Which of the following is the most serious adverse response to this drug, for which close monitoring is required?

a. Agranulocytosis
b. Cholestatic jaundice
c. Gout
d. Renal tubular necrosis
e. Rhabdomyolysis
f. Thyroid cancer

368. Parathyroid hormone causes which of the following?

a. Decreased active absorption of Ca from the small intestine
b. Decreased excretion of phosphate
c. Decreased renal tubular reabsorption of Ca
d. Decreased resorption of phosphate from bone
e. Increased mobilization of Ca from bone

369. A 60-year-old man with type 2 diabetes mellitus is treated with pioglitazone. The drug's anticipated ability to lower blood glucose levels is based on its ability to do which of the following?

a. Increase release of endogenous insulin
b. Cause glycosuria (increased renal glucose excretion)
c. Increase hepatic gluconeogenesis
d. Increase target tissue sensitivity to insulin
e. Block off intestinal carbohydrate absorption

370. A 27-year-old woman with endometriosis is treated with danazol. Which of the following is the most likely drug-induced side effect or adverse response for which you should be monitoring often?

a. Anemia from excessive vaginal bleeding
b. Abnormal liver function tests
c. Psychosis
d. Thrombocytopenia
e. Weight loss

371. Which of the following is a very atypical, if not unusually rare, finding associated with the abuse of anabolic steroids, as done by some athletes?

a. Anorexia
b. Decreased spermatogenesis
c. Depression
d. Feminization in males
e. Renal fluid retention

372. A 60-year-old man on long-term therapy with a drug develops hypertension, hyperglycemia, and decreased bone density. Blood tests indicate anemia. Stool samples initially were positive for occult blood and then developed a "coffee-grounds" appearance. Which of the following drugs is most likely responsible for the patient's symptoms?

a. Beclomethasone
b. Hydrochlorothiazide
c. Metformin
d. Pamidronate
e. Prednisone

373. Which adverse response or side effect is typical of those expected with administration of chlorpropamide?

a. Cutaneous flushing, headache, after consuming alcohol
b. Hyponatremia
c. Hypertonic (hyperosmolal) urine compared with normal
d. Reduced serum T_3 and T_4 levels, symptomatic hypothyroidism
e. Weight gain unrelated to effects on glycemic status

374. A 22-year-old woman has been sexually assaulted. She requests a postcoital contraceptive. Which of the following is the most appropriate drug, assuming no contraindications?

a. Ergonovine (or methylergonovine)
b. Mifepristone
c. Raloxifene
d. Ritodrine
e. Tamoxifen

375. A 53-year-old woman with type 2 diabetes mellitus is started on a sulfonylurea. Which of the following is one mechanism by which these drugs lower blood glucose levels?

a. Decrease insulin resistance by lowering body weight
b. Enhance renal excretion of glucose
c. Increase insulin synthesis
d. Promote glucose uptake by muscle, liver, and adipose tissue via an insulin-independent process
e. Release insulin from the pancreas

376. A patient with a history of type 2 diabetes mellitus presents in the emergency department. His complaints include nonspecific gastrointestinal symptoms, including nausea and vomiting. He states he is bloated and has abdominal pain. His appetite has been suppressed for several days. He has malaise and difficulty breathing. His liver is enlarged and tender; liver function tests indicate hepatic damage. Serum bicarbonate is low and lactate levels are high. Kidney function is falling rapidly.

The diagnosis is lactic acidosis, and the suspicion is that it was caused by an antidiabetic drug. Which of the following drugs is this patient most likely to be taking?

a. Acarbose
b. Glipizide
c. Glyburide
d. Metformin
e. Rosiglitazone

377. A 50-year-old woman at very high risk of breast cancer is given tamoxifen for prophylaxis. This drug does which of the following?

a. Blocks estrogen receptors in breast tissue
b. Blocks estrogen receptors in the endometrium
c. Increases the risk of osteoporosis
d. Raises serum LDL cholesterol and total cholesterol, lowers HDL
e. Reduces the risk of thromboembolic disorders

378. A patient has hyperthyroidism from a thyroid cancer, and the medical team concludes that oral radioiodine [sodium iodide 131 (^{131}I)] is the preferred treatment. The dosage is calculated correctly, and the drug is administered. Which of the following is also correct about this approach?

a. A β-adrenergic blocker should not be used for symptom control if or when ^{131}I is used
b. Hyperthyroidism symptoms resolve almost completely within 24 to 48 h after dosing
c. Many patients treated with ^{131}I develop metastatic nonthyroid cancers in response to the drug
d. Oral antithyroid drugs should be administered up to and including the day of ^{131}I administration
e. There is a very high incidence of delayed hypothyroidism after using ^{131}I

379. A woman goes into premature labor early enough that there are great concerns about inadequate fetal lung development and the risk of fetal respiratory distress syndrome. Ritodrine therapy is started to slow labor, but parturition seems imminent. What other adjunct should be administered prepartum, specifically for the purpose of reducing the risks and complications of the newborn's immature respiratory system development?

a. Albuterol (β_2 agonist)
b. Betamethasone
c. Ergonovine (or methylergonovine)
d. Indomethacin
e. Magnesium sulfate

380. A 50-year-old woman is recently diagnosed with type 2 diabetes mellitus. Exercise and diet do not provide adequate glycemic control, so drug therapy is needed. The physician contemplates prescribing metformin. Which of the following statements about this drug is correct?

a. Beneficial and unwanted actions are unaffected by liver function status
b. Lactic acidosis occurs frequently, but it is seldom serious
c. Metformin-induced hypoglycemia seldom occurs
d. Useful, as monotherapy, for both type 1 and type 2 diabetes
e. Weight gain is a common and unwanted side effect

381. You are doing summer volunteer work at a health clinic in a very poor region of the world. A 25-year-old man is diagnosed with vitamin D–resistant rickets. Aside from high-dose vitamin D and oral phosphate, an additional therapeutic approach might be to use which of the following drugs?

a. Calcitriol
b. Estrogen
c. Hydrochlorothiazide
d. Pamidronate
e. Prednisone

382. A 55-year-old postmenopausal woman develops weakness, polyuria, polydipsia, and significant increases of serum creatinine concentration. A computed tomogram (CT scan) indicates nephrocalcinosis. A drug is considered to be the cause. Which of the following drugs is most likely responsible?

a. Estrogens
b. Etidronate
c. Glipizide
d. Prednisone
e. Vitamin D

383. A 76-year-old man complains of progressive difficulty starting his stream on urinating, and having to get up at least once each night to urinate. Rectal examination reveals a generally enlarged, smooth-surfaced prostate. Prostatic serum antigen (PSA) titers are elevated. Urine flow increases, and prostate size decreases, in response to finasteride treatment. This drug's main mechanism of action involves which of the following?

a. α-adrenergic receptor blockade
b. Lowering serum testosterone levels
c. Steroid 5α-reductase inhibition
d. Testosterone receptor blockade
e. Testosterone synthesis inhibition

384. A recalcitrant patient with type 2 diabetes mellitus is noncompliant with medication and diet recommendations nearly all the time. However, he thinks he's smart enough to fool the physician into thinking otherwise: he takes his medication and eliminates nearly all carbohydrate intake for a few days before each clinic visit, knowing he will get a finger-stick for a spot check of serum glucose levels. The simplest, most cost-effective, and most informative way for the physician to assess for past noncompliance and long-term glycemic control would be to perform or measure which of the following?

a. Clinical lab assay of glucose in venous blood sample (rather than glucometer testing of blood from a finger stick)
b. Glucose tolerance test
c. HbA_{1C}
d. Serum levels of the antidiabetic drug
e. Urine ketone levels (in a sample donated at the time of clinic visit)
f. Urine glucose levels

385. Many therapeutic insulins are often modifications of "regular" insulin. The modifications include substituting some amino acids in the protein using recombinant DNA technology, conjugating insulin with NPH (neutral protamine Hagedorn), or combining it with zinc. For all these insulins, which of the following is the one common result of such changes?

a. Elimination of allergic responses
b. Enabling administration by either subcutaneous or intravenous routes
c. Modification of onsets, durations of action
d. Prevention of cellular K^+ uptake as glucose enters cells
e. Reactivation of endogenous (pancreatic) insulin synthesis
f. Selective effects on glucose metabolism, little/no effects on lipids

386. A woman wants a prescription for an oral contraceptive, and your choice is between an estrogen-progestin combination and a "minipill" (progestin only). A main difference is that, compared with the hormone combination products, progestin-only drugs:

a. Are associated with a higher risk of thromboembolism
b. Are directly spermicidal
c. Cause more menstrual irregularities (irregular cycle length, amenorrhea, spotting, etc.)
d. Have better contraceptive efficacy
e. Must be taken on an irregular cycle, rather than daily, so compliance is hindered

387. You have prescribed an oral agent to help control a patient's blood sugar because of type 2 diabetes. In explaining how the drug works, you describe it as a "starch blocker" that inhibits the intestinal uptake of complex carbohydrates in the diet. You advise also that flatus or some cramping or "grumbling sounds" in the belly may develop. Which of the following drugs best fits this description?

a. Acarbose
b. Any thiazolidinedione ("glitazone")
c. Glipizide
d. Metformin
e. Tolbutamide

388. The Yuzpe regimen is used for which of the following?

a. Acute management of thyrotoxicosis
b. Emergency contraception
c. Inducing pregnancy in women who have difficulty getting pregnant
d. Testing function of components of the hypothalamic-pituitary-adrenal cortical axis
e. Type 1 diabetes patients who are refractory to insulin

389. A woman who has been taking an oral contraceptive (estrogen + progestin) for several years is diagnosed with epilepsy and started on phenytoin. Which of the following is the most likely consequence of adding the phenytoin?

a. Agranulocytosis or aplastic anemia, requiring stopping both drugs immediately
b. Breakthrough seizures from increased phenytoin clearance
c. Phenytoin toxicity, significant and of fast onset
d. Profoundly increased risk of craniofacial abnormalities in the fetus
e. Reduced contraceptive efficacy
f. Thromboembolism from the estrogen component of the contraceptive.

390. A young sexually active woman with recurrent, moderate asthma is taking prednisone for suppression of airway inflammation and using two inhaled adrenergic bronchodilators: salmeterol for prophylaxis and albuterol for acute intervention (rescue therapy). She begins taking an oral contraceptive (estrogen-progestin combination). Which of the following is a potential interaction?

a. Contraceptive failure, pregnancy
b. Glucocorticoid withdrawal syndrome (Addisonian crisis)
c. Hypertensive crisis from enhanced adrenergic drug actions
d. Increased corticosteroid (prednisone) side effects
e. Increased risk of cardiac toxicity from the adrenergic agents
f. Recurrence of airway inflammation (corticosteroid effects antagonized)

391. A patient with Cushing's syndrome is being treated by X-irradiation of the pituitary. It may take several months of treatment for adequate symptomatic and metabolic improvement. Until that time, which of the following might be administered adjunctively to suppress glucocorticoid synthesis?

a. Cimetidine
b. Cortisol (massive doses)
c. Fludrocortisone
d. Ketoconazole
e. Spironolactone

392. A patient with type 1 diabetes is being treated with insulin glargine. What clinically important property sets this insulin apart from all the other insulins that might be used instead?

a. Blood levels, hypoglycemic effects, following injection are better described as a plateau rather as a definite "spike" or peak
b. Disulfiram-like reactions (acetadehyde accumulation from inhibited EtOH metabolism) more common, severe
c. Extremely fast onset, useful for immediate postprandial control of serum glucose elevations
d. Low/no risk of hypoglycemia if the patient skips several meals in a row
e. Sensitizes parenchymal cells to insulin (e.g., the administered insulin itself), not just provides insulin, thereby enhancing glycemic control

393. We prescribe bromocriptine for a woman with primary amenorrhea. Normal menstruation returns about a month after starting therapy. The drug worked by doing which of the following?

a. Blocking estrogen receptors, enhancing gonadotropin release
b. Increasing follicle-stimulating hormone (FSH) synthesis
c. Inhibiting prolactin release
d. Stimulating ovarian estrogen and progestin synthesis
e. Stimulating gonadotropin-releasing hormone (GnRH) release

394. A 54-year-old man with other well-treated medical disorders has erectile dysfunction. He takes a dose of sildenafil and shortly thereafter develops acute and severe hypotension. Upon arrival at the emergency department his blood pressure is very low, he is tachycardic, and an EKG shows changes indicative of acute myocardial ischemia. Which other medication was this man most likely taking?

a. Digoxin
b. Glipizide
c. Nitroglycerin
d. Propranolol
e. Testosterone

395. A patient with hypothyroidism following thyroidectomy will require lifelong hormone replacement therapy. Which one of the following agents generally would be most suitable?

a. Levothyroxine (T_4)
b. Liothyronine
c. Liotrix
d. Protirelin
e. Thyroid, desiccated

396. A patient develops marked skeletal muscle tetany soon after a recent thyroidectomy. This symptom can be reversed most quickly by administration of which of the following drugs?

a. Calcitonin
b. Calcium gluconate (CaG)
c. Plicamycin (mithramycin)
d. PTH (parathyroid hormone)
e. Vitamin D

397. A 40-year-old man with a symmetrically enlarged thyroid gland associated with elevated levels of T_3 and T_4 is treated with propylthiouracil (PTU). Which of the following is the principal mechanism of action of PTU?

a. Blocks iodide transport into the thyroid
b. Increases hepatic metabolic inactivation of circulating T_4 and T_3
c. Inhibits proteolysis of thyroglobulin
d. Inhibits thyroidal peroxidase
e. Releases T_3 and T_4 into the blood

Questions 398–401

There are many oral contraceptive (OC) combination products that can be prescribed, but they vary in terms of which drug is used to provide estrogen or progestin effects and the amounts (doses) or ratios of each ingredient. It is important, therefore, to choose the product that best meets the many needs of the patient, makes compliance as easy as possible, and minimizes side effects.

398. What is the main mechanism by which all the OCs exert their desired effects?

a. Acidify the cervical mucus, thereby making the mucus spermicidal
b. Displace/detach a fertilized egg from the endometrium
c. Inhibit nidation (implantation of a fertilized ovum)
d. Inhibit ovulation
e. Reduce uterine blood flow such that the fertilized ovum becomes hypoxic and dies

399. What is the most common estrogenic drug found in these products?

a. Ethinyl estradiol
b. Mestranol
c. Norethindrone
d. Norgestrel

400. Which side effect or adverse response that sometimes occurs during OC therapy is due to the *estrogen* component and generally reflects an estrogen excess in the prescribed drug?

a. Fatigue
b. Hypertension
c. Hypomenorrhea
d. Increased appetite
e. Weight gain

401. Your patient, who is taking an OC, has heard about and asks about the risk of thromboembolism as a result of taking these drugs. To reduce the risk of this potentially severe adverse hematologic response, but still provide reasonably effective contraception, you would prescribe which of the following?

a. A combination product with a higher estrogen dose
b. A combination product with a higher progestin dose
c. A combination product with a lower estrogen dose
d. A combination product with a lower progestin dose
e. An OC that contains only estrogen

402. A woman goes into premature labor, and the physician administers ritodrine. Which of the following is the main mechanism of action by which this drug slows or suppresses uterine contractions?

a. Blocks prostaglandin synthesis
b. Blocks uterine oxytocin receptors
c. Inhibits oxytocin release from the posterior pituitary
d. Inhibits oxytocin synthesis in the hypothalamus
e. Stimulates α-adrenergic receptors
f. Stimulates β_2-adrenergic receptors

403. A 27-year-old woman is diagnosed with hypercortism. To determine whether cortisol production is independent of pituitary gland control, you decide to suppress ACTH production by giving a high-potency glucocorticoid. Which of the following glucocorticoids is the best for this indication?

a. Dexamethasone
b. Hydrocortisone
c. Methylprednisolone
d. Prednisone
e. Triamcinolone

Endocrine System

Answers

356. The answer is d. (*Craig, pp 115, 749–750; Hardman, pp 260, 1574–1575; Katzung, p 637.*) In thyrotoxicosis, essentially the only effect of administering a β-adrenergic blocker—and it is an important effect, to be sure—is to provide prompt relief of both relatively innocuous manifestations of thyroid hormone excess, such as tremor, and those that are much more dangerous, including significant and potentially life-threatening increases in cardiac rate, contractility, and automaticity. Circulating thyroid hormone levels modulate the responsiveness of β-adrenergic receptors to their agonists (e.g., epinephrine, norepinephrine). When thyroid hormone levels are excessive, so is adrenergic receptor responsiveness. Therefore, we reduce the adrenergic consequences of the hormone excess using a β blocker. There are no effects on thyroid hormone levels or thyroid gland function or control.

357. The answer is b. (*Craig, p 773; Hardman, pp 1705–1706; Katzung, p 706.*) The most common side effect of the newer sulfonylureas (glyburide, glipizide, glimeperide) is hypoglycemia, and the relative incidence is higher than with any of the other drugs listed.

Normally insulin release peaks in response to a meal. That occurs even when there is a relative insulin deficiency (type 2 diabetes mellitus). Our hypothetical meal-skipping patient essentially fasts all day. His blood glucose levels will tend to fall as the meal-free interval progresses, and during this time physiologic insulin release would be relatively low. However, the newer sulfonylureas—glyburide, glipizide, glimeperide—act by causing insulin release, whether one has eaten or fasted. Thus, the hypoglycemic effect of the drug will enhance the tendency for hypoglycemia that accompanies fasting or that occurs with increased physical activity. This is likely to apply even in the presence of insulin resistance, which is common.

Acarbose is an α-glucosidase inhibitor. The main effect of that drug is a slowed rate of carbohydrate absorption from the gut. This blunts the insulin response to rising blood glucose levels. Because acarbose's effects center on inhibiting dietary carbohydrate absorption, the drug's effects will not occur in the absence of those foodstuffs. Indeed, effects are better when the drug is taken with or right before meals, and it seems to be more efficacious as the amount of carbohydrate in the meal increases.

Metformin does not directly increase or decrease insulin secretion. In contrast with the sulfonylureas, which are correctly classified as hypoglycemic drugs (i.e., they drive blood glucose levels down), the biguanides are *antihyperglycemic,* tending instead to keep blood glucose levels from going up.

Pioglitazone (a thiazolidinedione, or "glitazone" for short) sensitizes parenchymal cells (mainly adipocytes) to insulin and so reduces insulin resistance. (The glitazones apparently activate a nuclear peroxisomal proliferator-activated receptor, PPAR-γ, that participates in the cellular response to insulin.)

Because of the insulin-dependency of their actions, the intensity of the effects of a glitazone increase when insulin levels are high (e.g., postprandial) and diminish as insulin levels fall (e.g., fasting). Regardless, and unless a glitazone is prescribed with insulin or a sulfonylurea (common), the incidence of drug-induced hypoglycemia is very low.

Repaglinide, a meglitinide, seems to trigger pancreatic insulin release in the presence of sufficient (and high) blood glucose levels. However, when blood glucose levels are sufficiently low (as can occur during fasting or meal-skipping), that effect wanes and so the drug is not likely to cause or worsen hypoglycemia.

358. The answer is e. *(Hardman, pp 1733–1734; Katzung, pp 721, 727–730.)* Whether used for osteoporosis (prevention or management, men or women, idiopathic or drug-induced) or Paget's disease of the bone, bisphosphonates exert their effects on osteoclasts and osteoblasts. The drug is incorporated into bone. When drug-containing bone is resorbed by the osteoclasts, osteoclast function (and, so, subsequent bone resorption) is inhibited. The bisphosphonates also recruit osteoblasts, which then produce a substance that further inhibits osteoclast activity.

359. The answer is b. *(Craig, pp 758–760; Hardman, pp 1733–1734, 1738–1739; Katzung, p 721.)* Esophagitis, sometimes with esophageal ulcers, is the most worrisome adverse response. It is not due to any specific metabolic alteration causes by the bisphosphonates, but rather by direct, prolonged contact of the drug with the esophagus if the oral dose lodges there without passing quickly enough to the stomach. This is why the drug should not be administered to patients with esophageal disease, difficulty swallowing, or an inability to sit or stand up for at least 30 min (to help gravity bring the tablet to the stomach) after taking the drug. Otherwise, overall, the bisphosphonates cause remarkably few side effects in the vast majority of patients.

360. The answer is d. (*Craig, pp 758–760; Hardman, pp 1738–1739; Katzung, p 730.*) You should be able to deduce hyperparathyroidism as the answer by recalling that the bisphosphonates ultimately affect bone Ca^{2+} metabolism, and the parathyroid gland is the main regulator of serum Ca^{2+} levels. When a bisphosphonate is given to a patient with Paget's disease of the bone, after about a week the dramatic inhibition of bone resorption dramatically lowers serum Ca^{2+} levels (because an important portion of serum Ca^{2+} arises from bone that is being resorbed). When serum Ca^{2+} falls considerably, parathyroid hyperfunction can develop. The easiest way to prevent this is to administer dietary calcium supplements along with the bisphosphonate.

361. The answer is c. (*Craig, pp 650, 732; Hardman, pp 1441–1442, 1556; Katzung, pp 615, 687, 926.*) Leuprolide is a peptide that is related to GnRH or luteinizing hormone-releasing hormone (LHRH), and it is used to treat metastatic prostate carcinoma. By inhibiting gonadotropin release it induces a hypogonadal state; testosterone levels in the body fall significantly, and this appears to be the mechanism for suppression of the cancer.

362. The answer is c. (*Craig, p 760; Hardman, p 1733; Katzung, pp 721, 730.*) Calcitonin is useful in the therapy of Paget's disease of bone (osteitis deformans). Calcitonin therapy reduces urinary hydroxyproline excretion and serum alkaline phosphatase activity, and provides some symptomatic relief. Presumably, these effects result from the ability of calcitonin to inhibit bone resorption. Side effects of long-term therapy with this hormone can include nausea, edema of the hands, and urticaria. Resistance to the drug may develop after a while, presumably because neutralizing antibodies directed against it develop. Etidronate is a synthetic drug that is useful in Paget's disease. The compound is orally effective and lacks the antigenicity associated with calcitonin.

363. The answer is b. (*Craig, p 772; Hardman, pp 1703–1704; Katzung, pp 704–707.*) Glyburide is a second-generation sulfonylurea oral hypoglycemic. Of the main groups or chemical classes of oral antidiabetic agents, these are the ones typically associated with causing hypoglycemia, whether from overdose or as a rather expected response in some patients, particularly before meals. Sulfonylureas release insulin from the β cells of the pancreas (see Question 375 for more on this). Normally carbohydrates from a meal trigger insulin release; when blood glucose levels are low, as after the 18-h fast this patient experienced, physiologic insulin release would be low too. However, even in a fast-induced hypoglycemic state a sulfonylurea will release insulin and drive blood glucose down even further.

The elderly are particularly susceptible to sulfonylurea-induced hypoglycemia. Part of this may relate to diet. However, expected age-related falls of renal and/or hepatic function can reduce elimination of these drugs, thereby increasing their serum levels and their effects unless dosages are reduced accordingly.

This propensity for preprandial hypoglycemia is shared by the meglitinides—repaglinide and nateglinide—because they, too, increase pancreatic insulin release.

The thiazadolinediones (glitazones) seldom cause symptomatic hypoglycemia because they do not release insulin. The same applies to metformin, the biguanide; and acarbose (with, along with miglitol, is an α-glucosidase inhibitor). Because of a longer half-life, compared with glipizide, a sulfonylurea is more likely to cause preprandial hypoglycemia. Glipizide is contraindicated in patients with liver disease because it is metabolized in the liver. Care should be taken in the elderly because of their propensity to develop hypoglycemia, which is perhaps due to decreased hepatic and renal function that is evident in this patient population. Metformin, acarbose, and pioglitazone do not produce serious hypoglycemic reactions.

364. The answer is d. (*Craig, pp 699–700; Hardman, p 1765; Katzung, pp 655–656.*) Metyrapone, because it decreases serum levels of cortisol by inhibiting the 11β-hydroxylation of steroids in the adrenal, can be used to assess function of the pituitary-adrenal cortical axis. When metyrapone is given to normal persons, the adenohypophysis secretes more ACTH. This causes a normal adrenal cortex to synthesize increased amounts of 17-

hydroxylated steroids, which can be measured in the urine. However, patients who have disease of the hypothalamico-pituitary axis do not produce ACTH in response to metyrapone. As a result, we find no increased levels of the steroids in the urine. Before administering metyrapone we need to test responsiveness of the adrenal cortex to respond to administration of ACTH.

365. The answer is a. (*Craig, pp 774–775; Hardman, pp 1706–1707; Katzung, p 710.*) Acarbose, classified as an α-glucosidase inhibitor, slows the rate and extent of carbohydrate absorption from the intestines. (The related drug, miglitol, does the same.) The consequence of this for the hypoglycemic patient is that attempts to restore blood glucose levels by consuming sugar or sucrose-containing foods or beverages (e.g., orange juice is a popular choice) will be less effective—and certainly slower in terms of symptom relief. None of the other oral diabetes drugs have this mechanism of action and so will not hinder attempts to restore euglycemia when sugar is consumed.

366. The answer is e. (*Craig, pp 187–188; Hardman, pp 956, 1579, 1585; Katzung, pp 232–234, 630, 633.*) Amiodarone, an iodine-rich drug, has several actions that can lead to clinical hypothyroidism (or, less often and mainly in persons with iodine-deficient diets, hyperthyroidism). It inhibits a deiodinase (an enzyme that removes iodine on both the 5 and 5′ positions) that converts thyroxine to triiodothyronine (T_3), mainly in the liver. This process is the main contributor to the production of endogenous (circulating) T_3 that is used by most target tissues in the body. Inhibit this enzyme and the peripheral tissues have less T_3 to utilize, and signs and symptoms of hypothyroidism can ensue.

The excess iodine derived from metabolism of amiodarone may also contribute to the hypothyroidism. The mechanism is analogous to the way in which administering large doses of iodide are clinically useful for suppressing thyroid function in hyperthyroid individuals: iodide limits its own transport into follicular cells, and, acutely at least, high circulating levels of iodide inhibit thyroid hormone synthesis.

367. The answer is a. (*Craig, p 750; Hardman, p 1582; Katzung, p 633.*) The incidence of agranulocytosis due to propylthiouracil, or the related thio[n]amide, methimazole, is not rare. In addition, it may develop within the first few weeks of starting therapy, and so a "routine" blood test scheduled for several months or more after starting the drug may not catch it. However, if it is detected early (e.g., the patient promptly reports a sore throat or other flu-like symptoms) and the drug is stopped, it is usually spontaneously reversible. The most common side effect with the thioamides is urticaria. It may abate spontaneously or require symptomatic management with an antihistamine (either first or second generation) or with a corticosteroid.

None of the other responses listed are recognized as being associated with thioamides.

368. The answer is e. *(Craig, pp 755–756; Hardman, pp 1722–1724; Katzung, pp 716–717.)* Parathyroid hormone's main role is to maintain normal serum Ca^{2+} levels. When serum Ca^{2+} concentrations become sufficiently low, parathyroid hormone synthesis and release increase, and it helps restore a normocalcemic state by promoting (in concert with vitamin D) Ca^{2+} absorption from the intestines, promoting renal tubular Ca^{2+} reabsorption and phosphate excretion, and increasing mobilization of Ca^{2+} and phosphate from bone (i.e., bone resorption).

369. The answer is d. *(Craig, p 774; Hardman, p 1706; Katzung, pp 709–710.)* Pioglitazone, like all the glitazone oral antidiabetic drugs, works by increasing parenchymal cell responsiveness to insulin. The mechanism seems to involve activation of is peroxisome proliferator-activated receptors. This apparently increases transcription of insulin-responsive genes that control glucose (and lipid) metabolism and cellular glucose uptake via glucose transporters. The net effects include not only lowered plasma levels of glucose, but also fatty acids and (indirectly) of insulin. Given the necessary involvement of insulin in the drug's effects, it will not work (alone) for patients with type 1 diabetes. When used for patients who have type 2 diabetes, and who nonetheless require insulin, a thiazolidinedione can be a valuable adjunct that helps lower daily insulin requirements.

370. The answer is b. *(Katzung, pp 680–681.)* Danazol is a testosterone derivative used to treat endometriosis, and some of the side effects and adverse responses are those you would expect from testosterone itself: liver dysfunction, virilism (acne, hirsutism, oily skin, reduced breast size), and reductions in HDL cholesterol levels. Other reported adverse reactions include amenorrhea, weight gain, sweating, vasomotor flushing, and edema.

Nonetheless, danazol appears to be just as effective as an estrogen-progesterone combination for managing endometriosis, and relatively few patients have stoppped (or have had to stop) danazol treatment because of side effects or adverse reactions.

371. The answer is a. (*Craig, pp 408t, 419, 734; Hardman, pp 1637–1638, 1642; Katzung, pp 527, 683–686.*) Anorexia is not a typical finding with anabolic steroid abuse. Quite the contrary: appetite usually increases. Body weight increases too, due to several factors that include increased appetite (and food intake), renal fluid retention, and various metabolic changes, some of which lead to the increased muscle "bulking" and strength that steroid-abusing athletes often seek. (These same effects are among the ones sought when these drugs are prescribed, as for some debilitated patients.) Continued use of these anabolic/androgenic steroids can induce mood changes, including symptoms of depression or psychosis. The androgenic effects cause masculinization in women and may cause feminization in males. The latter effect is due to increased formation of estrogen. In addition, these steroids decrease testosterone synthesis by the testes and so may impair spermatogenesis. Anabolic steroids, used long enough and in sufficiently high doses, can cause serious hepatotoxicity; they can also increase the risk of cardiovascular diseases.

372. The answer is e. (*Craig, pp 693–694; Hardman, p 1667; Katzung, p 650.*) These findings are characteristic of what one would expect with long-term (and high dose) systemic glucocorticoid therapy (i.e., prednisone and many others, but not beclomethasone, which is given by oral inhalation and is not absorbed appreciably). Psychoses, peptic ulceration with hemorrhage (coffee-grounds stool, indicative of gastric bleeding) or without (possibly causing guaiac-positive stools), increased susceptibility to infection, edema, osteoporosis, myopathy, and hypokalemic alkalosis can occur. Other adverse reactions include cataracts, hyperglycemia, slowed lineal growth in children, and iatrogenic Cushing's syndrome.

Hydrochlorothiazide (and other thiazide and thiazide-like diuretics, such as chlorthalidone or metolazone) can increase blood glucose levels. However, they typically lower blood pressure (as evidenced by their widespread use as antihypertensives) and tend to raise, not lower, serum calcium levels (which would be inconsistent with the decreased bone density described in this man). None of the other drugs listed would cause a collection of findings consistent with what we described here.

373. The answer is a. (*Craig, p 772; Hardman, pp 1703–1704; Katzung, pp 705–706.*) Chlorpropamide is one of the older sulfonylurea oral hypoglycemic drugs and is one of the biggest offenders in terms of the frequency and severity of disulfiram-like reactions it can cause (by inhibiting oxidation of acetaldehyde, an intermediate in ethanol metabolism, by aldehyde dehydrogenase). Chlorpropamide differs from the rest—older or newer sulfonylureas—in some other important ways. It has the longest half-life (duration of action between 1 and 3 days, usually toward the longer). It seems to pose the highest risk of causing hypoglycemia. And it tends to enhance the effects of ADH on the collecting ducts of the nephron and/or enhance ADH release from the posterior pituitary. Greater effects (or levels) of ADH impair renal conservation of water. This leads to formation of large volumes of dilute urine; the extra free water loss may cause weight loss and tends to cause hypernatremia, not the opposite. Chlorpropamide (and the other sulfonylureas) cause no frequent or significant alterations of thyroid hormone status or thyroid function.

374. The answer is b. (*Craig, pp 701, 709; Hardman, pp 679, 1622–1623; Katzung, pp 656, 680.*) Mifepristone is a synthetic drug used as an abortifacient or postcoital contraceptive. Although the drug blocks glucocorticoid receptors, that effect does not account for its use or effects in the context described here. Here the actions arise from blocking uterine progesterone receptors. They include detachment of the conceptus from the uterine wall, softening and dilation of the cervix, and increased myometrial contraction that expels the conceptus. (The latter arises from both a drug-induced increase of local prostaglandin synthesis and greater myometrial responsiveness to them.) If mifepristone fails to induce expulsion of the fetus, misoprostol is usually given to increase uterine contractions further. (Estrogens used alone or in combination with progestins have also proven effective in postcoital contraception.)

Ergonovine and methylergonovine are ergot compounds that cause uterine contraction, and are used postpartum to control bleeding by increasing uterine tone. They are abortifacient drugs, but not used for postcoital contraception. Ralxoifene and tamoxifen are estrogen receptor agonists or antagonists (which effects occurs depends on the tissue) that are used to treat certain estrogen-dependent breast cancers.

Ritodrine is a β_2-adrenergic agonist used to slow uterine contractions and reduce uterine tone in premature labor.

375. The answer is e. (*Craig, pp 771–772; Hardman, pp 1701–1703; Katzung, pp 704–706.*) Recall that the sulfonylureas simplistically fall into two main classes, based largely on how long they have been used: the so-called first-generation agents, such as tolbutamide and chlorpropamide, and the newer second-generation drugs, glipizide, glyburide, and limepiride. Whether older or newer, these drugs mainly lower blood glucose levels by enhancing insulin release from the β cells of the pancreas. The mechanism involved binding to and blocking an ATP-sensitive K^+ channel on β cell membranes. This depolarizes the membrane, and resulting Ca^{2+} influx triggers insulin release. The mechanistic dependence on insulin release, of course, explains why these drugs are ineffective in type 1 diabetes.

Other probable actions of the sulfonylureas include reduced serum glucagons levels and increased binding of insulin to parenchymal tissue cells.

376. The answer is d. (*Craig, pp 773–774; Hardman, p 1705; Katzung, p 708.*) Metformin (a biguanide) poses the greatest risk, of all the antidiabetic drugs, of causing lactic acidosis. Although the overall risk of lactic acidosis from this drug is low, should it occur, mortality is quite common. Alcohol consumption or renal or hepatic disease increase the risk of lactic acidosis associated with metformin.

Acarbose, an α-glucosidase inhibitor (blocks starch uptake from the gut), the sulfonylureas (older ones such as tolubtamide or newer ones such as glipizide and glyburide), and rosiglitazone (and other glitazones, e.g., pioglitazone) are not associated with lactic acidosis (unless they are co-administered with metformin).

377. The answer is a. (*Craig, pp 649–650, 707, 709–710; Hardman, pp 1440–1441, 1613–1614; Katzung, pp 679–680, 916–917.*) Tamoxifen is often referred to as a selective estrogen receptor modifier (SERM). It blocks estrogen receptors in some tissues and stimulates them in some others. The drug can be used to prevent or treat estrogen-dependent breast cancers, and it works as an estrogen receptor antagonist there. A receptor-agonist action also accounts for one of the drug's more distressing and common side effects, hot flashes. In contrast, the drug activates estrogen receptors in the uterus, increasing the risk of endometrial cancers. Other estrogen-activating (estrogen-like) consequences include a reduced risk of osteoporosis, desirable changes in serum cholesterol profiles (reduced LDL and total cholesterols; increased HDL), and an increased risk of thromboembolic events. The related drug, raloxifene, is largely tamoxifen-like with one main exception: it does not activate uterine estrogen receptors, and so does not increase the risk of endometrial cancers.

378. The answer is e. (*Craig, pp 750–752; Hardman, pp 1586–1589; Katzung, p 637.*) Hypothyroidism is the most common disadvantage or limitation of using ^{131}I to treat hyperthyroidism. No matter how accurately the dose is calculated, according to some studies about 8 of 10 treated patients develop symptomatic hypothyroidism (that needs to be treated) by 10 or more years after treatment. It results, of course, from excessive thyroid cell destruction.

Substantive symptom relief from ^{131}I takes from several weeks to a couple of months to develop (although blood chemistries change somewhat faster). Until a euthyroid state develops, drugs such as β-adrenergic blockers or oral antithyroid drugs may be needed for symptom control. Oral antithyroid drugs can be given before ^{131}I treatment, but they should be stopped for a couple of days before radiotherapy so as not to prevent radioiodine uptake into the gland. Cancers, metastatic or not, occurring in the thyroid or elsewhere, are rare after ^{131}I therapy.

379. The answer is b. (*Craig, p 696; Katzung, p 650.*) We would give betamethasone to enhance fetal surfactant synthesis and suppress airway inflammation, thereby lessening the chance or severity of fetal respiratory distress syndrome at birth. (The action probably involves stimulating synthesis of fibroblast pneumocyte factor, which then stimulates surfactant synthesis by pneumocytes in the fetus. Recall that surfactant lowers alveolar surface tension, thereby reducing the likelihood of alveolar collapse and its consequences on gas exchange.)

Note: Other corticosteroids, especially dexamethasone, could be used. However, betamethasone is preferred because it binds less to plasma proteins than cortisol and most other glucocorticoids, allowing more steroid to cross the placenta.

Even though albuterol is used as a bronchodilator (e.g., for asthma or

COPD), it is classified, pharmacologically, precisely as we classify ritodrine, a relatively selective β₂ agonist. With the ritodrine being given already, administering albuterol would be pointless. In obstetrics, ergonovine or methylergonovine are given postpartum; their strong uterine contracting effects are used to reduce postpartum bleeding. Aside from being contraindicated before delivery, they have no pulmonary effects of the sort we want. Indomethacin is sometimes used to slow premature labor. It works by blocking synthesis of prostaglandins that have oxytocic activity, but prostaglandin synthesis inhibition also causes closure of the ductus arteriosus (which, in this setting, would be unwanted). Magnesium sulfate would not cause the desired pulmonary effects; it is used in obstetrics to prevent seizures in preeclampsia/eclampsia. The drug has tocolytic activity, but the jury is out on just how effective and safe the drug is when used to suppress uterine contractions.

Note: Three pharmaceutical preparations of surfactant are now available: calfactant, beractant, and poractant alfa. They are given to neonates with respiratory distress syndrome by direct intratracheal instillation.

380. The answer is c. (*Craig, pp 773–774; Hardman, pp 1705–1706; Katzung, p 708.*) Metformin, classified as a biguanide, "sensitizes" peripheral cells to insulin, thereby facilitating glucose uptake and utilization, and suppresses release of glucose from the liver and into the blood. It is largely ineffective in the absence of insulin and so is approved only for type 2 diabetes (used alone or in conjunction with such other drugs as a sulfonylurea or insulin).

Most patients taking metformin lose weight. This is probably due to an appetite-suppressing effect (leading to reduced caloric intake), rather than because of a specific effect on some metabolic reaction(s) or anorexia secondary to GI side effects.

The drug seldom causes hypoglycemia. Rather than actively driving down blood glucose levels (as, say, insulin does), metformin acts as if it caps physiologic rises of glucose concentrations. (Thus, it has been described as being an *antihyperglycemic* drug, rather than a hypoglycemic agent.)

Metformin is not metabolized by the liver, but liver dysfunction is one contraindication. That's mainly because of the risks of the drug's most important adverse effect, lactic acidosis, which is rare but often fatal when it does occur: impaired liver function impairs lactate elimination and favors its accumulation to toxic levels.

However the main primary cause of the lactic acidosis is renal insufficiency (serum creatinine > 1.5 mg/dL in men, 1.4 mg/dL in women), whether caused by renal disease or by renal hypoperfusion (ischemia, as might occur with heart failure and/or hypotension).

381. The answer is a. *(Craig, p 760; Hardman, pp 1720–1721, 1731–1732; Katzung, pp 717, 726, 728–729.)* Recall that vitamin D_3 is hydroxylated to 25-OH D_3 (calcifediol). Calcifediol is then hydroxylated in the kidney to the most active form of vitamin D, which is 1,25-dihydroxyvitamin D (calcitriol).

Given as a drug, calcitriol rapidly elevates serum Ca levels by enhancing the intestinal absorption of Ca. It is indicated in vitamin D deficiency, particularly in patients with chronic renal failure or renal tubular disease, hypoparathyroidism, osteomalacia, and rickets. Serum phosphate levels usually increase with prolonged treatment.

382. The answer is e. *(Craig, pp 459–460; Hardman, p 1729; Katzung, pp 717–718.)* Overmedication with vitamin D may lead to a toxic syndrome called *hypervitaminosis D.* The initial symptoms can include weakness, nausea, weight loss, anemia, and mild acidosis. As the excessive doses are continued, signs of nephrotoxicity can develop, such as polyuria, polydipsia, azotemia, and eventually nephrocalcinosis. In adults, osteoporosis can occur. Also, there is CNS impairment, which can result in mental retardation and convulsions.

383. The answer is c. *(Craig, p 732; Hardman, p 1646; Katzung, pp 688, 1030.)* Finasteride competitively inhibits steroid 5-reductase, the enzyme necessary for synthesis of the active form of testosterone (dihydrotestosterone) in the prostate. Testosterone synthesis and circulating testosterone levels don't fall in response to the drug. PSA titers will, however. [Recall, by the way, that the α-adrenergic blockers (e.g., prazosin) provide symptomatic relief in some men with BPH by relaxing smooth muscle in the urethra,, bladder neck, and prostate capsule. Their effects do not involve testosterone synthesis or cellular responses to the hormone.]

384. The answer is c. *(Craig, p 768; Hardman, pp 1691–1692; Katzung, p 703.)* Serum glucose reacts nonenzymatically with hemoglobin to form glycated hemoglobin products (e.g., Hb A_{1C}). The rate of Hb A_{1C} formation is related to ambient glucose levels, and the amount of Hb A_{1C} measured in any given blood sample reflects the average blood glucose levels over the last 2 to 3 months. Thus, although the patient's serum glucose levels may be acceptable after a couple of days' fast, Hb A_{1C} measurements give the big picture about how good glycemic control was on a more long-term (and more important) timeline. Note that although measuring HbA_{1C} gives important information about the long-term, it does not provide any information about day-to-day fluctuations in glucose levels or what's happening "right now", and such information is important to optimal control of diabetes and its symptoms. Nonetheless, regular, periodic checks of Hb A_{1C} should be part of the monitoring for every patient with diabetes (type 1 or 2), not so much as a way to assess for noncompliance as to make sure that the current treatment plan with which the patient is complying is working. It is a common and relatively inexpensive assay.

Having the clinical lab measure glucose in a venous blood sample won't give any additional or meaningful information: hand-held glucometers, used properly, are remarkably accurate. Glucose tolerance tests, even those done with oral glucose, will provide little historic information, and they are expensive. Few clinical labs are set up to measure serum concentrations of most oral antidiabetic drugs, and the cost for these nonstandard tests would be quite expensive. Measuring urine ketone levels are of no benefit for our purposes. All that they might prove is that our patient has fasted for several days. Urine glucose monitoring is not very enlightening either. Recall that glucose appears in the urine only when serum concentrations exceed a renal threshold for reabsorption (around 180 mg/dL or so). A glucose-free urine sample, then, would only indicate that serum glucose levels are below the threshold: they still could be unacceptably high, or normal, or low, and you would never know just by urine testing.

385. The answer is c. (*Craig, pp 765–766, 768–770; Hardman, pp 1692–1695; Katzung, pp 696–701.*) Insulin modifications, whether by rDNA technology or by physical means (e.g., modification with zinc or NPH) alter onsets and durations of action.

[Recall that regular insulin, given by SC injection, has an onset of about 30 min, peaks in about 3 h, and has a duration of about 7 to 8 h. Lispro and aspart insulins work faster, peak earlier, and have the shortest durations (rapid/short); lente and NPH insulins ("intermediate-acting") have onsets, times to peak, and durations longer than regular insulins; and ultralente insulin and insulin glargine have the slowest onsets (4 to 6 h), with durations that are on par with lente and NPH.]

In general, the modified *human* insulins rarely cause allergic responses (not the case with porcine lente and NPH insulins), but the problem is not prevented altogether, particularly with NPH insulins: the protamine used to modify either the human or porcine insulins, which are then called NPH insulins, is a large (and potentially antigenic) protein. Beyond that, however, the modifications yield clinically useful pharmacokinetic—not biochemical—changes.

386. The answer is c. (*Craig, pp 706–712; Hardman, pp 1623–1627; Katzung, pp 673–679.*) Progestin-only oral contraceptives ("minipills") are associated with a higher risk of menstrual irregularities than the more common estrogen-progestin preparations. That is largely due to the lack of estrogen. However, the absence of estrogen also lowers the risk of thromboembolic disorders. Progestin-only formulations are, overall, less effective in terms of preventing pregnancy than combination products; like combination products they lack definitive spermicidal effects (but they thicken cervical mucus, retard sperm motility in that way, and reduce the likelihood of nidation), and their administration schedule is continuous—every day, rather than the cyclic schedule used for combination products.

387. The answer is a. (*Craig, pp 774–775; Hardman, pp 1706–1707; Katzung, pp 710–711.*) Acarbose, and the newer related drug, miglitol, act in intestinal brush border cells to inhibit monosaccharide formation from complex carbohydrates and oligosaccharides. They do so by inhibiting α-glucosidases in the brush border of intestinal cells. The effect is optimal, of course, when carbohydrates are present in the gut: i.e., during and right after a meal. Thus, the drug should be taken with meals. Its main effect will be a slowing of carbohydrate absorption and a blunting of typical postprandial rises of blood glucose. GI side effects, mainly those described in the question, are the most common ones with acarbose. Used alone, hypoglycemia is rare; however, the drug is often used as an adjunct to a sulfonylurea, and their propensity for causing hypoglycemia is not reduced by acarbose. Very high doses of acarbose may raise serum transaminases, usually reflecting some hepatic dysfunction caused by the drug.

388. The answer is b. *(Hardman, p 1624.)* The Yuzpe is a method of emergency contraception that involves administering two doses of an estrogen-progestin oral contraceptive (several brand name formulations of oral contraceptives can be used). One dose is taken as soon as possible after intercourse, but certainly within 72 h, and the earlier the greater the risk of contraception; a second dose is taken 12 h later. There's a high incidence of nausea and vomiting associated with the drugs, so we usually premedicate the patient with a suitable antiemetic before giving the drugs.

389. The answer is e. *(Craig, pp 36–37, 378, 713; Hardman, pp 1609, 1621; Katzung, pp 1119, 1122.)* Phenytoin is one of several agents that can enhance the hepatic metabolism of oral contraceptives (especially the estrogen component), leading to reduced OC levels and unintended pregnancy (contraceptive failure). It is also one that interacts by inducing synthesis of hormone-binding globulins: more hormone molecules are bound to the protein, and so less free (active) drug is in the circulation. Several other common anticonvulsants interact with the same potential outcome, especially barbiturates (including phenobarbital, mephobarbital, and primidone), carbamazepine, and oxcarbazepine. Be sure to recall that rifampin (and rifabutin) and protease inhibitors (ritonavir, others) are also important interactants with OCs via a metabolism-inducing mechanism. Finally, some antibiotics (e.g., tetracyclines) interact with OCs, but here the mechanism differs: the antibiotics suppress gut flora that participate in enterohepatic recycling of the OCs. When the bacteria are suppressed, OCs that are secreted into the gut are lost in the feces, rather than being reabsorbed.

390. The answer is d. *(Craig, p 713; Hardman, pp 1609, 1621; Katzung, p 1119.)* Combination oral contraceptives (presumably the estrogen component) can impair the hepatic metabolism of several drugs, prednisone and several glucocorticoids among them. The most likely outcome is an increase in the number and/or severity of expected corticosteroid-associated side effects, including weight gain and alterations of carbohydrate, lipid, and protein metabolism. Thus, we need to monitor for this and reduce corticosteroid doses downward as needed. Because we have centered this patient scenario on asthma, we should add that oral contraceptives also inhibit clearance and increase the risk of toxicity from, theophylline.

391. The answer is d. (*Craig, pp 700–701; Hardman, pp 1302, 1674–1675; Katzung, pp 687–688.*) Ketoconazole, traditionally used as an antifungal agent (see the chapter, "Anti-Infectives"), is one of the most efficacious inhibitors of corticosteroid synthesis. It is not a primary therapy for pituitary tumors/Cushing's syndrome, but is a useful adjunct. The main problem associated with this drug is the risk of hepatotoxicity and the potential for interactions with some other drugs. An alternative to ketoconazole is aminoglutethimide, which also interferes with synthesis of all the adrenal steroids.

Cimetidine, the H_2 histamine blocker that is well known as an inhibitor of P450-mediated metabolism of many drugs, would be of no benefit. Massive doses of cortisol, although theoretically "reasonable" (feedback suppression of pituitary function), would be of little help in terms of regulating the pituitary's activity and clearly would aggravate signs and symptoms of adrenal corticosteroid excess that we already have. Fludrocortisone has intense mineralocorticoid activity and is the only drug indicated for replacement therapy in chronic mineralocorticoid deficiencies. Spironolactone blocks aldosterone receptors; it would counteract only the aldosterone-related responses to corticosteroid excess and would not have any effects on adrenal corticosteroid synthesis.

392. The answer is a. (*Craig, p 769; Katzung, p 700.*) Insulin glargine is a genetically engineered insulin that is poorly (but adequately) soluble at physiologic pH values. The drug dissolves and enters the bloodstream slowly and in such away that there is more of a stable plateau than a well-defined spike in blood levels and effects. This plateau is rather, and remarkably, consistent over the typical 24-h duration following a SC injection. Thus, the drug is better able than most other insulins for maintaining round-the-clock control of blood glucose levels, but less able to suppress the postprandial elevation of glucose that is necessary for some patients. Insulin glargine's onset and duration of action are comparable to such preparations as NPH insulins or lente insulins. It is what happens in between, temporally, that distinguishes this drug from the rest.

393. The answer is c. (*Craig, pp 369, 769; Hardman, p 1551; Katzung, pp 275, 277, 452.*) Primary amenorrhea is associated with hyperprolactinemia. Women who are amenorrheic from hyperprolactinemia also often present with galactorrhea and infertility. Bromocriptine, a dopamine receptor agonist, inhibits prolactin release. The site of action is the pituitary, and it involves the same site and mechanism by which dopamine, released from the hypothalamus, normally suppresses prolactin release. Some causes of hyperprolactinemia, in both men and women, include pituitary cancer, hypothalamic dysfunction, and some drugs (e.g., antipsychotics, estrogens). Recall that bromocriptine, by virtue of its central dopaminergic activity, is sometimes used to help correct the dopamine-ACh imbalance that underlies Parkinson's disease.

394. The answer is c. *(Craig, pp 738–740; Hardman, pp 850–851, 1303; Katzung, p 189.)* This is the interaction (and one that can be fatal) between sildenafil, tadalafil, or vardenafil, and organic nitrovasodilators (e.g., and perhaps especially, nitroglycerin). It occurs because both interactants cause vasodilation through a nitric oxide-cGMP-dependent mechanism, and the combination causes greater than additive effects of each agent alone. It is also an interaction that should be foremost in the mind of any physician who prescribes one of these wildly popular drugs for erectile dysfunction. For more complete comments on the mechanisms and manifestations of the interaction, check the answer to Question 213 (cardiovascular chapter).

395. The answer is a. *(Craig, pp 748–749; Hardman, pp 1576–1578; Katzung, pp 630, 634–636.)* Levothyroxine is usually considered the first choice for long-term maintenance therapy of hypothyroidism, such as that which occurs after thyroidectomy or radiation therapy of the thyroid. Once absorbed, we get the slow-onset and rather steady, long-lasting effects of the T_4. In addition, much of the administered T_4 is physiologically deiodinated in the tissues to T_3, "automatically" providing usually adequate levels and effects of this more rapidly and shorter-acting hormone without the need to administer T_3 (liothyronine) separately.

If the patient develops profound hypothyroidism (e.g., myxedema), some clinicians may still prefer T_3 for its prompt effects. However, in this instance too, T_4 is generally regarded as the preferred way to replace both hormones and reestablish a euthyroid state (administered with corticosteroids for myxedema coma). Desiccated thyroid products are outmoded for managing hypothyroidism. Protirelin is a synthetic tripeptide, chemically identical to thyrotropin-releasing hormone (TRH), that is used to diagnose some thyroid disorders.

396. The answer is b. *(Craig, pp 754–756; Hardman, pp 1718–1720; Katzung, p 724.)* We're dealing with hypocalcemia in this patient with tetany postthyroidectomy, because the parathyroid gland was damaged or removed during the surgery. Administration of intravenous calcium gluconate would immediately correct the tetany. Parathyroid hormone is appropriate, but it has a slower onset of action that would not be of much help in a tetanic state. We would then probably use vitamin D and dietary modifications for long-control of serum calcium levels. Calcitonin is a hypocalcemic antagonist of parathyroid hormone. (Note that calcitonin or calcitriol will raise serum calcium levels faster than vitamin D, but in this emergent situation they will not work fast enough, which is why we need direct administration of ionic calcium.) Plicamycin (mithramycin) is used to treat Paget's disease and hypercalcemia. The dose employed is about one-tenth the amount used for plicamycin's cytotoxic action.

397. The answer is d. *(Craig, p 750; Hardman, p 1581; Katzung, pp 631–632.)* Propylthiouracil, a thioamide use to manage many patients with hyperthyroidism, has three main actions. It inhibits peroxidase, and in doing so inhibits oxidation of inorganic iodide to iodine, and the iodination of tyrosine. It also blocks coupling of iodotyrosines and inhibits deiodination of T_4 to T_3 in the periphery.

398. The answer is d. *(Craig, pp 704–707; Hardman, pp 1624–1625; Katzung, p 673–675.)* There are two main mechanisms by which OCs exert their main effects. Arguably the most important is inhibition of ovulation. This prevents (or reduces the risk of) fertilization, a process that must come before such others as impairing nidation (which implicitly means the ovum has been fertilized). The other is thickening of cervical mucus. That effect, mainly caused by the progestin component, provides a physical (rather than metabolic or pH-dependent) barrier that slows or stops sperm motility. It is not a spermicidal effect, per se.

399. The answer is a. *(Craig, p 708; Hardman, pp 1623–1624; Katzung, p 674.)* Ethinyl estradiol and mestranol are the estrogens found in combination OCs, and in the vast majority of products available ethinyl estradiol is the one you will find. Norethindrone (mainly, and less often norgestrel and other drugs, including ethynodiol diacetate and desogestrel) are the ingredients that provide the progestin component of the products.

400. The answer is b. (*Craig, pp 709–711; Hardman, pp 1625–1626; Katzung, p 675.*) Hypertension, which may occur (and usually transiently) in response to OCs, is mainly due to estrogen excess. Fatigue, weight gain (usually triggered by increased appetite), and hypomenorrhea are mainly associated with progestin excess. Hypomenorrhea may also be due to inadequate estrogen levels in the combination product. Unusually frequent menses—hypermenorrhea—tends to be related to too little progestin in the product.

401. The answer is c. (*Craig, p 710; Hardman, pp 1610, 1625–1626; Katzung, pp 673–678.*) Thromboembolism associated with OC administration is attributed to the estrogen component in these products. If thromboembolism is a concern, then one approach to reducing the risk would be selecting a product with a lower—not higher—estrogen dose. Even that may not be sufficient, long term. Progestins seem to have little impact on the development of thrombotic/embolic disorders during OC therapy, and so increasing or decreasing progestin content will do little more than nothing for most patients. Smoking is a major risk factor for thromboembolism, especially for women taking an oral contraceptive, so it's essential to encourage the patient to quit (or not start) smoking. There are no OCs that contain estrogen only [unlike the case with progestin-only OCs—the so-called minipills (Question 386)].

402. The answer is f. (*Craig, p 720; Hardman, p 231; Katzung, pp 135–138.*) Ritodrine, a predominantly β_2-selective adrenergic agonist, slows uterine contractions by that action. The sequence of events following binding of ritodrine to its receptor includes increased myometrial cAMP formation, activation of cAMP-dependent protein kinase, and extrusion of Ca^{2+} from smooth-muscle cells such that contractile force is reduced. There are no effects on oxytocin synthesis or release, nor on hypothalamic or pituitary function. Ritodrine's effects are not at all like those of ergot compounds (e.g., methylergonovine), which induce uterine contraction by a mechanism that involves α-adrenergic receptor activation. Be sure to understand that despite the classification of ritodrine as a "β_2-selective adrenergic agonist," or as a uterine relaxant, the drug can activate all β-adrenergic receptors and cause a host of unwanted side effects or adverse responses that include tachycardia (direct and reflexly, in response to reduced blood pressure), pulmonary edema, and myocardial ischemia. This very effective drug is contraindicated in eclampsia or severe eclampsia. In these situations the goal is to deliver the fetus (the definitive cure for eclampsia), not prolong labor.

403. The answer is a. *(Craig, pp 692, 693; Hardman, pp 1673–1674; Katzung, pp 647, 649–650.)* Of the drugs listed, dexamethasone is by far the most potent in terms of relative glucocorticoid effects. The dexamethasone suppression test has several uses: it allows not only complete suppression of pituitary ACTH production, but also accurate measurement of endogenous corticosteroids, such as 17-ketosteroids, in the urine. The small amount of dexamethasone present contributes minimally to this measurement.

Anti-Infectives

Antibacterials	Antivirals
Antimycobacterials	Antiprotozoals
Antifungals	

Questions

DIRECTIONS: Each item contains a question or incomplete statement that is followed by possible responses. Select the **one best** response to each question.

404. A 19-year-old being treated for leukemia develops a fever. You give several agents that will cover bacterial, viral, and fungal infections. Two days later, he develops acute renal failure. Which of the following drugs was most likely responsible?

a. Acyclovir
b. Amphotericin B
c. Ceftazidime
d. Penicillin G
e. Vancomycin

405. A 26-year-old woman with acquired immunodeficiency syndrome (AIDS) develops cryptococcal meningitis. She refuses intravenous medication. Which of the following antifungal agents is the best choice for oral therapy of the meningitis?

a. Amphotericin B
b. Fluconazole
c. Ketoconazole
d. Metronidazole
e. Nystatin

406. An adult patient is being treated with a parenteral aminoglycoside for a serious *Pseudomonas aeruginosa* infection. They require immediate surgery. They are premedicated with midazolam. A dose of succinylcholine is administered for intubation, with skeletal muscle paralysis maintained during surgery with pancuronium. Balanced anesthesia is maintained with nitrous oxide, isoflurane, and oxygen. Which of the following is the most likely outcome of having the aminoglycoside "on board" in the perioperative setting along with all these other drugs?

a. Acute hepatotoxicity from an aminoglycoside-isoflurane interaction
b. Antagonism of midazolam's amnestic and sedative effects
c. Enhanced aminoglycoside toxicity to host cells
d. Increased or prolonged response to neuromuscular blockers
e. Reduced risk of catecholamine-induced cardiac arrhythmias

407. A patient on antimicrobial therapy develops the following signs and symptoms that ultimately are found to be drug-induced: cough, dyspnea, and pulmonary infiltrates; neutropenia and bleeding tendencies; and paresthesias. Which of the following is the most likely cause of this patient's symptoms?

a. Amoxicillin
b. Azithromycin
c. Ciprofloxacin
d. Isoniazid
e. Nitrofurantoin

408. A patient requires an antibiotic that is most effective against *P. aeruginosa*. Which of the following is the quinolone of choice?

a. Ciprofloxacin
b. Enoxacin
c. Lomefloxacin
d. Norfloxacin
e. Ofloxacin

409. A 59-year-old woman is diagnosed with tuberculosis (TB). Before prescribing a drug regimen, you take a careful medication history because one of the drugs commonly used to treat TB induces microsomal cytochrome P450 enzymes in the liver. Which drug is it?

a. Ethambutol
b. Isoniazid
c. Pyrazinamide
d. Rifampin
e. Vitamin B$_6$

410. A patient is being treated with an antibiotic for a vancomycin-resistant enterococcal infection. They consume an over-the-counter medication containing ephedrine and develop a significant spike of blood pressure that leads to a pounding headache. They are transported to the hospital. As part of the work-up, blood tests indicate some bone marrow suppression. Which of the following antibiotics is most likely associated with this clinical picture?

a. Azithromycin
b. Ciprofloxacin
c. Erythromycin estolate
d. Gentamicin
e. Linezolid

411. A child who previously was healthy develops bacterial meningitis. Assuming no specific contraindications, which of the following is the drug of choice?

a. Ceftriaxone
b. Erythromycin
c. Penicillin G
d. Penicillin V
e. Procaine penicillin

412. In patients with hepatic coma, or portal-systemic encephalopathy, decreases in the production and absorption of ammonia from the gastrointestinal (GI) tract will be beneficial. Which of the following is the antibiotic of choice in this situation?

a. Cephalothin
b. Chloramphenicol
c. Neomycin
d. Penicillin G
e. Tetracycline

413. A patient has a severe infection caused by anaerobic bacteria. The first-year house officer writes an order for gentamicin. This approach is likely to have unwanted clinical outcomes because anaerobes:

a. Cannot metabolize the aminoglycosides, which are all prodrugs, to their bactericidal free radical forms
b. Cannot oxidatively metabolize aminoglycosides to moieties that are nontoxic to host cells
c. Lack molecular oxygen that is a prerequisite for drug binding to the 50S subunit of bacterial ribosomes
d. Lack the ability to transport aminoglycosides from the extracellular milieu
e. Synthesize more and more active resistance factors than do aerobic bacteria

414. The main reason that such agents as clavulanic acid, sulbactam, or tazobactam are added to some proprietary (manufactured) penicillin combination products is to:

a. Add antibiotic activity against *Pseudomonas* and many *Enterobacter* species
b. Facilitate antibiotic penetration into the central nervous system and cerebrospinal fluid
c. Inhibit cell wall transpeptidases
d. Inhibit inactivation of penicillin by β-lactamase-producing bacteria
e. Inhibit the normally significant hepatic metabolism of the penicillin
f. Reduce the risk and/or severity of allergic reactions in susceptible patients

415. A patient with active tuberculosis is being treated with isoniazid (INH) and ethambutol as part of the overall regimen. Which of the following is the main reason for including the ethambutol?

a. To facilitate entry of the INH into the mycobacteria
b. To facilitate penetration of the blood-brain barrier
c. To retard the development of organism resistance
d. To slow renal excretion of INH to help maintain effective blood levels
e. To retard absorption after intramuscular injection

416. As part of a multidrug attack on a patient's infection with *Mycobacterium tuberculosis,* a physician plans to use an aminoglycoside antibiotic. Which one of the following is most active against the tubercle bacillus and seems to be associated with the fewest problems with resistance or typical aminoglycoside-induced adverse effects?

a. Amikacin
b. Kanamycin
c. Neomycin
d. Streptomycin
e. Tobramycin

417. We are starting therapy for an established HIV infection in a 28-year-old man. The drugs are ritonavir, saquinavir, zidovudine, and didanosine. We are obviously using two protease inhibitors and two nucleoside reverse transcriptase inhibitors (NRTIs). Which of the following is the main purpose of using the ritonavir?

a. Help maintain adequate saquinavir levels by inhibiting its metabolism
b. Induce the metabolic activation of the NRTIs, which are prodrugs
c. Prevent the likely development of hypoglycemia
d. Reduce, or hopefully eliminate, saquinavir-mediated host toxicity
e. Serve as the main, most active, inhibitor of viral protease in this combination

418. A 55-year-old man has an infection with *Legionella pneumophila.* Assuming no contraindications, which of the following is the drug of choice?

a. Chloramphenicol
b. Erythromycin
c. Lincomycin
d. Penicillin G
e. Streptomycin

419. A 45-year-old man with recurrent asthma is being treated with oral theophylline and prednisone, supplemented with an adrenergic bronchodilator (e.g., albuterol), inhaled "as needed." He has been exposed to *Haemophilus influenzae* by a family member, and is started on rifampin for prophylaxis against getting the infection himself. Which of the following is the most likely outcome of adding the rifampin?

a. Failure of rifampin prophylaxis due to induction of its metabolism by the theophylline
b. Increased risk of theophylline toxicity
c. Loss of asthma control, onset of asthma signs and symptoms
d. Rapid development of cholestatic jaundice and liver failure from acute rifampin toxicity
e. Sudden sodium and fluid retention, weight gain, from impaired prednisone metabolism

420. Which of the following is the most effective agent in the treatment of *Rickettsia, Mycoplasma,* and *Chlamydia* infections?

a. Bacitracin
b. Gentamicin
c. Penicillin G
d. Tetracycline
e. Vancomycin

421. A patient with tuberculosis is started on isoniazid (INH). The physician starts therapy with vitamin B_6 at the same time. The main reason for giving the vitamin B_6 is that it:

a. Is a cofactor required for activity of INH
b. Prevents some adverse effects of INH therapy
c. Potentiates the antitubercular activity of the INH
d. Inhibits metabolism of INH, thereby increasing INH blood levels
e. Facilitates INH renal excretion, thereby protecting against nephrotoxicity

422. You are taking an initial health history from a 22-year-old woman who just moved to your town. She is remarkably fit and healthy, but is wearing two hearing aids for binaural (bilateral) high-frequency hearing loss. You inquire about the possible reason(s) for this. She says she lost most of her hearing after receiving an antibiotic for a severe infection when she was 19, but cannot recall the specific drug. Which of the following drugs was most likely responsible for her hearing loss?

a. Aminoglycoside (e.g., gentamicin)
b. Cephalosporin, first-generation
c. Cephalosporin, third-generation
d. Fluoroquinolone (e.g., ciprofloxacin)
e. Penicillin

423. Streptomycin and other aminoglycosides inhibit bacterial protein synthesis by binding to which of the following?

a. 30S ribosomal particles
b. DNA
c. mRNA
d. Peptidoglycan units in the cell wall
e. RNA polymerase

424. Which cephalosporin would have increased activity against anaerobic bacteria such as *Bacteroides fragilis?*

a. Cefaclor
b. Cefoxitin
c. Cefuroxime
d. Cephalexin
e. Cephalothin

425. Amantadine, used prophylactically against influenza A_2, is thought to act by:

a. Preventing production of viral capsid protein
b. Preventing virion release
c. Preventing penetration of the virus into the host cell
d. Preventing uncoating of viral DNA
e. Causing lysis of infected host cells by release of intracellular lysosomal enzymes

426. A 30-year-old man with a 2-year history of chronic renal failure requiring dialysis consents to transplantation. A donor kidney becomes available. He is given cyclosporine to prevent transplant rejection. Which of the following is the most likely adverse effect of this drug?

a. Bone marrow depression
b. Nephrotoxicity
c. Oral and GI ulceration
d. Pancreatitis
e. Seizures

427. Narrow spectrum penicillins—both penicillinase-sensitive and -resistant—have relatively poor activity against gram-negative bacteria. In general, that is because resistant gram-negative bacteria:

a. Actively transport any absorbed penicillin back to the extracellular space
b. Have an outer membrane that serves as a physical barrier to the penicillins
c. Lack a surface enzyme necessary to metabolically activate the penicillins
d. Lack penicillin-binding proteins
e. Metabolically inactivate these penicillins by mechanisms not involving β-lactamase

428. A patient with a *P. aeruginosa* infection is receiving intravenous gentamicin. The aminoglycoside blood levels are well above the minimum inhibitory concentration (MIC), but the clinical response is not satisfactory. A new medication order calls for adding a penicillin, administered in a separate IV line to avoid a physical incompatibility. If this order is carried out, which of the following will occur?

a. The aminoglycoside will inactivate the penicillin
b. The aminoglycoside will chemically neutralize and abolish the effects of the penicillin
c. The patient is likely to develop *Clostridium difficile* colitis (superinfection)
d. The penicillin will enhance the bacterial response to the aminoglycoside
e. The penicillin will increase the risk of aminoglycoside nephrotoxicity
f. The risk of inducing resistance to both drugs increases dramatically

429. A patient's history notes a documented severe (anaphylactoid) reaction to a penicillin. What other antibiotic or class is likely to cross-react and so should be avoided in this patient?

a. Aminoglycosides
b. Azithromycin
c. Cephalosporins
d. Erythromycin
e. Linezolid
f. Tetracyclines

430. A man who has been at the local tavern, drinking alcohol heavily, is assaulted. He is transported to the hospital. Among various findings is an infection for which prompt antibiotic therapy is indicated. Given his high blood alcohol level, which antibiotic(s) should be avoided because of a high potential of causing a serious disulfiram-like reaction that might provoke ventilatory or cardiovascular failure? Assume that were it not for the alcohol consumption, the antibiotic prescribed would be suitable for the infectious organisms that have been detected.

a. Amoxicillin
b. Cefoperazone or cefotetan
c. Erythromycin ethylsuccinate
d. Linezolid
e. Penicillin G

431. Which property or action is shared by the penicillins, the cephalosporins, and amphotericin B?

a. Act, though various mechanisms, on cell walls or membranes of susceptible organisms
b. Contraindicated in immunocompromised patients
c. Interact with many drugs by inducing their hepatic metabolism
d. Leukopenia (increased white cell counts) is a common side effect
e. Nephrotoxicity precludes use in patients with impaired renal function

432. Compared with virtually all the other penicillins, ticarcillin poses a greater risk of which of the following?

a. Acute renal failure
b. Bronchoconstriction, bronchospasm, asthma
c. Fever, arthralgia, and other signs of a lupus-like syndrome
d. Hypertension, hypervolemia, and bleeding
e. Inducing penicillinase and causing resistance

433. Members of the rifamycin antibiotic family (e.g., rifampin) are involved in a significant number of drug interactions because they:

a. Displace other drugs from their plasma protein-binding sites
b. Induce resistance to many other drugs by stimulating antibody formation
c. Induce the hepatic microsomal drug-metabolizing enzymes
d. Markedly increase glomerular filtration rates and excretion of the interactants
e. Reduce oral absorption and bioavailability of many drugs via a pH-dependent action in the stomach

434. Compared with most other cephalosporins, the administration of cefmetazole, cefoperazone, or cefotetan is associated with a higher incidence of which of the following?

a. Acute heart failure
b. Acute renal failure
c. Bleeding tendencies in patients taking warfarin
d. Hypertension
e. Ototoxicity
f. Severe allergic reactions in patients with mild penicillin allergies

Questions 435–436

The next two questions (435 and 436) relate to a patient receiving antimicrobial drug therapy and who develops antibiotic-associated pseudomembranous colitis (AAPMC).

435. Given the relative risks of AAPMC, which of the following drugs is most likely to have caused it?

a. Amoxicillin
b. Azithromycin
c. Clindamycin
d. Metronidazole
e. Trimethoprim plus sulfamethoxazole

436. The patient develops profuse, watery diarrhea, fever, abdominal pain, and leukocytosis. *C. difficile* infection in the gut is confirmed. Preferred antimicrobial therapy for this antibiotic-associated pseudomembranous colitis is which of the following?

a. Amoxicillin
b. Azithromycin
c. Clindamycin
d. Metronidazole
e. Trimethoprim plus sulfamethoxazole

437. A 30-year-old woman develops a severe *P. aeruginosa* infection. The physician chooses to treat it with amikacin, not with gentamicin. Amikacin differs from gentamicin mainly in that it:

a. Does not require monitoring of blood levels during therapy
b. Exerts significant bactericidal effects against anaerobes too
c. Has broadest spectrum against gram-negative bacilli
d. Lacks ototoxic potential
e. Protects against typical aminoglycoside nephrotoxicity

438. A patient with an infectious disease routinely takes their antimicrobial medication with milk or other dairy products in an attempt to reduce stomach upset from the drug. This is most likely to lead to therapeutic failure if the drug is which of the following?

a. Aminoglycoside
b. Antimycobacterial drug, specifically isoniazid
c. Cephalosporin, first generation
d. Cephalosporin, third generation
e. Penicillin
f. Tetracycline

439. A patient with an opportunistic infection with *Pneumocystis carinii* is receiving a combination of sulfamethoxazole (SMZ) and trimethoprim (TMP). The mechanism by which this combination exerts its desired effects—and does so better than if just one of the drugs was administered—is which of the following?

a. The combination exerts significant antiviral activity, thereby reducing the risk of opportunistic *P. carinii* infections during antiviral therapy with other medications
b. The SMZ permeabilizes bacterial cell walls, allowing better penetration of the TMP
c. They inhibit sequential steps in bacterial synthesis of tetrahydrofolic acid
d. TMP inhibits normal transmission of resistance factors directed against SMZ
e. TMP kills gut flora that otherwise would reduce oral bioavailability of the SMZ

440. When considering all the main antibacterial drugs that work by inhibiting protein synthesis in one way or another, virtually every one exerts bacteriostatic actions. Which differs in that the usual outcome of therapeutic serum levels is bactericidal?

a. Aminoglycosides
b. Clindamycin
c. Erythromycins
d. Linezolid
e. Tetracyclines

441. A patient with AIDS is treated with a combination of agents, one of which is zidovudine. This drug exerts its main effects by inhibiting which of the following?

a. Nonnucleoside reverse transcriptase
b. Nucleoside reverse transcriptase
c. RNA synthesis
d. Viral particle assembly
e. Viral proteases

442. A 39-year-old man with aortic insufficiency and a history of multiple antibiotic resistances is given a prophylactic intravenous dose of antibiotic before surgery to insert a prosthetic heart valve. As the antibiotic is being infused, the patient becomes flushed over most of his body. Which of the following antibiotics is most likely responsible?

a. Erythromycin
b. Gentamicin
c. Penicillin G
d. Tetracycline
e. Vancomycin

443. An 86-year-old man complains of cough and blood in his sputum for the past 2 days. On admission, his temperature is 103°F. Physical examination reveals rales in his right lung, and x-ray examination shows increased density in the right middle lobe. A sputum smear shows many gram-positive cocci, confirmed by sputum culture as penicillinase-producing *Staphylococcus aureus*. Which of the following agents should be given?

a. Ampicillin
b. Carbenicillin
c. Mezlocillin
d. Oxacillin
e. Ticarcillin

444. Which of the following drugs is primarily used in pneumonia caused by *P. carinii*?

a. Carbenicillin
b. Metronidazole
c. Nifurtimox
d. Penicillin G
e. Pentamidine

Questions 445–446

The numbered questions below describe a patient with a stated infection, and a drug that is given for it. Select the letter, from the options below, that correctly states the mechanism by which the antimicrobial drug works against the stated organism. Each letter may be used once, more than once, or not at all.

Select the process that is directly *inhibited* by the drug given to the patients described below:

a. Cell-wall synthesis
b. Protein synthesis
c. Folic acid synthesis
d. Topoisomerase II (DNA gyrase)
e. DNA polymerase

445. A 39-year-old woman with a history of chronic UTI develops a new infection with *Escherichia coli* that is sensitive to levofloxacin.

446. A 25-year-old woman with a sinus infection caused by *Haemophilus influenzae* is treated with trimethoprim-sulfamethoxazole.

447. The main reason for avoiding chloramphenicol in the vast majority of infectious diseases is an unacceptably high incidence of causing which of the following?

a. Aplastic anemia
b. Hepatotoxicity
c. Interstitial nephritis
d. Pulmonary fibrosis
e. Torsade de pointes or ventricular fibrillation

448. A 27-year-old woman has just returned from a trip to Southeast Asia. Over the past 24 h she has developed shaking, chills, and a temperature of 104°F. A blood smear reveals *Plasmodium vivax*. Which of the following agents should be used to eradicate the extraerythrocytic phase of the organism?

a. Chloroguanide
b. Chloroquine
c. Primaquine
d. Pyrimethamine
e. Quinacrine

449. A young boy presents with infestation with *Taenia saginata* (tapeworm). Which of the following is the most appropriate drug to administer?

a. Ceftriaxone
b. Chloroquine
c. Mebendazole
d. Niclosamide
e. Primaquine

450. Ampicillin and amoxicillin are in the same group of penicillins. However, compared with ampicillin, amoxicillin differs in which of the following ways?

a. Has better oral bioavailability, particularly when taken with meals
b. Is effective against penicillinase-producing organisms
c. Is a broad-spectrum penicillin
d. Does not cause hypersensitivity reactions
e. Has great antipseudomonal activity

451. A jaundiced 1-day-old premature infant with an elevated free bilirubin is seen in the premature baby nursery. The mother had received an antibiotic combination for a urinary tract infection (UTI) 1 week before delivery. Which of the following is the most likely cause of the baby's kernicterus?

a. A fourth-generation cephalosporin
b. An aminopenicillin (e.g., amoxicillin)
c. Azithromycin
d. Erythromycin
e. A sulfonamide
f. A tetracycline

452. A sputum culture of a 65-year-old man with pneumonia is positive for β-lactamase-positive staphylococci. Which of the following is the best choice of penicillin therapy in this patient?

a. Ampicillin
b. Carbenicillin
c. Oxacillin
d. Penicillin G
e. Ticarcillin

453. A 35-year-old woman complains of itching in the vulval area. Hanging-drop examination of the urine reveals trichomonads. Which of the following is the preferred treatment for the trichomoniasis?

a. Doxycycline
b. Emetine
c. Metronidazole
d. Pentamidine
e. Pyrimethamine

454. A 40-year-old man is HIV-positive with a cluster-of-differentiation-4 (CD4) count of 200/mm^3. Within 2 months he develops a peripheral white blood cell count of 1000/mm^3 and a hemoglobin of 9.0 mg/dL. Which of the following drugs most likely caused the hematologic abnormalities?

a. Acyclovir
b. Dideoxycytidine
c. Foscarnet
d. Rimantadine
e. Zidovudine

455. A 75-year-old man has a fever of 104°F. He develops a cough that produces blood-tinged sputum with gram-positive cocci in clusters. A chest x-ray shows increased density in the right upper lobe. Which penicillin is likely to fail to treat this infection adequately?

a. Cloxacillin
b. Dicloxacillin
c. Nafcillin
d. Oxacillin
e. Ticarcillin

456. A 50-year-old man with type 2 diabetes develops an external otitis from which *Pseudomonas* organisms are cultured. Topical therapy with polymyxin is effective. The drug's efficacy was due to its ability to:

a. Disrupt membrane permeability
b. Form reactive products that interfere with DNA replication
c. Inactivate bacterial protein sulfhydryl groups
d. Inhibit cell-wall synthesis
e. Inhibit protein synthesis by binding to tRNA

457. A patient will be started on primaquine to treat active *Plasmodium vivax* malaria, specifically to target the hepatic forms of the parasite. Before you administer the drug you should screen the patient to assess their relative risk of developing which of the following "most common and severe" adverse responses to the primaquine?

a. Cardiac conduction disturbances
b. Hemolytic disease
c. Nephrotoxicity
d. Retinopathy
e. Seizures, convulsions

Anti-Infectives

Answers

404. The answer is b. (*Craig, pp 597–598; Hardman, pp 1298–1299; Katzung, pp 792–794.*) Amphotericin B, given intravenously, often alters kidney function. The most common and most easily detected manifestation of this is decreased creatinine clearance. If this occurs, the dose must be reduced. Amphotericin B also commonly increases potassium (K^+) loss, leading to hypokalemia; and can cause anemia and neurologic symptoms. A liposomal preparation of amphotericin B may reduce the incidence of renal and neurologic toxicity. Vancomycin may cause renal damage, but the overall incidence is lower, the severity less.

405. The answer is b. (*Craig, pp 598–599; Hardman, pp 1304–1305, 1147, 1296; Katzung, p 797.*) Fluconazole penetrates into cerebrospinal fluid, where it is exerts good antifungal activity against *Cryptococcus neoformans*. When it is given orally, blood levels are almost as high as when it is given parenterally. Amphotericin is administered intravenously and even when given intrathecally does not appear to be highly effective in fungal meningitis.

406. The answer is d. (*Craig, pp 541–542; Hardman, p 1230; Katzung, pp 440, 767–768.*) Aminoglycosides, at sufficiently high serum levels, can cause skeletal neuromuscular blockade in their own right. This probably arises from a combination of effects: inhibition of neuronal ACh release and perhaps direct blockade of nicotinic receptors on skeletal muscle. This would add to and prolong the effects of both neuromuscular blockers the patient has received. In addition, isoflurane and other halogenated hydrocarbon volatile liquid anesthetics have some neuromuscular blocking effects in their own right—but not to a degree that is sufficient to obviate the need for succinylcholine and/or nondepolarizing blockers when skeletal muscle paralysis is indicated. So here we have a combination of drugs that affect skeletal muscle activation.

The greatest concern, of course, would be the prolongation of neuromuscular blockade. A "greater degree" of paralysis is largely inconsequential, so long as ventilation is supported. It is the prolonged blockade—and especially the *return* of skeletal muscle weakening and ventilatory insufficiency after mechanical ventilation has been discontinued and additional doses of aminoglycoside are given—which poses the greatest risk if the patient had already been taken off ventilatory support.

(Note, too, in your studies, that some other antimicrobials seem to have some skeletal neuromuscular blocking activity, including polymyxin B and clindamycin.)

You should recall that although such agents as isoflurane and other halogenated hydrocarbon volatile liquid anesthetics may potentiate the effects of a neuromuscular blocker, once they are eliminated (that occurs rather rapidly when inhalation is stopped) there is no added risk of prolonged or greater skeletal muscle weakness or paralysis.

We should add that in settings (e.g., hospitals) where the overall incidence of aminoglycoside resistance is low (or in the absence of documented resistance to a particular aminoglycoside in a particular patient), tobramycin or gentamicin is usually the aminoglycoside of choice. Amikacin should be reserved for situations where there is proven resistance to the alternatives.

As with other aminoglycosides, periodic monitoring of peak and trough serum levels is essential to help insure optimal antibiotic effects while reducing the risk of ototoxicity and nephrotoxicity—both of which can be caused by any aminoglycoside (although with varying relative risks). No aminoglycoside has "nephroprotective" effects.

Finally, no aminoglycoside can kill anaerobes.

407. The answer is e. (*Craig, pp 64, 521; Hardman, pp 1181–1185; Katzung, p 829.*) Although several of the antimicrobial agents listed here can cause one (or perhaps two) of the adverse responses noted here, nitrofurantoin is the most likely cause. GI side effects (anorexia, nausea, vomiting) are the most common side effects caused by this drug, which is still widely used for managing acute lower urinary tract infections (e.g., from many strains of *E. coli*, staphylococci, streptococci, *Neisseria, Bacteroides*). However, the drug can also cause acute or subacute pulmonary reactions such as those described, various hematologic reactions (in particular, leukopenia and thrombocytopenia), and peripheral sensory and motor neuropathies.

Amoxicillin—and most other penicillins—may cause central neurotoxicity if present at extraordinarily high serum levels. Beyond that, allergic reactions are the most important adverse responses. Pulmonary, hematologic, and peripheral neuropathic adverse responses are not associated with these drugs.

Azithromycin's profile of adverse effects is quite similar to that of erythromycin and other macrolides, and that profile does not include the signs and symptoms noted here (GI upset, mild to severe, are the most common complaints, and azithromycin may be ototoxic, a property not shared by other macrolides).

Ciprofloxacin (or other fluoroquinolones) is not likely to cause any of the adverse responses noted. They are quite well tolerated and cause a variety of side effects that, in general, are mild. If one were to recall one "unique" toxicity, it would be alterations of collagen metabolism that may lead to tendon rupture.

Isoniazid can cause peripheral neuropathy (mainly from a drug-induced pyridoxine deficiency) and hepatotoxicity. Pulmonary and bleeding problems are not at all common in terms of drug-induced problems.

408. The answer is a. (*Craig, pp 519–520; Hardman, p 1183; Katzung, pp 777–780.*) Ciprofloxacin is highly effective against *P. aeruginosa*. Others in the fluroquinolone class have less activity toward *P. aeruginosa*, although they are effective against many other common gram-negative organisms.

409. The answer is d. (*Craig, pp 37, 559; Hardman, pp 1163, 1250, 1279, 1303; Katzung, p 1123.*) Rifampin induces cytochrome P450 enzymes, which causes a significant increase in elimination of drugs, such as oral contraceptives, anticoagulants, ketoconazole, cyclosporine, and chloramphenicol. It also promotes urinary excretion of methadone, which may precipitate withdrawal.

410. The answer is e. (*Katzung, p 762.*) There are several pieces of information you should link together to help arrive at the answer, for which a relatively new drug is the correct answer. (1) Although linezolid has several uses, it is best reserved for vancomycin-resistant enterococci (VRE) and methicillin-resistant *S. aureus* (MRSA) infections. (It's seldom a first-line antibiotic because of the risk of resistance.) (2) Linezolid is occasionally linked to bone marrow suppression that is usually reversible upon discontinuation of the drug. (Granted, such other antibiotics as chloramphenicol pose greater risks of bone marrow suppression, but this property is nonetheless associated with linezolid.) (3) The third piece of evidence is the rise of blood pressure in response to ephedrine, a mixed-acting sympathomimetic that works, in part, by releasing neuronal norepinephrine. Linezolid has monoamine oxidase inhibitory activity (albeit relatively weak compared with traditional MAO inhibitors). Piece these three lines of evidence together and the only reasonable choice is linezolid.

411. The answer is a. (*Craig, pp 531–533; Katzung, pp 745–746.*) Penicillins were used in the treatment of meningitis because of their ability to pass across an inflamed blood-brain barrier. The third-generation cephalosporin, ceftriaxone, is preferred because it is effective against β-lactamase producing strains of *H. influenzae* that may cause meningitis in children.

412. The answer is c. (*Craig, pp 539, 540; Katzung, p 770.*) Neomycin, an aminoglycoside, is not significantly absorbed from the GI tract. After oral administration, the intestinal flora is suppressed or modified and the drug is excreted in the feces. This effect of neomycin is used in hepatic coma to decrease the coliform flora, thus decreasing the production of ammonia and reducing levels of free nitrogen in the bloodstream. Other antimicrobial agents (e.g., tetracycline, penicillin G, chloramphenicol, and cephalothin) do not have the potency of neomycin in causing this effect.

413. The answer is d. (*Craig, pp 539–540; Hardman, pp 1221–1222; Katzung, pp 764–767.*) Aminoglycosides, which are mainly used for parenteral therapy of severe infections from aerobic gram-negative bacilli (e.g., *E. coli, Serratia, Klebsiella*), require oxygen in order for the drug to be transported across the bacterial cell membrane. Such incorporation is necessary for these drugs to exert their bactericidal effects, which arise from binding to the 30S subunit of susceptible bacteria. Ultimately the aminoglycoside-ribosomal binding leads to premature termination of bacterial protein synthesis and the formation of abnormal bacterial proteins. Such abnormal proteins ultimately insert into the bacterial cell membrane, causing leakiness and cell death.

The aminoglycosides are not prodrugs, and so metabolism (whether aerobic or otherwise) is not necessary for the formation of an active drug; formation of an oxygen free radical or an aminoglycoside free radical has nothing to do with their antibiotic effects. Moreover, metabolism by host cells is not an important process in the elimination of aminoglycosides, nor of reducing host cell toxicity (e.g., to the kidneys or auditory nerve). Renal excretion is the main route of elimination for these drugs, which explains why renal function is such an important consideration in dosing adjustments.

Clearly, both aerobic and anaerobic bacteria can elaborate resistance factors (or develop resistance in other ways) to a variety of antibiotic classes. From a clinical viewpoint, the presence or absence of molecular oxygen is not a crucial or even relevant issue in this matter, however.

414. The answer is d. *(Craig, p 530; Hardman, pp 1214–1215; Katzung, pp 747–788.)* These agents are inhibitors of penicillinase (β-lactamase) and are used in conjunction with β-lactamase-sensitive penicillins to potentiate their activity. These drugs are found in several brand-name fixed-dose penicillin combination products (amoxicillin and clavulanic acid; sulbactam with ampicillin; tazobactam with piperacillin). Clavulanic acid is an irreversible inhibitor. These agents do not, per se, add activity against *Pseudomonas* or *Enterobacter* (an activity already possessed by piperacillin but not by ampicillin or amoxicillin). Likewise, they have no intrinsic effect to facilitate entry into the CNS or CSF. They do not inhibit hepatic metabolism of the penicillins, and you should recall that renal excretion (not metabolism) is the main pathway for penicillin elimination. Importantly, the penicillinase inhibitors have absolutely no impact on the risks or severities of allergic reactions to penicillins.

415. The answer is c. *(Craig, p 560; Hardman, pp 1279–1280; Katzung, pp 785–786.)* An important problem in the chemotherapy of TB is bacterial drug resistance. For this reason, concurrent administration of two or more drugs should be employed to delay the development of resistance. Ethambutol is often given along with INH for this purpose. Streptomycin or rifampin may also be added to the regimen to delay even further the development of drug resistance.

416. The answer is d. *(Craig, pp 541, 560; Hardman, pp 1231, 1280–1281, 1285; Katzung, p 786.)* Streptomycin is bactericidal for the tubercle bacillus organism. Other aminoglycosides (e.g., gentamicin, tobramycin, neomycin, amikacin, and kanamycin) have activity against this organism but are seldom used clinically because of toxicity or development of resistance.

417. The answer is a. (*Craig, pp 590–592; Hardman, pp 1369–1371; Katzung, pp 816–819.*) Ritonavir is a powerful inhibitor of the liver's P450 system. Ritonavir is used in combination with saquinavir solely to inhibit saquinavir's metabolism, thereby keeping serum concentrations in a therapeutic range longer. Ritonavir does have protease inhibitory activation, but in this combination it is the saquinavir that is causing the main therapeutic effect. The protease inhibitors do not cause hypoglycemia, nor does ritonavir reduce the ability of saquinavir to alter serum glucose levels. In fact, whether used alone or in combination, the protease inhibitors typically cause hyperglycemia (and may cause clinical diabetes mellitus), and quite often raise serum cholesterol and triglycerides levels too.

The NRTIs (zidovudine, didanosine) are, indeed, prodrugs that must be metabolically activated to the triphosphate form in order to serve as a substrate for reverse transcriptase. However, the protease inhibitors do not facilitate that metabolism.

418. The answer is b. (*Craig, p 548; Hardman, pp 1251, 1254; Katzung, pp 758–760.*) Erythromycin, a macrolide antibiotic, was initially designed to be used in penicillin-sensitive patients with streptococcal or pneumococcal infections. Erythromycin has become the drug of choice for the treatment of pneumonia caused by *Mycoplasma* and *Legionella*.

419. The answer is c. (*Craig, pp 37, 559; Hardman, p 1279; Katzung, p 1123.*) Rifampin is an excellent example of a drug that induces the hepatic metabolism of many other drugs, thereby lowering blood levels (and effects) of its interactants. Theophylline and corticosteroids are among them. Thus, as a result of the interaction we would expect decreases—not increases—in the effects of theophylline and/or of the prednisone. Both are susceptible to the metabolizing-inducing effects of rifampin.

With the expected decline in blood levels of both the oral bronchodilator (theophylline) and the anti-inflammatory drug (prednisone), it is likely that control of the patient's asthma will be lost and symptoms will appear.

Absorbed rifampin is rapidly eliminated in the bile and undergoes enterohepatic recirculation. However, there is no reason to suspect that either the theophylline, the corticosteroid, or their combination would have effects on rifamycin elimination. Likewise, these drugs do not increase the risk of rifampin-induced hepatotoxicity, which is quite rare unless the patient is taking other hepatotoxic drugs or has pre-existing liver disease.

420. The answer is d. (*Craig, pp 545–546; Katzung, pp 755–758.*) Tetracycline is one of the drugs of choice in the treatment of *Rickettsia, Mycoplasma,* and *Chlamydia* infections. The antibiotics that act by inhibiting cell-wall synthesis have no effect on *Mycoplasma* because the organism does not possess a cell wall; penicillin G, vancomycin, and bacitracin will be ineffective. Gentamicin has little or no antimicrobial activity with these organisms.

421. The answer is b. (*Craig, pp 558–559; Hardman, pp 1276–1277; Katzung, pp 782–784.*) Isoniazid (INH) inhibits cell-wall synthesis in mycobacteria. Increasing vitamin B_6 levels prevents complications associated with this inhibition, including peripheral neuritis, insomnia, restlessness, muscle twitching, urinary retention, convulsions, and psychosis, without affecting the antimycobacterial activity of INH.

422. The answer is a. (*Craig, pp 541–542; Hardman, pp 1227–1229; Katzung, pp 767–768.*) Aminoglycosides (gentamicin, tobramycin, others) are classic examples of ototoxic drugs, and they can affect both branches of the eighth cranial nerve.

The risks of aminoglycoside-induced ototoxicity (and nephrotoxicity) are among the reasons why it is important to keep an eye on peak and trough drug levels during therapy, adjust dosages accordingly, and avoid concomitant use of other ototoxic drugs. That is because the hearing loss is blood level–dependent (as opposed to being an idiosyncratic or allergic reaction). Aminoglycoside-induced ototoxicity is usually irreversible. The risk and severity of hearing loss from aminoglycosides are increased if they are administered with other ototoxic drugs (below).

Recall that there are two main forms of drug-induced ototoxicity. Cochlear toxicity includes hearing loss, tinnitus ("ringing in the ears"), or occasionally both. Hearing loss may also occur with loop diuretics (particularly ethacrynic acid), *cis*-platinum, and the vinca alkaloids (anticancer drugs). These drugs are intrinsically ototoxic; use one or more of them together or with an aminoglycoside and the risk of ototoxicity increases greatly.

Tinnitus (usually reversible) is typically associated with such drugs as aspirin (and, possibly, some other NSAIDs) and quinidine.

The other main form of ototoxicity is vestibular toxicity, which is typically manifest as balance and gait problems, vertigo, and nausea resulting from vestibular apparatus dysfunction.

Nephrotoxicity may develop during or after the use of an aminoglycoside. It is generally more common in the elderly when there is preexisting renal dysfunction. In most patients, renal function gradually improves after discontinuation of therapy. Aminoglycosides rarely cause neuromuscular blockade that can lead to progressive flaccid paralysis and potential fatal respiratory arrest. Hypersensitivity and dermatologic reactions occasionally occur following use of aminoglycosides.

None of the other antibiotics listed are linked to ototoxicity, whether from excessive blood levels or due to a hypersensitivity or true allergic reaction. Azithromycin (not an answer choice) is, however, another antibiotic for which there is growing evidence of a link to sudden onset hearing loss. The mechanism is unknown, and the incidence is neither dose-dependent nor predictable.

423. The answer is a. (*Craig, pp 538–539; Hardman, pp 1221–1222; Katzung, p 764.*) The bactericidal activity of streptomycin and other aminoglycosides involves a direct action on the 30S ribosomal subunit, the site at which these agents both inhibit protein synthesis and diminish the accuracy of translation of the genetic code. Proteins containing improper sequences of amino acids (known as *nonsense proteins*) are often nonfunctional.

424. The answer is b. (*Katzung, p 745.*) Cefoxitin and cefmetazole are suitable for treating intraabdominal infections, which are caused by mixtures of aerobic and anaerobic gram-negative bacteria like *B. fragilis*. Cefoxitin alone has been shown to be as effective as the traditional therapy of clindamycin plus gentamicin.

425. The answer is d. (*Craig, p 575; Hardman, pp 1328–1329; Katzung, p 824.*) Amantadine's mechanism of action involves inhibition of uncoating of the influenza A viral DNA. The primary target is the membrane M2 protein. The drug does not affect penetration and DNA-dependent RNA polymerase activity. Amantadine both reduces the frequency of illness and diminishes the serologic response to influenza infection. The drug has no action, however, on influenza B. As a weak base, amantadine buffers the pH of endosomes, thus blocking the fusion of the viral envelope with the membrane of the endosome.

426. The answer is b. (*Craig, p 659; Hardman, p 1469; Katzung, pp 589, 941.*) Nephrotoxicity may occur in almost three-quarters of patients treated with cyclosporine. Regular monitoring of blood levels can reduce the incidence of adverse effects.

427. The answer is b. (*Craig, pp 527–530; Hardman, pp 1190–1193; Katzung, pp 734–736.*) Both susceptible and resistant gram-negative and gram-positive bacteria have penicillin-binding proteins (PBPs). Resistance to the narrow spectrum penicillins by gram-negative bacteria arises from the presence of an outer membrane with pores that are too small to allow adequate penetration of the drug and access to the PBPs. Thus, we are dealing with what amounts to a physical barrier to the drug.

Most penicillins (with few exceptions, such as bacampicillin) are active in the form in which they are administered (i.e., they are not prodrugs), and so no subsequent metabolic activation is required.

428. The answer is d. (*Craig, p 540; Hardman, pp 1221–1222, 1231–1232; Katzung, p 768.*) The rationale behind this combination is that penicillins essentially weaken the cell walls of susceptible bacteria, which in turn facilitates access of the aminoglycoside to its site of action, the bacterial ribosomes. This usually provides better antibiotic response than with either antibiotic used alone, and with the aminoglycoside, serum levels aren't necessarily so high that they are more likely to cause ototoxicity, nephrotoxicity, or other adverse responses.

You should also recall at least two other things: (1) the penicillin in this combination is usually an extended-spectrum penicillin, such as ticarcillin; and (2) as we specifically noted in the question, the administration of these drugs is by separate IV lines. That is because if the two drugs were mixed together in sufficiently high concentrations, the penicillin may chemically inactivate the gentamicin.

429. The answer is c. (*Craig, pp 530–531, 533; Hardman, pp 1203–1205; Katzung, p 747.*) Unless there are no reasonable alternatives, cephalosporins should be avoided for patients with prior severe responses to penicillins because of their cross-reactivity. None of the other drugs or drug groups listed here cross-react in penicillin-sensitive patients.

430. The answer is b. (*Craig, p 533; Hardman, pp 1212–1213; Katzung, p 375, 1112.*) Cefoperazone (third-generation cephalosporin) or cefotetan (second-generation) inhibit aldehyde dehydrogenase and cause accumulation of acetaldehyde (as does disulfiram), and so can cause all the typical and potentially serious consequences of a disulfiram-like reaction. Cefmetazole, a second-generation cephalosporin, also causes a similar adverse interaction with alcohol. (Note that these three cephalosporins are also the ones that are associated with vitamin K-related bleeding problems, as addressed in Question 434.)

Erythromycin (whether administered as the base or one of the common salts, e.g., ethylsuccinate, estolate, or stearate) can inhibit the hepatic P450 system sufficient to cause adverse interactions with (excessive effects of) such drugs as warfarin, carbamazepine, and theophylline. However, based on current evidence there is no specific inhibition of aldehyde dehydrogenase, nor resulting accumulation of acetaldehyde, that would correctly qualify as a disulfiram-like interaction.

Amoxicillin, penicillin G, and other penicillins do not participate in disulfiram-like reactions.

Linezolid inhibits monoamine oxidase (MAO), albeit weakly, and so can trigger potentially significant adverse interactions in persons receiving such sympathomimetics as cocaine, ephedrine, or pseudoephedrine. However, the drug does not inhibit alcohol metabolism or cause the adverse responses noted in this question.

431. The answer is a. (*Craig, pp 527, 531, 596–597; Hardman, pp 1190–1192, 1298; Katzung, pp 734, 742, 793.*) Penicillins, cephalosporins, and amphotericin B exert their desired clinical effects by altering the structure or function of cell walls of susceptible organisms. Penicillins interfere with bacterial cell wall synthesis: their β-lactam structures bind to and inhibit normal enzymatic function of transpeptidases that provide susceptible bacteria with cell walls that are capable of maintaining an osmotically stable intracellular milieu. Cephalosporins, by virtue of their β-lactam ring, work in essentially the same way. Amphotericin B (a polyene antifungal drug) binds to ergosterol in the fungal cell membrane; the ultimate outcome is increased cell permeability. Nonetheless, the ultimate effect is osmotic instability of the organism, leading to cell death.

Neither penicillins, cephalosporins, or amphotericin B are contraindicated in patients with immunodeficiencies. Indeed, they may play a key role in managing opportunistic infections in such patients.

They do not induce the metabolism of other drugs, or interact in most of the typical pharmacokinetic ways. They do not trigger leukopenia.

Amphotericin B can cause decreased platelet counts and leukopenia, but this is rare. The most common hematologic adverse response to this drug is a normochromic, normocytic anemia. Penicillins and cephalosporins do not share these properties.

Finally, you should know that amphotericin B is clearly nephrotoxic. When given intravenously, renal dysfunction is the most serious and most common long-term manifestation of this antifungal drug's toxic spectrum. Penicillins and cephalosporins are not nephrotoxic.

(You might also want to recall that the new lipid formulations of amphotericin B—amphotericin B colloidal dispersion, liposomal amphotericin B, and a lipid complex of the drug—apparently cause much less nephrotoxicity than conventional amphotericin B formulations. That is probably because these newer formulations alter distribution of the antifungal drug such that renal concentrations, and so the nephrotoxic potential, are lower.)

432. The answer is d. (*Craig, pp 530–531; Hardman, pp 1203–1206; Katzung, pp 741–742.*) There are several main reasons for the greater propensity for cardiovascular and bleeding problems with ticarcillin. The drug is available as a disodium salt, and we often need to administer large doses of the drug. The added sodium load can increase blood volume and blood pressure. In addition, ticarcillin seems to have antiplatelet activity. This, alone, can cause a slight increase in the risk of spontaneous or excessive bleeding, and it appears that the risks are much greater if the ticarcillin is given to a patient already taking antiplatelet drugs or drugs that impair coagulation or platelet function by other mechanisms.

Ticarcillin is no more nephrotoxic than other penicillins (low). It is not contraindicated for asthmatics, nor does it (or other penicillins) cause signs or symptoms of asthma other than those that would be expected with allergic responses to any penicillin. None of the penicillins induce penicillinase (β-lactamase).

433. The answer is c. *(Craig, pp 37, 559; Hardman, pp 1278–1279; Katzung, pp 551, 785, 1123.)* Rifampin and other rifamycins are noteworthy for their ability to induce the hepatic P450 enzyme system, increasing the metabolism of other drugs. Because most of the documented interactants with rifampin are inactivated by metabolism, the consequence of that interaction is a reduced response to the interactant. None of the other answers given are correct, because rifampin does not possess those properties.

434. The answer is c. *(Craig, p 533.)* Cefmetazole and cefotetan, both second-generation cephalosporins, and cefoperazone (third generation) can interfere with hepatic vitamin K metabolism, leading to what amounts to a deficiency of vitamin K–dependent clotting factor activity. Because this is the general mechanism by which warfarin exerts its anticoagulant effects, combined use of one of these cephalosporins can cause further (and potentially dangerous) prolongations of the International Normalized Ratio (or prothrombin time); the clinical consequence can be spontaneous, prolonged, or excessive bleeding. One should also be cautious when these cephalosporins are given to patients taking aspirin or other antiplatelet drugs (e.g., clopidogrel) or thrombolytics.

Although most cephalosporins are excreted unchanged by the kidneys, renal failure (especially severe and acute) seldom occurs with these or other cephalosporins. There is no link between administration of even high doses of these cephalosporins (or others) with the development of acute heart failure. Hypertension (or other substantial changes of blood pressure) are not associated with cephalosporins, nor are these drugs ototoxic.

Although a history of severe allergic reactions to penicillins requires caution when considering a cephalosporin (indeed, cephalosporins should be avoided, if possible, in such patients), there is nothing unique about cefmetazole, cefoperazone, or cefotetan in this context. None of the cephalosporins are contraindicated for patients with mild allergic reactions due to penicillins.

435. The answer is c. *(Craig, p 549; Hardman, p 1258; Katzung, pp 760–761.)* More so than just about any other antibiotic, clindamycin is associated with the highest risk of AAPMC (*C. difficile* superinfection). Thus, it is mainly reserved for certain anaerobic infections located outside the CNS (susceptible anaerobes include B. *fragilis, Fusobacterium,* and *Clostridium perfringens,* plus anaerobic streptococci).

436. The answer is d. (*Craig, p 608; Katzung, pp 828, 877–878.*) Among the indications for metronidazole is management of C. *difficile* (and other clostridia) infections, including AAPMC. Many other obligate anaerobes will respond, as will various types of intestinal or systemic amebiasis infections (the drug is generally used adjunctively with iodoquinol for gut infections—symptomatic amebiasis); and for giardiasis and *Trichomonas vaginalis* infections (generally the drug of choice).

An alternative (or adjunct) to metronidazole in the setting of AAPMC would be vancomycin.

None of the other drugs listed would be suitable. As noted in the previous question, clindamycin would be wholly inappropriate as it is the most likely cause of the AAPMC to begin with.

437. The answer is c. (*Craig, pp 539–541; Hardman, p 1233; Katzung, p 770.*) Amikacin stands out among all the aminoglycosides in two main ways: it has the broadest spectrum against gram-negative bacilli, and it is least susceptible to bacterial enzymes that inactivate aminoglycosides and lead to resistance. (Recall that among gram-negative bacteria, genetic information that codes for the production of these inactivating enzymes is transferred via R factors.)

438. The answer is f. (*Craig, p 545; Hardman, pp 1242–1243; Katzung, p 756.*) Tetracyclines interact with many polyvalent metal cations such that their absorption from the gut (i.e., bioavailability) is reduced. The extent of this reduction can be clinically significant, i.e., leading to inadequate blood levels and effects of the antibiotic.

Calcium is, of course, abundant in dairy products, some OTC antacid products, and in supplements touted for "bone health." Other metals that can interact with tetracyclines by this mechanism include iron, magnesium, aluminum, and zinc. Note that one or several of these interactants are typically found in antacid products, multivitamin/mineral supplements, and even (the trend is growing) in some (mineral-) fortified foods, such as cereals, and citrus juices.

Although foods (in general) may interfere with the oral absorption of several other antibiotics, the cation-antibiotic interaction is specific for and important to the tetracyclines.

439. The answer is c. (*Craig, pp 518–519; Hardman, pp 1176–1177; Katzung, pp 775–776.*) SMZ and TMP act on sequential steps in the synthesis of tetrahydrofolic acid in susceptible bacteria. Sulfamethoxazole (and sulfonamides in general) inhibit incorporation of *para*-aminobenzoic acid (PABA) into folic acid. Trimethoprim then inhibits dihydrofolate reductase, the enzyme that (in the presence of NADPH) converts dihydrofolate into tetrahydrofolate. This leads to the bacteriostatic effect in susceptible organisms, and a clinical response that is better than with either drug used alone.

Note that this mechanism accounts for the selectively toxic effect on microbes, as opposed to host cells, because (a) mammalian cell dihydrofolate reductases are largely insensitive to the effects of TMP and (b) host cell viability is not dependent on tetrahydrofolate synthesis (they use "preformed" folic acid, i.e., folate from the diet) and so they are unaffected by the sulfonamide.

Neither SMZ nor TMP, alone or in combination, exerts antiviral activity. Moreover, none of the other mechanisms listed apply.

440. The answer is a. (*Craig, pp 538–539; Hardman, pp 1221–1222; Katzung, pp 764–767.*) Of all the protein synthesis inhibitors, only the aminoglycosides routinely cause bacterial death, not just suppression of growth or replication.

441. The answer is b. (*Craig, pp 586–587; Hardman, p 1353; Katzung, pp 810–813.*) Zidovudine competitively inhibits HIV-1 nucleoside reverse transcriptase. It is also incorporated in the growing viral DNA chain to cause termination. Each action requires activation via phosphorylation of cellular enzymes. Zidovudine decreases the rate of clinical disease progression and prolongs survival in HIV-infected patients.

442. The answer is e. (*Craig, pp 553–554; Hardman, p 1264; Katzung, p 749.*) This "red man" syndrome is characteristically associated with vancomycin. It is thought to be caused by histamine release. Prevention consists of a slower infusion rate and pretreatment with antihistamines.

443. The answer is d. (*Craig, pp 529–530; Hardman, pp 1147, 1193–1194.*) Unlike the other listed drugs, oxacillin is resistant to penicillinase. The other four agents are broad-spectrum penicillins, whereas oxacillin is generally specific for gram-positive microorganisms. Use of penicillinase-resistant penicillins should be reserved for infections caused by penicillinase-producing staphylococci.

444. The answer is e. *(Craig, p 609; Hardman, p 1110; Katzung, pp 879–881.)* Both trimethoprim-sulfamethoxazole and pentamidine are effective in pneumonia caused by *P. carinii*. This protozoal disease usually occurs in immunodeficient patients, such as those with AIDS. Nifurtimox is effective in trypanosomiasis and metronidazole in amebiasis and leishmaniasis, as well as in anaerobic bacterial infections. Penicillins are not considered drugs of choice for this particular disease state.

445. The answer is d. *(Craig, pp 519–521; Hardman, pp 1179–1182; Katzung, pp 777–780.)* Bacterial DNA gyrase is composed of four subunits, and levofloxacin binds to the strand-cutting subunits, inhibiting their activity.

446. The answer is c. *(Craig, pp 517–518; Hardman, pp 1176–1177; Katzung, pp 775–777.)* Trimethoprim inhibits dihydrofolic acid reductase. Sulfamethoxazole inhibits *p*-aminobenzoic acid (PABA) from being incorporated into folic acid by competitive inhibition of dihydropteroate synthase. Either action inhibits the synthesis of tetrahydrofolic acid.

447. The answer is a. *(Craig, pp 59, 546–547; Hardman, pp 1248–1250; Katzung, p 755.)* Hematologic toxicity is by far the most important adverse effect of chloramphenicol. The toxicity consists of two types: (1) bone marrow depression (common) and (2) aplastic anemia (rare). Chloramphenicol can produce a potentially fatal toxic reaction, the "gray baby" syndrome, caused by diminished ability of neonates to conjugate chloramphenicol, leading to high serum concentrations of the drug.

448. The answer is c. *(Craig, p 614; Hardman, p 1084; Katzung, pp 864–867.)* Primaquine is effective against the extraerythrocytic forms of *P. vivax* and *P. ovale*. It is used to eradicate plasmodia from the liver, and in doing so it not only provides a cure but also helps prevent relapse. Chloroquine would not be used because it is effective only in the erythrocytic phase of the malarial parasites' life spans: it will not work against the exoerythrocytic forms of malaria parasites, nor can it serve as primary prevention. This 4-aminoquinoline derivative is a weak base that selectively concentrates in infected red blood cells. There it probably interferes with the ability of plasmodia to convert heme—a toxin to the parasite—to nontoxic metabolites.

449. The answer is d. (*Craig, pp 622, 625; Hardman, p 1133; Katzung, p 892.*) Niclosamide exerts its effect against cestodes by inhibition of mitochondrial oxidative phosphorylation in the parasites. The mechanism of action is also related to its inhibition of glucose and oxygen uptake in the parasite.

450. The answer is a. (*Craig, pp 528–531; Hardman, pp 1201–1202; Katzung, p 756.*) Amoxicillin and ampicillins are aminopenicillins. Amoxicillin absorption is affected less by the presence of food, so the bioavailability is better. Amoxicillin is inactivated by β-lactamases and has a narrow spectrum of activity toward certain gram-positive and gram-negative organisms, but not *Pseudomonas*. Because it is a penicillin, hypersensitivity reactions are possible.

451. The answer is e. (*Craig, p 517; Hardman, pp 1161, 1176; Katzung, p 775.*) Sulfonamides cross the placenta and enter the fetus in concentrations sufficient to produce toxic effects. They compete with and displace bilirubin from plasma protein binding sites, raising free bilirubin levels and causing the jaundice and other manifestations of kernicterus. For the same reason, sulfonamides should also not be given to neonates, especially premature infants. This woman should not have been given the sulfonamide, whether alone or in combination with trimethoprim.

452. The answer is c. (*Hardman, pp 1147, 1193–1194; Katzung, pp 736, 740–741.*) Oxacillin is classified as a penicillinase-resistant penicillin that is relatively acid-stable and, therefore, is useful for oral administration. Major adverse reactions include penicillin hypersensitivity and interstitial nephritis. With the exception of methicillin, which is no longer used, all penicillinase-resistant penicillins are highly bound to plasma proteins. Oxacillin has a very narrow spectrum and is used primarily as an antistaphylococcal agent.

453. The answer is c. (*Craig, pp 607–608; Hardman, p 1106; Katzung, pp 877–878.*) Metronidazole penetrates all tissues and fluids of the body. Metronidazole's spectrum of activity is limited largely to anaerobic bacteria—including *B. fragilis*—and certain protozoa. It is considered to be the drug of choice for trichomoniasis in females and carrier states in males, as well as for intestinal infections with *Giardia lamblia.*

454. The answer is e. (*Craig, pp 586–587; Hardman, pp 1354–1355; Katzung, pp 810–813.*) One of zidovudine's major adverse effects is bone marrow depression that appears to be dose- and length-of-treatment-dependent. The severity of the disease and a low CD4 count contribute to the bone marrow depression.

455. The answer is e. (*Craig, pp 529–530; Hardman, pp 1194, 1196, 1202–1203.*) Ticarcillin (which is quite similar to carbenicillin in many clinically relevant ways) has a high degree of potency against *Pseudomonas* and *Proteus* organisms, but is inactivated by penicillinase produced by various bacteria, including most staphylococci. Oxacillin, cloxacillin, nafcillin, and dicloxacillin are all penicillinase-resistant and are effective against staphylococci.

456. The answer is a. (*Craig, p 554; Hardman, p 1262; Katzung, pp 829, 1016.*) Polymyxins disrupt the structural integrity of the cytoplasmic membranes by acting as cationic detergents. On contact with the drug, the permeability of the membrane changes. Polymyxin is often applied in a mixture with bacitracin and/or neomycin for synergistic effects. Bacitracin, cycloserine, cephalothin, and vancomycin inhibit cell-wall synthesis.

457. The answer is b. (*Craig, p 614; Hardman, p 1084; Katzung, pp 871–782.*) Hemolysis is the most common and serious adverse response to primaquine. The risk is clearly highest in patients who have red cell deficiencies in glucose-6-phosphate dehydrogenase, a heritable trait and one that can be screened for before giving the drug. [This G6PD deficiency is more common in blacks, and whites with darker skin (e.g., some from certain regions of the Middle East or the Mediterranean countries).] Regardless of the results of pretreatment screening, periodic blood counts should be done, and the urine checked for unusual darkening (indicating the presence of hemoglobin from lysed red cells), during treatment.

Note: If you answered "retinopathy," you were probably thinking about chloroquine, because that adverse response (accompanied by visual changes) is associated with that "other main" antimalarial drug.

Cancer Chemotherapy and Immunosuppressants

Cell cycle, cell cycle specificity
Alkylating agents
Anticancer hormones and their
   antagonists
Antitumor antibiotics

Antimetabolites
Plant alkaloids
Immunomodulators
Immunosuppressants

Questions

DIRECTIONS: Each item contains a question or incomplete statement that is followed by possible responses. Select the **one best** response to each question.

458. Which phase of the cell cycle is resistant to most chemotherapeutic agents, i.e., those that are classified as phase-specific?

a. G_0
b. G_1
c. G_2
d. M
e. S

Questions 459–463

The next 5 questions relate to a patient with advanced Hodgkin's disease. He is placed on combination therapy with vincristine, mechlorethamine, procarbazine, and prednisone (the so-called MOPP regimen).

459. Which of the following is the main mechanism by which the vincristine is exerting its intended effects?

a. Alkylating DNA, causing cross-links between parallel DNA strands
b. Blocking microtubular assembly and mitosis during M-phase
c. Inhibiting topoisomerase, preventing repair of DNA strand breaks
d. Intercalating in DNA strands, thereby preventing DNA replication by mRNA
e. Stabilizing assembled microtubular arrays, thereby preventing mitosis

460. Which of the following is the main mechanism by which the mechlorethamine exerts its cell killing?

a. Alkylating DNA, causing cross-links between parallel DNA strands
b. Blocking microtubular assembly and mitosis during M-phase
c. Inhibiting topoisomerase, preventing repair of DNA strand breaks
d. Intercalating in DNA strands, thereby preventing DNA replication by mRNA
e. Stabilizing assembled microtubular arrays, thereby preventing mitosis

461. Which of the following is the most likely adverse response to occur as a result of the vincristine?

a. Nephrotoxicity, renal dysfunction or failure
b. Neutropenia
c. Peripheral sensory and motor neuropathy
d. Pulmonary damage
e. Thrombocytopenia, bleeding

462. Which of the following is the most likely main role of the prednisone in this therapeutic plan?

a. Counteracting fluid overload from chemotherapy-induced renal dysfunction
b. Counteracting hyperglycemia caused by the other agents
c. Exerting direct cytotoxic actions, independent of the other agents
d. Forcing cancer cells into more responsive phases of the cell cycle
e. Preventing opportunistic infections
f. Suppressing emesis and vomiting

463. When the patient was first seen, the oncology team used the Karnofsky scale as part of their initial evaluation and will use it again as treatment progresses. This scale is used to describe or attempt to quantify which of the following?

a. The number and severity of expected drug-induced side effects or adverse responses
b. The number of chemotherapy drugs and adjuncts likely to be needed
c. The patient's overall health, morbidity, ability for self-care, before and in response to therapy
d. The predicted responsiveness of the tumor to specific classes of anticancer drugs
e. The step-wise or sequential plan for actually administering the anticancer drugs or drug classes

Questions 464–465

464. A 47-year-old woman with choriocarcinoma is treated with very high doses of methotrexate (MTX). You anticipate significant host cell toxicity in response to the high MTX dose, and so immediately after giving the anti-cancer drug you administer which of the following?

a. Deferoxamine
b. Leucovorin
c. N-acetylcysteine
d. Penicillamine
e. Vitamin K

465. While reviewing charts in a general medicine clinic you see that another patient, 55 years old and with no history of cancer at all, is also taking methotrexate. The drug is most likely being given to manage which of the following conditions?

a. Asthma or emphysema
b. Hyperthyroidism
c. Hyperuricemia or clinical gout
d. Myasthenia gravis
e. Rheumatoid arthritis or psoriasis

Questions 466–467

466. A cancer patient receives prophylactic allopurinol before a course of chemotherapy. Which of the following is the main purpose of doing this?

a. Facilitate host cell detoxification of the chemotherapeutic drug, thereby reducing host cell toxicities
b. Inhibit the potential for DNA repair, by topoisomerases, that otherwise might lead to chemotherapy failure
c. Potentiate the action of a nitrogen mustard or nitrosourea to bind to (cross-link) purine moieties in DNA strands
d. Prevent myelosuppression and related blood dyscrasias
e. Reduce the risk of hyperuricemia and its main consequences (renal damage, gout) that can occur with a massive cell kill

467. Allopurinol should be avoided, or reduced doses of the chemothera-peutic agent given, if the anticancer drug is which of the following?

a. Bleomycin
b. Cisplatin
c. Cyclophosphamide
d. Doxorubicin
e. Mercaptopruine

468. A cancer patient develops severe, irreversible cardiomyopathy because the maximum lifetime dose of an anticancer drug was exceeded. Which of the following is most likely responsible for this patient's symptoms?

a. Asparaginase
b. Bleomycin
c. Cisplatin
d. Cyclophosphamide
e. Doxorubicin
f. Vincristine

469. A patient with Wilms' tumor is receiving a chemotherapeutic agent that is described as working by intercalating into DNA strands, and that is efficacious regardless of which stage of the cell cycle the tumor cells are in. Which of the following agents best fits this description?

a. Anastrozole
b. Cytarabine
c. Dactinomycin (actinomycin D)
d. Fluorouracil
e. Tamoxifen

Questions 470–471

A 41-year-old woman is admitted to the outpatient area of the hematology-oncology center for her first course of adjuvant chemotherapy for metastatic breast cancer following a left modified radical mastectomy and axillary lymph node dissection for infiltrating ductal carcinoma of the breast. Two biopsies were positive for cancer.

Following premedication with dexamethasone and ondansetron, she will receive combination chemotherapy with doxorubicin, cyclophosphamide, and fluorouracil. Premedications include intravenous ondansetron and dexamethasone.

470. Twenty-four hours after the first course of chemotherapy she will start a 10-day regimen with filgrastim. Which of the following is the purpose of giving that drug?

a. Control of nausea and emesis
b. Potentiate the anticancer effects of the chemotherapeutic agents
c. Prevent doxorubicin-induced cardiotoxicity
d. Reduce the risk/severity of chemo-induced neutropenia, and related infections
e. Stimulate the gastric mucosa to repair damage caused by the chemotherapy drugs

471. Which of the following is the purpose of administering ondansetron?

a. Activate cancer cells to move out of G_0 and into a more responsive, actively replicating cell cycle phase
b. Block estrogen receptors, thereby enhancing the efficacy of the cyclophosphamide
c. Prevent cardiotoxicity caused by one of the anticancer drugs in the combination
d. Prevent metabolism of adrenal cortical androgens to estrogens, which would facilitate breast tumor growth
e. Suppress chemotherapy-induced nausea and vomiting

472. A 42-year-old woman is diagnosed with metastatic breast cancer. You consider use of tamoxifen, raloxifene, toremifene, or fulvestrant. Why might fulvestrant be the best choice, all other factors being equal?

a. Exerts antiplatelet, rather than thrombotic, effects
b. Lacks ability to cause hot flashes or other disturbing side effects
c. Lower risk of causing endometrial cancer
d. Provides clinical cure, rather than palliation, in all patients
e. Significantly improves mineral density in, strength of, long bones

473. A 30-year-old woman being treated for ovarian cancer develops high frequency hearing loss and declining renal function in response to anti-cancer drug therapy. Which of the following drugs is the most likely cause?

a. Bleomycin
b. Cisplatin
c. Doxorubicin
d. 5-Fluorouracil
e. Paclitaxel

474. The oncology team has treated many patients with acute lympho-cytic leukemia using a combination of drugs. One drug tends to cause a high incidence of lumbar and abdominal pain, significant increases of serum amylase and transaminase activity, and other symptoms of hepatic and/or pancreatic dysfunction. Some patients developed serious hypersen-sitivity reactions upon drug administration, and there have been occasional sudden deaths. Which of the following drugs best fits this description?

a. 6-mercaptopurine
b. Asparaginase
c. Doxorubicin
d. Methotrexate
e. Vincristine

Questions 475–477

A 45-year-old woman has had a heart transplant. She receives cyclosporine as part of the immunosuppressant regimen.

475. Which of the following is the main mechanism of cyclosporine's immunosuppressant effects?

a. Blocks the CD3 site on T lymphocytes, blocks all T cell functions
b. Directly destroys proliferating lymphoid cells
c. Directly inhibits B and T lymphocyte proliferation
d. Inhibits calcineurin and resulting IL-2 synthesis that is necessary for B and T cell proliferation
e. Lyses antigen-activated lymphocytes, reduces responsiveness of T lymphocytes to IL-1, reduces IL-2 production by lymphocytes and monocytes

476. Which of the following are the most common and worrisome adverse responses associated with cyclosporine therapy?

a. Cardiotoxicity and hepatotoxicity
b. Hepatotoxicity and nephrotoxicity
c. Hypotension and pulmonary fibrosis
d. Nephrotoxicity and infection risk
e. Thrombosis and pulmonary embolism or ischemic stroke

477. Which of the following drugs can interact with cyclosporine and reduce its serum levels and immunosuppressant effects, thereby rendering the patient more vulnerable to graft rejection unless we make appropriate drug/dosage adjustments?

a. Erythromycin
b. Gentamicin
c. Grapefruit juice
d. Indomethacin
e. Ketoconazole
f. Trimethoprim-sulfamethoxazole

478. A patient with chronic myelogenous leukemia (CML) is being treated with imatinib (STI571), a relatively new drug for this disorder. With this particular drug you should anticipate which of the following?

a. A high rate of therapeutic failure, and the need to switch to interferons α-2a and -2b
b. Hypotension and hypovolemia due to significant drug-induced diuresis
c. Interactions with other drugs that depend on or affect the cytochrome P450 system
d. Significant toxicity to normal host cells due to profound inhibition of tyrosine kinase
e. Thrombocytosis, with a high risk of intravascular clotting

479. As a rule, large (and older) solid tumors are more difficult to eradicate when chemotherapy is started because:

a. Growth fraction slows, more cells enter G_0
b. Higher tumor blood flow washes away anticancer drugs faster
c. P-glycoprotein activity decreases as tumors get older
d. Their higher metabolic rate makes them less vulnerable to chemotherapeutic agents
e. Topoisomerase activity (ability to self-repair DNA strand damage) increases with tumor size

480. A man has prostate cancer that will be treated with leuprolide. Which of the following drugs must be used adjunctively when we start chemotherapy?

a. An aromatase inhibitor (e.g., anastrozole)
b. Flutamide
c. Prednisone or another potent glucocorticoid
d. Tamoxifen
e. Testosterone

Cancer Chemotherapy and Immunosuppressants

Answers

458. The answer is a. (*Craig, pp 630–631; Hardman, pp 1386–1388; Katzung, pp 900–902.*) The G_0 phase is the resting or dormant stage of the cell cycle. No cell division takes place. This phase is, overall, the most resistant to chemotherapeutic agents because most of the (phase-specific) anticancer drugs produce their lethal effects quickest and best on cells that are actively proliferating, whether synthesizing or preparing to synthesize DNA, or to undergo mitosis. Good examples of drugs that are reasonably effective against cells in G_0 (or any other phase) are the alkylating agents (e.g., cyclophosphamide) and several of the antitumor antibiotics (e.g., dactinomycin, doxorubicin).

Obviously, not all cancer cells present will be in a more vulnerable stage of the cell cycle (i.e., not in G_0), but some will be. This provides one rationale for combining a cycle-nonspecific agent with a cycle-specific one: attack as many cancer cells as possible, no matter where in the cycle they may be. This concept also provides a reason why cycle-specific agents are often administered in repeated courses over an extended time (as opposed to a single dose): repeating the dose increases the chance that we will eventually catch more cells as they enter into a more responsive part of the cycle.

459-b. (*Craig, pp 639, 648; Hardman, pp 1417–1419; Katzung, p 911*); **460-a** (*Craig, pp 639, 640; Hardman, p 1394; Katzung, pp 902–905*) Vincristine and the other vinca alkaloids bind to tubulin and impair microtubular assembly, preventing mitosis (M-phase-specific).

Mechlorethamine, like cyclophosphamide (and carmustine and several others), is an alkylating agent. They are called bifunctional alkylating agents because they can covalently bind to DNA in two places ("nucleophilic attack"), thereby forming cross-links between two adjacent strands or between two bases in one strand. This ultimately disrupts DNA and RNA synthesis or may cause strand breakage. Cyclophosphamide (which can be considered the prototype of the alkylating agents) is actually a pro-drug—it requires metabolic activation in order for its effects to occur. Cyclophosphamide (and other alkylating agents) are cell cycle-nonspecific, although their efficacy is greater when cells are not in G_0.

Bleomycin, dactinomycin, and doxorubicin are good examples of drugs that intercalate in DNA strands. Thus, the altered DNA no longer serves as an adequately precise template for eventual synthesis of more functional DNA and RNA. They are classified as antitumor antibiotics.

Etoposide and topotecan are examples of drugs that inhibit topoisomerase II. The consequence is inhibited ability of affected cells to repair DNA strand breaks. This stops the cell cycle in G_2.

The taxoids (e.g., paclitaxel) impairs mitosis, but by stabilizing assembled microtubules rather than by exerting a vinca alkaloid-like inhibition of microtubular assembly.

461. The answer is c. *(Craig, p 648; Hardman, pp 1418–1419; Katzung, p 911.)* Vincristine is one of relatively few cytotoxic anticancer drugs that does not cause bone marrow suppression (and all the potential consequences of that) as its main toxicity. Rather, it causes neuropathies involving both sensory and motor nerves. Paresthesias are a common example of the former (hearing loss can also occur); muscle weakness and obtunded reflexes are examples of the latter. Important note: Vincristine differs from the other two vinca alkaloids, vinblastine and vinorelbine, which *do* cause bone marrow suppression (and not neuropathies) as their main dose-limiting toxicity.

462. The answer is f. *(Craig, p 635; Hardman, pp 1032–1033.)* Although the precise mechanism isn't known, corticosteroids (prednisone, methylprednisolone, or dexamethasone) are useful in suppressing nausea and vomiting associated with chemotherapy. Although they may be used as the sole agents, more likely they are used as adjuncts to more traditional antiemetics (e.g., ondansetron, a serotonin antagonist; dronabinol, a cannabinoid; or prochlorperazine, a phenothiazine that works as a central dopamine antagonist). Even though antiemetic therapy is generally short term, you should realize that even if the prednisone were given long term, or in very high doses, it would not "counteract fluid overload" because these drugs tend to cause renal fluid and electrolyte retention; nor would they counteract hyperglycemia, because glucocorticoids tend to raise blood glucose levels; nor will they prevent infection, because, if anything, these drugs can suppress the immune responses and render the patient more susceptible to infection. The prednisone will not alter cell cycling nor exert direct cytotoxic effects.

463. The answer is c. (*Katzung, p 928.*) The Karnofsky scale, more properly called the Karnofsky Performance Scale, is a way of providing a semi-quantitative measure of the patient's overall health before and in response to chemotherapy. A "score" of 100% means the patient is essentially normal in terms of activities of daily living (independent, able to work and provide complete self-care, etc.). At the other extreme, a score of 10 would be assigned to a very moribund patient with disease progressing so quickly and severely that death is imminent. A score of 0 indicates a dead patient.

464. The answer is b. (*Craig, pp 643–644; Hardman, pp 1399–1404, 1512; Katzung, pp 907–908.*) This essential technique to reduce host cell toxicity in response to MTX therapy is known as leucovorin rescue. Methotrexate, a folic acid analog/antimetabolite, can be curative for women with choriocarcinoma and is also useful for non-Hodgkin's lymphomas and acute lymphocytic leukemias in children. The drug kills responsive cancer cells by inhibiting dihyrofolate, an enzyme necessary for forming tetrahydrofolic acid (FH_4). The FH_4, in turn, is critical for eventual synthesis of DNA, RNA, and proteins. Inhibition of thymidylate synthesis is probably the single most important consequence in the overall reaction scheme.

Some cancer cells are resistant to MTX because they lack adequate mechanisms for transporting the drug intracellularly. These include some head and neck cancers and osteogenic sarcomas. In such cases we need to give very large doses of MTX to establish a high concentration gradient that essentially "drives" it into the cells. Unfortunately, normal host cells depend on folate metabolism, they take up MTX well, and they will be affected.

To protect normal cells we administer leucovorin (also called citrovorum factor or folinic acid) right after giving the MTX. It is taken up by the normal cells, bypasses the block induced by the MTX, and so spares normal cell metabolism. The leucovorin does not spare cancer cells: just as they cannot take up MTX well, they cannot take up the rescue agent and save themselves from cytotoxicity.

Leucovorin rescue is not done "automatically" in every case when MTX is given. When low MTX doses are used leucovorin may be withheld until and unless blood counts show evidence of MTX-induced bone marrow suppression. However, it is quite usually given along with MTX when MTX doses are very high (as in severe or MTX-resistant cases), and host toxicity is very probable.

The main adverse responses to MTX, regardless of the purpose for which it is given, include bone marrow suppression, pulmonary damage (infiltrates, fibrosis), stomatitis, and lesions elsewhere in the GI tract. High doses can be nephrotoxic (risk reduced by maintaining adequate hydration and alkalinizing the urine). MTX is also teratogenic.

Recall that deferoxamine is used to treat iron poisoning (it is an iron chelator). N-acetylcysteine is mainly used either as a mucolytic (mucus-thinning) drug for certain pulmonary disorders or as an antidote for acetaminophen poisoning. Penicillamine is mainly a copper chelator, used for copper poisoning or Wilson's disease. Vitamin K is used for deficiency states, for combating excessive effects of warfarin, or for managing bleeding disorders in newborns of mothers who have been taking certain drugs (e.g., anticonvulsants such as phenytoin) during pregnancy.

465. The answer is e. (*Craig, pp 432–433; Hardman, p 718; Katzung, p 588.*) The main uses of MTX for conditions other than responsive cancers are management of rheumatoid arthritis (RA) and psoriasis. Doses and dosage schedules differ from those typically used for cancers.

MTX is one of many disease-modifying antirheumatic drugs (DMARDs), which are often called slow-acting antirheumatic drugs (SAARDs) because their onset of symptom relief is much slower than traditional NSAIDs (salicylates and other first-generation COX-1/-2 inhibitors, or second-generation/COX-2 inhibitors, i.e., the "coxibs").

Nonetheless, although the onset is considered slow, meaningful symptom relief usually occurs with as little as 3 to 4 weeks of therapy—faster than the other DMARDs. (Other typical first-choice DMARDs are sulfasalazine and hydroxychoroquine, which unlike MTX, have no cancer-related uses.) All the potential side effects, adverse responses, and contraindications that apply to using MTX for cancer apply to the drug's use for RA or psoriasis (Question 464).

466. The answer is e. (*Craig, pp 445–446; Hardman, p 722; Katzung, pp 598–599.*) Hyperuricemia is associated with many cancers and is a common outcome of massive cell kills induced by chemotherapeutic drugs. The uric acid is derived from cellular purine degradation, eventually formed from hypoxanthine and xanthine via xanthine oxidase, the key enzyme that is inhibited by allopurinol. Recall that renal damage (and other damage, such as gout) is due to uric acid's poor solubility in body fluids, especially at low pH.

Allopurinol has no effect on the P450 system or on cellular transitions from one phase of the cell cycle to another. There is no effect on DNA synthesis or repair, or any direct cytoprotective effect on myeloid or other tissues.

467. The answer is e. (*Craig, pp 446, 644; Hardman, pp 722, 1471; Katzung, p 909.*) Mercaptopurine and other thiopurines are purine antimetabolites that are metabolically inactivated (detoxified) by xanthine oxidase. This purine degradation pathway of metabolism not only leads to formation of uric acid, but also is important to reducing host cell toxicity to the thiopurines. Thus, concomitant use of allopurinol increases the risk of host cell toxicity. Note that azathioprine (an inhibitor of B and T lymphocyte proliferation, and typically used as an immunosuppressant) is metabolized to mercaptopurine. As a result, it too is an interactant with allopurinol.

The metabolism of the other drugs listed is not xanthine oxidase–dependent.

468. The answer is e. (*Hardman, p 1428; Katzung, pp 913–914.*) Doxorubicin, an antitumor antibiotic, is cardiotoxic, and the risk for and severity of cardiomyopathy is dose-related. [There is a maximum recommended lifetime (cumulative) dose for this drug, and if it is exceeded the risk of cardiac damage rises significantly.]

Asparaginase, used only for acute lymphocytic leukemia, tends to cause mainly pancreatitis, hepatic dysfunction, and allergic/hypersensitivity reactions. The main organ-specific toxicity of bleomycin, also an antitumor antibiotic, is pulmonary damage that presents initially usually as pneumonitis. It occurs in about 1 of 10 patients treated with this drug. In some cases the pulmonary damage will progress to pulmonary fibrosis that is, of course, irreversible.

Cisplatin's main dose-limiting toxicity is renal damage, which can be prevented somewhat by ensuring that the patient is adequately hydrated and producing adequate amounts of urine. Diuretics may be used as adjuncts. The goal is to minimize accumulation of the nephrotoxic drug in the renal tubules and urine. (A related drug, oxaliplatin, tends to cause peripheral sensory neuropathies and does so in most patients who receive this drug.)

Cyclophosphamide has no particular organ-specific toxicity. Rather, main manifestations of toxicity involve rapidly growing cells such as those in the bone marrow, intestinal tract mucosae, and hair follicles.

Vincristine's major dose-limiting toxicity is peripheral nerve damage: motor, sensory, and in some cases autonomic. It probably arises in a manner related to the drug's anticancer effect: inhibition of microtubular function—or, in the case of nerves, neurotubules—as a result of drug binding to tubulin.

469. The answer is c. (*Craig, pp 647–648; Hardman, pp 1425–1426; Katzung, pp 913–914.*) Dactinomycin intercalates between and eventually binds to DNA base pairs. This distortion of the DNA chains makes the DNA an unsuitable template for RNA polymerase, and ultimately RNA and protein synthesis is inhibited. Dactinomycin is phase-nonspecific.

Anastrozole is a relatively new aromatase inhibitor. This is an oral agent used for postmenopausal women with early or advanced breast cancer. In postmenopausal women, the major source of estrogen (which supports growth and replication of estrogen-dependent tumors) is adrenal androgens. Those androgens are metabolized by aromatase to estrogens. As a result, anastrozole depletes estrogens and can arrest tumor cell growth.

Cytarabine (also called cytosine arabinoside) is a pyrimidine analog (antimetabolite) that is metabolized to the active moiety, ara-CTP. The ara-CTP becomes incorporated into DNA, with the main ultimate effect being suppression of DNA synthesis. It is highly specific for cells in S-phase.

Fluorouracil, also an antimetabolite, inhibits thymidylate synthetase through its active metabolite, 5-fluoro-2'-dxoyuridine-5'-monophosphate (FdUMP). It is not phase-specific, but its activity depends on cells not being in the G_0 stage.

Tamoxifen is used for breast cancers. It blocks estrogen receptors on the breast cancer cells (for which the main physiologic agonist is estradiol). Recall that tamoxifen is classified as a selective estrogen receptor modifier (SERM). Although it blocks estrogen receptors on responsive breast cancer cells and is therapeutic for them, it acts as an estrogen receptor agonist in the uterus. Thus, one of the main risks of therapy with tamoxifen is endometrial hyperplasia that may lead to endometrial cancer. Because the drug acts as an estrogen receptor agonist in some tissues and an antagonist in others, risk-benefit ratios must be considered carefully. The beneficial effects in active breast carcinoma may outweigh the risks of inducing endometrial disease. However, the preventative use in the absence of breast cancer has a much lower benefit:risk ratio.

470. The answer is d. *(Craig, pp 639, 653; Hardman, pp 1386, 1443; Katzung, pp 539, 919.)* Filgrastim, also known as granulocyte colony-stimulating factor (GCSF), enhances neutrophil production. One use, therefore, is to prevent neutropenia and infection associated with bone marrow depression from cancer chemotherapy. (Hint: Look at the generic name, filgrastim: *granulocyte stim*ulating.)

The drug lacks antiemetic effects, potentiates the chemotherapeutic actions of no drug, has no effect on the gastric mucosa or on doxorubicin-mediated cardiotoxicity.

471. The answer is e. *(Craig, p 477; Hardman, pp 1029–1033; Katzung, pp 271–272, 1049–1052.)* Ondansetron is used to control nausea and vomiting, which are common consequences of chemotherapy. It is a serotonin 5-HT$_3$ receptor antagonist, working primarily in the chemoreceptor trigger zone and afferent vagal nerves in the upper GI tract. It is probable that the dexamethasone, which was also given to our patient, was also given for antiemetic effects.

Note that serotonin antagonists such as ondansetron (and dopamine receptor antagonists such as prochlorperazine) have the broadest antiemetic spectrums (and clinical uses) of all the main antiemetic drug classes. They are useful for controlling not only emesis associated with chemotherapy, but also that which arises in radiation therapy and in many common postoperative settings.

Ondansetron has no effect on the cell cycle, nor does it have any effect on estrogen receptors or estrogen metabolism (as from androgens, which is important in postmenopausal women and is a process that can be inhibited by such drugs as anastrozole, an aromatase inhibitor). Ondandsetron has no effect on chemotherapy-induced cardiotoxicity (which, in the drug combination noted here, would be a property of the doxorubicin).

472. The answer is c. *(Craig, pp 649, 707, 711–712; Katzung, pp 917, 926, 961.)* Fulvestrant is associated with a much lower risk of causing endometrial pathology, including cancer. It is a "pure" estrogen antagonist. That effect, in breast tissue, is what accounts for the drug's beneficial effects in some patients with metastatic, estrogen-supported, breast cancer. In contrast, tamoxifen, raloxifene, and toremifene are classified as selective estrogen receptor modifiers (SERMs). Although they block estrogen receptors in breast tissue (just as fulvestrant does), they also have estrogenic (agonist) activity in some other tissues, notably the uterus. There they can cause endometrial proliferation, hyperplasia, and (apparently) an increased risk of endometrial cancer. (For more information, see the answers to Question 377 in the chapter, "Endocrine System" and Question 469.)

Because fulvestrant lacks estrogen agonist activity, it will not enhance bone mineralization nor favorably modify cholesterol profiles, as the SERMs tend to do. The SERMs slightly increase the risk of thromboembolism. Fulvestrant may too, but it also lacks any ability to prevent platelet aggregation or thromboembolism. Hot flashes are fairly common with any of these drugs.

473. The answer is b. (*Craig, pp 651–652; Hardman, pp 1433–1434; Katzung, pp 905–907.*) Cisplatin, which is sometimes classified along with traditional alkylating agents, is unique among all the common anticancer agents in terms of the relative incidence of hearing loss and nephrotoxicity.

(You are correct in associating vincristine with hearing loss, but nephrotoxicity is very rare; in contrast, you may have recalled that methotrexate can cause nephrotoxicity, but it does not cause hearing loss, and it is indicated for a variety of cancers, but not ovarian.)

Bleomycin's main targeted toxicity is the lungs (pulmonary infiltrates, fibrosis, etc.). Doxorubicin, as noted above, is cardiotoxic. The drug is mainly used for testicular carcinomas, squamous cell cancers, and lymphomas. 5-FU, a pyrimidine antimetabolite, is used for a variety of solid tumors. However, peripheral neuritis or neuropathy (and, especially, hearing loss) or renal damage are uncommon; rather, we are faced with a relatively high incidence of bone marrow suppression and oral and GI mucosal damage. Paclitaxel is a microtubular stabilizing drug (and plant alkaloid). It is considered first-line for some patients with advanced ovarian cancer or non-small-cell lung cancers, causes dose-dependent bone marrow suppression and peripheral neuropathy, and a fairly high incidence of acute infusion-related hypersensitivity reactions (probably due to the vehicle in which the drug is delivered).

474. The answer is b. (*Craig, pp 639, 649; Hardman, pp 1431–1432; Katzung, p 918.*) Asparaginase is an enzyme that catalyzes the hydrolysis of serum asparagine to aspartic acid and ammonia. Major toxicities from asparaginase are related to antigenicity (it is a foreign protein, and some fatal anaphylactic reactions have occurred), pancreatitis, and a 50% incidence of some hepatic dysfunction based on the presence of elevated serum transaminases. The drug, which is largely G_1 phase-specific, is not cytotoxic to cells other than leukemic lymphoblasts. Host (and other cells) can synthesize and replace asparagine that has been hydrolyzed by the drug; the lymphoblasts cannot, and so they are killed.

475. The answer is d. (*Craig, p 659; Hardman, pp 1465–1468; Katzung, pp 940–941.*) Cyclosporine acts on helper T lymphocytes. First it binds to cyclophilin and then inhibits calcineurin, which is important in the synthesis of cytokines, including IL-2. These cytokines are necessary for proliferation of B cells and cytolytic T cells (also called cytotoxic T cells, or CD8 cells). Tacrolimus works by a mechanism that is largely similar to that of cyclosporine, but its initial intracellular binding site is not cyclophilin, but rather another protein.

Muromonab-CD3 is the immunosuppressant that blocks the CD3 site on T lymphocytes. Cyclophosphamide exerts direct toxic effects on proliferating lymphoid cells. Azathioprine, which is metabolically activated to mercaptopruine, inhibits B and T lymphocyte proliferation by inhibiting DNA synthesis. Glucocorticoids, at high doses, lyse antigen-activated lymphocytes and reduce IL-2 production by lymphocytes and macrophages.

476. The answer is d. (*Craig, p 659; Hardman, p 1469; Katzung, p 941.*) Nephrotoxicity, or at least some clinically significant degree of renal dysfunction, occurs in about 8 of 10 patients receiving cyclosporine. It is typically dose-dependent and, particularly in renal transplant patients, could be due to either the drug (too much) or to rejection. Infection occurs about as often as renal dysfunction. Cyclosporine can cause hepatotoxicity, but the incidence is far lower than that of renal responses or infection. Blood pressure changes can occur, but with cyclosporine the change usually involves increased pressure, and it is common. Cardiac or pulmonary toxicities and thromboembolism due to the drug itself are extremely uncommon.

477. The answer is f. (*Craig, pp 36–37; Hardman, pp 1229, 1256, 1303, 1469.*) TMP-SMZ induces cyclosporine metabolism and can cause dramatic reductions of the immunosuppressant's desired effects. Other common drugs that interact in this way, causing essentially the same outcome, are phenytoin, phenobarbital, carbamazepine (all common anticonvulsants), and rifampin (or rifabutrin). Macrolide antibiotics (e.g., erythromycin), amphotericin B (which can also aggravate renal damage), and the azole antifungals can profoundly inhibit cyclosporine metabolism. (Ketoconazole is sometimes administered with cyclosporine intentionally for this effect. The required reduction of cyclosporine dosage reduces the cost of cyclosporine therapy, but of course ketoconazole is not an innocuous drug.) A compound in grapefruit juice dramatically reduces first-pass metabolism of cyclosporine, too. (Indeed, the clinical significance of this "grapefruit juice effect" was first discovered, or at least appreciated, in studies of cyclosporine pharmacokinetics and responses.)

Gentamicin and indomethacin (and other aminoglycosides and NSAIDs) are examples of drugs that can increase the risk of nephrotoxicity.

478. The answer is c. (*Craig, p 653; Katzung, pp 841–842, 948, 970, 978–979.*) One of several problems with imatinib therapy is that it is a substrate and rather powerful inhibitor of several cytochromes (CYP3A4, 2C9, and 2D6), which are important for the metabolism of many other drugs—warfarin, theophylline, and many others—whose actions can be increased excessively if dosages are not adjusted accordingly. Conversely, imatinib is a target of interactions by this mechanism. Phenytoin, carbamazepine, barbiturates, and rifampin are examples of drugs that can induce imatinib metabolism and reduce the clinical response to it; and such drugs as azole antifungals and erythromycin can reduce imatinib's clearance and increase the risk of toxicity.

Because of the issue of drug interactions, a high frequency of adverse responses, limited use (see below), and even cost, imatinib is generally reserved for use after a trial of interferons has proven inadequate. The reverse—using imatinib first—usually isn't done.

Hypotension and hypovolemia are not what one would expect with this drug. Rather, we see a rather high incidence of fluid retention that may not only affect blood pressure, but also cause such other problems as ascites, pericardial and pleural effusions, and possibly pulmonary edema. Likewise, thrombocytosis is the opposite of what typically occurs: thrombocytopenia and bleeding problems, plus neutropenia and an increased risk of infection are fairly common.

You should recall that chronic myelogenous leukemia cells do synthesize an abnormal constituitively active tyrosine kinase (Bcr-Abl) that is involved in (abnormal) protein phosphorylation. It is that aberrant tyrosine kinase—not ones found in normal host cells—that is affected by the drug and that confers selectivity for the drug's actions. Thus, tyrosine kinase inhibition does not seem to account for the adverse effects of this drug on host cells.

479. The answer is a. (*Craig, pp 631–632; Hardman, pp 1387–1388; Katzung, pp 900–901.*) Gompertzian analysis (a plot of the log of the number of cancer cells in a tumor vs. time) shows that after a tumor has reached a certain size, the rate of tumor growth (and "overall metabolic rate") slows (lower growth fraction or, stated differently, the longer it takes for the tumor to double in size). This slowed growth is partially due to more cells entering the G_0 (resting) phase of the cell cycle, where responsiveness to many chemotherapeutic agents is low. (One reason for this is the sheer size of the tumor as related to blood flow and the delivery of nutrients that the rapidly dividing cells need. Reduced nutrient and oxygen delivery not only reduces cell replication, but also delivery of the chemotherapeutic agents.)

P-glycoprotein activity does not necessarily decrease with time or tumor size. However, even if it did, that would predict *increased* responsiveness to most anticancer drugs, because it is P-glycoprotein that normally pumps drugs *out* of the cancer cell. Self-repair mechanisms, as by topoisomerase, is not a factor in explaining reduced vulnerability of very large tumors.

480. The answer is b. (*Craig, pp 650, 732; Hardman, pp 1442, 1645; Katzung, pp 688, 917, 926.*) Flutamide, one of three androgen receptor blockers used for managing prostate cancer, is used as an adjunct to leuprolide. Leuprolide acts like gonadotropin-releasing hormone (GnRH; or luteinizing hormone-releasing hormone). When leuprolide therapy is started, it stimulates release of interstitial cell–stimulating hormone from the pituitary, thereby increasing testosterone production and supporting tumor growth. It is only with continued exposure to leuprolide that GnRH receptors become desensitized, and the eventual inhibition of testosterone production (and, thereby, support of tumor growth) occurs. Flutamide, by blocking androgen receptors, prevents the potential worsening of the tumor in the early phase of leuprolide therapy when testosterone levels rise. Even when leuprolide's pituitary-desensitizing effects occur, androgens that can support prostate tumor growth will come from the adrenal gland. Their effects, too, are blocked by the flutamide.

Toxicology

Air pollutants, toxic gases
Alcohols, ethylene glycol
Antidotes for common drugs

Chemical warfare agents
Heavy metals
Poisonings of unknown cause

Questions

DIRECTIONS: Each item contains a question or incomplete statement that is followed by possible responses. Select the **one best** response to each question.

481. Your patient is a firefighter who attempted to extinguish a car fire. She had a leak in her protective air mask. She develops cyanide poisoning from the combustion of plastic. Aside from rendering symptomatic, supportive care, which of the following might be administered to combat the cyanide poisoning?

a. Ammonium chloride
b. Deferoxamine
c. Dimercaprol (BAL; British anti-Lewisite)
d. Mannitol
e. Pralidoxime
f. Sodium thiosulfate

482. A patient has taken a potentially lethal dose of acetaminophen. The current preferred antidotal involves administration of a drug that:

a. Alkalinizes the urine to facilitate acetaminophen excretion
b. Causes metabolic acidosis to combat the toxic metabolite's metabolic alkalosis
c. Inhibits hepatic oxidative metabolism to inhibit formation of acetaminophen's toxic metabolite
d. Inhibits synthesis of superoxide anion radical and hydrogen peroxide
e. Is rich in sulfhydryl (–SH) groups

483. A patient who receives a rapid IV injection of a drug develops hypocalcemic tetany. Which of the following is the most likely cause?

a. Deferoxamine
b. Dimercaprol
c. Edetate disodium (Na$_2$EDTA)
d. N-acetylcysteine
e. Penicillamine

484. Alkalinization of the urine with sodium bicarbonate is a useful, if not essential, adjunct to other therapies in treating poisoning with which of the following drugs?

a. Amphetamine
b. Aspirin (acetylsalicylic acid)
c. Cocaine
d. Morphine
e. Phencyclidine

485. A 3-year-old girl ingests 30 tablets of aspirin, 325 mg each. Which of the following antidotes should be administered as part of the initial treatment plan?

a. Activated charcoal
b. Deferoxamine
c. Dimercaprol
d. Na$_2$EDTA
e. Penicillamine

486. A 50-year-old man has been consuming large amounts of alcohol (ethanol) on an almost daily basis for many years. One day, unable to find any ethanol, he ingests a large amount of methanol (wood alcohol) that he found in his garage. Which of the following is the most likely consequence of this?

a. Atrioventricular conduction defect
b. Blindness
c. Bronchospasm
d. Delirium tremens
e. Metabolic alkalosis

487. A 15-year-old boy attempts suicide with a liquid that he found in his parents' greenhouse. His dad used it to get rid of "varmints" around the yard. The toxin causes intense abdominal pain, skeletal muscle cramps, projectile vomiting, and severe diarrhea that leads to fluid and electrolyte imbalances, hypotension, and difficulty swallowing. On examination he is found to be volume depleted and is showing signs of a reduced level of consciousness. His breath smells "metallic." Which of the following probably accounts for these symptoms?

a. Arsenic (As)
b. Cadmium (Cd)
c. Iron (Fe)
d. Lead (Pb)
e. Zinc (Zn)

488. A 60-year-old man has been using a kerosene space heater and candles to keep warm in the winter. He is transported to the hospital with complaints of severe headaches, nausea, dizziness, and a diminution in vision. He has a decreased arterial blood oxygen (O_2)-carrying capacity without a change in the P_{O_2}. Which of the following most likely accounts for these findings?

a. Carbon monoxide (CO)
b. Methane
c. Nitrogen dioxide
d. Ozone
e. Sulfur dioxide

Questions 489–490

A 5-year-old boy consumed a liquid from a container in the family garage. He presents with central nervous system (CNS) depression, obtunded reflexes, and ventilatory depression. A blood sample indicates profound metabolic acidosis. A check of the urine reveals crystals that are presumed to be oxalate.

489. Which of the following is the most likely cause of the poisoning?

a. A halogenated hydrocarbon from a can of spray paint
b. An insecticide
c. Ethylene glycol
d. Gasoline
e. Paint thinner

490. Among other things, which of the following is the preferred drug to administer for this poisoning?

a. Allopurinol
b. Atropine
c. Ethanol
d. Lorazepam
e. Syrup of ipecac

Questions 491–492

A 22-year-old girl is brought to the emergency department by a friend. They had been at a bar for about an hour, and then the patient suddenly became drowsy but was still conscious. She fell and cut her head, and she says "yes, it hurts." Her ventilatory rate and depth are depressed, but not to a worrisome degree. Her patellar reflexes are blunted and she is ataxic. She responds slowly to questions, but is unable to recall anything that happened after arriving at the bar. Her friend stated that the patient had only one cocktail and hadn't been drinking before they went out.

491. Based on this presentation, it is most likely that someone "spiked" the patient's drink with which of the following drugs?

a. A barbiturate
b. A benzodiazepine
c. An opioid
d. Chloral hydrate
e. Cocaine
f. Pure (grain) alcohol

492. Which of the following should you administer first, specifically to confirm or reject your suspected diagnosis and hopefully to normalize the patient's vital signs?

a. Activated charcoal
b. Caffeine
c. Flumazenil
d. Naloxone
e. Oxygen

Questions 493–495

A mother calls to report that her 6-year-old child appears to have swallowed a large but unknown amount of an over-the-counter sleep aid about 5 h ago. The product contained only one active drug.

493. Which of the following is the most likely active drug in the product?
a. Atropine
b. Diphenhydramine
c. Fexofenadine
d. Loperamide
e. Pseudoephedrine

494. Assuming your reasoned guess about the cause of poisoning was correct, which of the following would you expect to find, upon physical exam, to confirm your hunch?

a. Fever; clear lungs; absence of bowel sounds; urinary retention, dry, flushed skin; mydriasis and photophobia; bizarre behavior
b. Irritability (CNS stimulation); uncontrolled diarrhea and urination
c. Miosis with little/no papillary response to bright lights; tachycardia; piloerection; spontaneous micturition; lack of response to painful stimuli
d. Profuse sweating; hypothermia; bounding pulse; hypertension
e. Skeletal muscle weakness or paralysis; profound hypomotility of gut and bladder smooth muscle; bronchospasm

495. Your suspicion is confirmed, but the poisoning progresses quickly. The child develops seizures, for which you administer lorazepam and phenytoin, IV. Which of the following drugs might be of specific help to correct the underlying problems and, ultimately, many of the symptoms?
a. Flumazenil
b. Naloxone
c. Physostigmine
d. Pralidoxime (2-PAM)
e. Sodium bicarbonate

Questions 496–497

Recent occupational health studies in several heavily populated urban areas have revealed an astonishingly large number of homes that have lead-based paint and children living in them. However, a number of environmental poisons that could lead to acute or chronic poisoning have also been found there.

496. Which of the following signs and symptoms would be consistent with chronic exposure to toxic levels of inorganic lead?

a. Anorexia and weight loss; weakness, especially of extensor muscles (e.g., wrist drop); recurrent abdominal pain
b. Gingivitis, discolored gums, loosened teeth, or stomatitis; tremor of the extremities; swollen parotid or other salivary glands
c. Hallucinations, insomnia, headache, generalized CNS irritability
d. Hyperventilation in response to metabolic acidosis; hypotension; abdominal pain, diarrhea, brown or bloody vomitus; pallor or cyanosis
e. Severe, watery diarrhea; garlicky or metallic breath; encephalopathy, hypovolemia and hypotension

497. Assume that lab tests are positive for chronic lead exposure in a child. Lead levels are significantly elevated, but symptoms fortunately are mild and not at all imminently life-threatening. Which of the following is the most appropriate chelator for reducing his body load of excessive and potentially toxic lead?

a. Ca-Na$_2$-EDTA
b. Deferoxamine
c. Dimercaprol
d. N-acetylcysteine
e. Penicillamine
f. Succimer

498. A patient presents with food poisoning that is attributed to botulism (botulinus toxin poisoning). Which of the following is a correct characteristic, finding, or mechanism associated with this toxin?

a. Complete failure of all cholinergic neurotransmission
b. Favorable response to administration of pralidoxime
c. Impairment of parasympathetic, but not sympathetic, nervous system activation
d. Massive overstimulation of all structures having muscarinic cholinergic receptors
e. Selective paralysis of skeletal muscle

499. Physostigmine is the antidote for poisoning with antimuscarinic drugs (e.g., atropine). Another AChE inhibitor, neostigmine, is not suitable. That is because neostigmine cannot overcome the adverse effects of the antimuscarinic drug in or on which of the following?

a. Central nervous system (e.g., the brain)
b. Exocrine glands
c. Heart
d. Skeletal muscle
e. Smooth muscle

500. A terrorist drops a vial of "nerve gas" into a crowded subway at rush hour. The patients are brought to the nearest emergency centers and are given atropine. Which of the following effects of the nerve gas will not be beneficially affected by the antidote?

a. Bradycardia
b. Bronchospasm
c. Excessive lacrimal, mucus, sweat, and salivary secretions
d. GI hypermotility, fluid and electrolyte loss from profuse diarrhea
e. Skeletal muscle hyperfunction or paralysis

501. A patient develops status epilepticus from an unknown poisoning. Which of the following is the most appropriate *first* IV drug to give?

a. Carbamazepine
b. Lorazepam
c. Phenobarbital
d. Phenytoin
e. Valproic acid

Toxicology

Answers

481. The answer is f. (*Craig, p 66; Hardman, pp 1892–1893; Katzung, p 992.*) Cyanide reacts with Fe(III) in mitochondrial cytochrome oxidase, inhibiting oxidative phosphorylation. The shift in metabolism from aerobic to glycolytic soon leads to not only ATP depletion, but also severe lactic acidosis.

Cyanide normally reacts with endogenous sulfur-containing compounds, mainly thiosulfate, and under catalysis by rhodanese forms relatively less toxic thiocyanate that is formed and excreted in the urine. In cyanide poisoning, endogenous sulfur-containing substrate stores are quickly depleted. We manage this, then, by IV infusion of an aqueous sodium thiosulfate solution. (This is the same approach we use for "therapeutic cyanide poisoning," as can arise when nitroprusside doses are too great.)

Ammonium chloride would be ineffective and may actually make matters worse by exacerbating metabolic acidosis. Deferoxamine, an iron chelator, would be of no benefit in terms of signs, symptoms, or their causes or consequences. Dimercaprol is a heavy metal (mainly lead) chelator that would be of no benefit. Mannitol, an osmotic diuretic that is sometimes used to hasten the renal excretion of some toxins (via "forced diuresis"), would not alleviate or shorten signs and symptoms. Pralidoxime is a cholinesterase reactivator that is effective only for poisoning with organophosphate insecticides, nerve gases (sarin, soman), or other drugs that cause profound and largely permanent inactivation of acetylcholinesterase.

482. The answer is e. (*Craig, pp 66, 314; Hardman, pp 434, 704–705; Katzung, pp 988–989.*) We give N-acetylcysteine for acetaminophen poisoning and use it because it is a sulfhydryl-rich drug that, if given soon enough and properly enough, can prevent hepatic necrosis. At safe blood levels, the major pathways of acetaminophen elimination involve glucuronidation and sulfation. When these pathways are overwhelmed, as occurs with acetaminophen poisoning, a cytochrome P450–dependent pathway attempts to handle the metabolic load. So long as ample hepatocyte stores of glutathione (a –SH compound) are available, cytotoxicity will not occur. However, severe poisoning depletes –SH stores, and so a hepatotoxic metabolite (probably an hydroxylated product or N-acetyl-benzoiminoquinone) attacks key cellular macromolecules. That leads to hepatic necrosis.

N-acetylcysteine basically sacrifices itself to react with the toxic metabolite, thereby sparing –SH groups on key hepatocyte macro-molecules.

Alkalinization of the urine is of no benefit with acetaminophen poisoning, as it is with severe salicylate poisoning (because raising urine pH reduces tubular reabsorption of salicylate and increases its excretion). Superoxide anion radical, or hydrogen peroxide, are not directly involved in the cytotoxicity.

483. The answer is c. (*Hardman, pp 1867–1868; Katzung, pp 532, 977–981, 994.*) Disodium EDTA, a calcium chelator that is used to treat severe, acute hypercalcemia, causes hypocalcemic tetany on rapid IV administration. This effect of Na_2EDTA is not observed on slow infusion (15 mg/min) because extracirculatory calcium stores are available to prevent a significant reduction in plasma calcium levels. When $CaNa_2EDTA$ is given IV (it is sometimes used to diagnose or treat lead poisoning), hypocalcemia does not develop, even when large doses are required.

The other drugs listed do not cause hypocalcemia. Dimercaprol [British anti-Lewisite (BAL)], another chelator, is used to treat arsenic and Hg poisoning, as well as in certain cases of Pb poisoning in children. Penicillamine, mainly used as a copper chelator, is the drug of choice in treating Wilson's disease (chronic copper poisoning). It is also used sometimes to chelate mercury and lead. N-acetyl-L-cysteine is an antidote used in the treatment of overdosage with acetaminophen to prevent hepatotoxicity.

484. The answer is b. (*Craig, p 42; Hardman, pp 702–703; Katzung, pp 579, 581–582, 988, 991.*) Alkalinizing the urine with sodium bicarbonate interferes with the renal tubular reabsorption of organic acids (such as aspirin and phenobarbital) by increasing the ionized form of the drug in the urine (per the Henderson-Hasselbach equation). This increases their net excretion. Note that another consequence of severe aspirin (salicylate) toxicity is a combined metabolic plus respiratory acidosis. So in addition to enhancing urinary excretion of salicylate, the administration of sodium bicarbonate also tends to counteract the fall of blood pH.

Excretion of organic bases (such as amphetamine, cocaine, phencyclidine, and morphine) would be reduced by alkalinizing the urine (or, conversely, enhanced by acidifying the urine).

485. The answer is a. (*Craig, pp 312–313; Hardman, p 77; Katzung, pp 987, 991.*) Activated charcoal, a fine, black powder with a high adsorptive capacity, is considered to be a valuable agent in the treatment of many kinds of drug poisoning—but primarily if administered early on and followed by gastric lavage. Drugs that are well adsorbed by activated charcoal include primaquine, propoxyphene, dextroamphetamine, chlorpheniramine, phenobarbital, carbamazepine, digoxin, and aspirin. Mineral acids, alkalies, tolbutamide, and other drugs that are insoluble in acidic aqueous solution are not well adsorbed. Charcoal also does not bind Ca, lithium (Li), or Fe.

The other antidotes listed in the question are metal chelators and play no role in managing aspirin (salicylate) poisoning, nor poisoning with any substances other than the metals they chelate.

486. The answer is b. (*Craig, pp 64, 66; Hardman, pp 78, 438, 1886; Katzung, pp 375–377, 989, 993.*) Methanol is metabolized by the same enzymes used to metabolize ethanol, but the products are different: formaldehyde and formic acid. Headache, vertigo, vomiting, abdominal pain, dyspnea, and blurred vision can occur. However, the most dangerous (or at least permanently disabling) consequence in severe cases is hyperemia of the optic disc that can lead to blindness. The rationale for administering ethanol to treat methanol poisoning is fairly simple. Ethanol has a high affinity for alcohol and aldehyde dehydrogenases and competes as a substrate for those enzymes, reducing metabolism of methanol to its more toxic intermediates. Important adjunctive treatments include hemodialysis to enhance removal of methanol and its products and administration of systemic alkalinizing salts (e.g., sodium bicarbonate) to counteract metabolic acidosis. Administration of systemic acidifying substances such as ascorbic acid would aggravate the condition.

487. The answer is a. (*Craig, pp 64, 66t, 68; Hardman, pp 1862–1865; Katzung, pp 974–975, 977–979.*) Arsenic is a constituent of fungicides, herbicides, and pesticides. Symptoms of acute toxicity include tightness in the throat, difficulty in swallowing, and stomach pains. Projectile vomiting and severe diarrhea can lead to hypovolemic shock, significant electrolyte derangements, and death. Chronic poisoning may cause peripheral neuritis, anemia, skin keratosis, and capillary dilation leading to hypotension. Dimercaprol [British anti-Lewisite (BAL)] is the main antidote used for arsenic poisoning.

488. The answer is a. (*Craig, pp 66–67; Hardman, pp 1878–1882; Katzung, pp 959–961, 992.*) Carbon monoxide has an affinity for hemoglobin that is about 250 times greater than that of O_2. It therefore binds to hemoglobin (forming carboxyhemoglobin) and reduces the O_2-carrying capacity of blood. The symptoms of poisoning are due to tissue hypoxia; they progress from headache and fatigue to confusion, syncope, tachycardia, coma, convulsions, shock, respiratory depression, and cardiovascular collapse. Carboxyhemoglobin levels below 15% rarely produce symptoms; above 40%, symptoms become severe. Treatment includes establishment of an airway, supportive therapy, and administration of 100% (or hyperbaric) O_2. Sulfur dioxide, ozone, and nitrogen dioxide are mucous membrane and respiratory irritants. Methane is a simple asphyxiant.

489. The answer is c. (*Craig, p 66; Hardman, p 1887; Katzung, p 993.*) These are among the classic findings with ethylene glycol (antifreeze) ingestion. It is initially oxidized by alcohol dehydrogenase and then further metabolized to oxalic acid and other products. Oxalate crystals can be found in various tissues of the body, but they are eliminated in the urine, where they can be detected relatively easily. Renal failure can occur because of tubular blockade by the crystals. There will be a significant anion gap indicative of the metabolic acidosis and the presence of unmeasured anions accompanying it [anion gap = $(Na^+ + K^+) - (HCO_3^- + Cl^-)$; we would also see this with methanol poisoning].

490. The answer is c. (*Hardman, pp 438, 1887; Katzung, p 993.*) We give ethanol to inhibit the first step in the metabolism of ethylene glycol and, thereby, prevent further formation of oxalate and other products. Muscarinic receptor activation and purine degradation play no role in this poisoning, so atropine or allopurinol are irrational. Lorazepam would be indicated if seizures develop, but giving it (or any other CNS depressant) early on is premature and more likely to aggravate CNS depression than to help. Syrup of ipecac, an emetic, would increase the risk of ethylene glycol aspiration, increase absorption, and do more harm than good. Gastric lavage would be indicated, however.

491. The answer is b. (*Hardman, p 409; Katzung, pp 358, 361–362, 413, 989, 993.*) Arguably the most important tip-off in this presentation is the antegrade amnesia, which (among other things) is rather unique to a benzodiazepine. The most likely benzodiazepine used was rohypnol (flunitrazepam, better known as "roofies" on the street and by those who use it as a date-rape drug). Unless this patient were a very atypical responder, it is unlikely that any of the other CNS depressants—a barbiturate, an opioid, chloral hydrate—would cause the same responses. She's had one drink yet still feels pain from her head gash. She apparently hasn't had enough alcohol to be so obtunded that she doesn't feel pain, and a barbiturate is likely to enhance the sensation of pain.

Chloral hydrate is still used medically, mainly as a sedative for children. However, it is not as readily available as the illicit benzodiazepines; it does not cause antegrade amnesia (important to the perpetrator, because he or she anticipates no recall of what happened by the victim), but it is not readily available, and it simply doesn't have the "reputation" as a preferred date-rape drug among those who use such drugs.

492. The answer is c. (*Craig, pp 296, 357t; Hardman, pp 412, 629; Katzung, pp 359–360, 989, 993.*) On the basis of the clinical presentation, hopefully you have narrowed down your suspected cause to either an opioid or a benzodiazepine and pieced together enough information that you believe the culprit is the benzodiazepine. You administer flumazenil, and a prompt restoration of normal ventilation would confirm the diagnosis. That assumes, of course, that the cause of the syndrome was solely or largely due to a benzodiazepine. If other CNS depressants had been consumed in sufficient quantities, the benzodiazepine antagonist may cause little, if any, improvement.

Ordinarily, ventilatory stimulants (analeptics, such as caffeine) or generalized or specific depressants (barbiturates, opioids) should not be used to manage ventilatory symptoms.

Administering activated charcoal, and performing gastric lavage, would be appropriate. However, it would do nothing to point to a diagnosis, nor quickly reverse or antagonize the progression of signs and symptoms.

493-b *(Craig, pp 361, 455, 457; Hardman, pp 421–422, 653, 655; Katzung, pp 1065, 1067, 1072);* **494-a** *(Craig, pp 138t–139; Hardman, pp 167, 653; Katzung, pp 111–115, 264–267, 990);* **495-c** *(Craig, pp 126–128, 130; Hardman, p 189; Katzung, pp 105–106, 118, 267, 989–990.)* These three questions may seem unfair, because arriving at the correct answer for the second and third depends heavily on knowing the answer to the first one; and that requires some knowledge of what drugs are found in common OTC medications. Nonetheless, that is clinical reality.

Most OTC sleep aids contain a first-generation antihistamine (sedating agent, almost always an ethanolamine, either diphenhydramine or the very similar drug, doxylamine). The preponderant signs and symptoms of toxicity arise not from any histamine receptor-blocking activity, but from intense antimuscarinic (atropine-like) effects, plus dose-dependent CNS depression that ultimately (and early on, in children) can lead to seizures. The signs and symptoms described in answer a for Question 494, therefore, include many that you will see in "atropine poisoning." Aside from symptomatic and supportive care, including the use of traditional drugs for status epilepticus, physostigmine (the nonquaternary, centrally and peripherally acting acetylcholinesterase inhibitor) may be life-saving. It will certainly help reverse many of the central and peripheral signs and symptoms of the overdose.

As far as the other possible choices for the causative agent go: You won't find atropine in OTC products, although the related agents, belladonna alkaloids, are found in a few marketed for respiratory tract or GI symptoms, but not as sleep aids; fexofenadine, a second-generation (nonsedating) antihistamine is available in OTC allergy remedies (as are several related drugs); loperamide, an opioid derivative, is found in OTC medications for short-term relief of diarrhea; and pseudoephedrine, a mixed-acting sympathomimetic (adrenergic agonist) is an active ingredient in many OTC oral nasal decongestant products. Signs and symptoms of overdose with those drugs (aside from the belladonna alkaloids) are very different from those of diphenhydramine, and management of overdoses is very different too.

496. The answer is a. *(Craig, p 68; Hardman, pp 1853–1855; Katzung, pp 971–974.)* The presentation of chronic lead exposure, as from being exposed to (or even eating) older lead-based paints, differs from the typical presentation of acute organic lead poisoning (answer c), which usually arises from sniffing leaded gasoline (and just about all gasolines nowadays are organic lead-enriched). Answer b, with the predominant gingival/head/neck signs and symptoms, is typical of chronic or acute mercury intoxication. Answer d, with the hyperventilation, GI disturbances (including discolored vomitus) and pallor, is what you are likely to encounter in acute iron poisoning (as from a consuming ferrous sulfate supplements in large doses). A characteristic breath (garlicky or metallic), profuse diarrhea, encephalopathy, and hypotension (answer e) are typical of acute inorganic arsenic poisoning (see Question 487). Knowing more about the patient's history and environment will help immensely in sorting out what the "most likely" cause of intoxication is.

497. The answer is f. (*Craig, p 66; Hardman, pp 1856–1857; Katzung, pp 972–974, 979.*) Succimer (a more polar salt of dimercaprol) would be the choice, given the proof of lead poisoning and the lack of acute symptoms and the fact that our patient is a child. Succimer is easy to give orally and is tolerated far better than the alternatives: Ca-Na$_2$-EDTA, penicillamine (traditionally viewed as a copper chelator, but it also chelates lead), or dimercaprol itself. Although the heavy metal chelation profiles for succimer are not drastically different from those of dimercaprol, the fact that succimer is more polar (and, therefore, less likely to enter cells) seems to account for far fewer and milder side effects than those of dimercaprol (especially with respect to risks of tachycardia and hypertension).

498. The answer is a. (*Craig, pp 66–67, 94, 340–341; Hardman, pp 127, 143; Katzung, pp 90, 444, 1107.*) Botulinus (botulinum) toxin prevents release of acetylcholine (from storage vesicles) by virtually all cholinergic nerves. Thus, there is no activation of any cholinergic receptors, whether nicotinic or muscarinic. Noteworthy findings, then, include an inability to activate all postganglionic neurons (sympathetic and parasympathetic), no physiologic release of epinephrine from the adrenal medulla, and flaccid skeletal muscle paralysis due to failure of ACh release from motor nerves. The cause of death is ventilatory failure because the intercostal muscles and diaphragm are nonfunctional.

Pralidoxime is a cholinesterase reactivator, an antidote for poisonings with "irreversible" cholinesterase inhibitors such as soman, sarin ("nerve gases"), and many organophosphorus insecticides. Because no ACh is being released in botulinus poisoning, "reactivation" of the enzyme that normally metabolizes the neurotransmitter is irrelevant (and ineffective).

499. The answer is a. (*Craig, pp 126–130; Hardman, pp 179, 183–184, 186; Katzung, pp 101–102, 105–106, 989–990.*) Physostigmine is basically the only clinically useful AChE inhibitor that gets into the brain, a major target of atropine/antimuscarinic poisoning. That is because it lacks the quaternary (charged at virtually all pH values likely to be found in a living person) structure that nearly all the other common alternatives possess, and lacking that structure it can cross the blood-brain barrier.

Alternatives such as neostigmine, pyridostigmine, and others, will combat peripheral effects of atropine poisoning, just as physostigmine will. Unfortunately, some of the CNS manifestations (e.g., severe fever, leading to seizures) contribute greatly to the morbidity and mortality associated with high doses of antimuscarinics, and the quaternary agents simply will not combat them in the CNS.

By the way, basically the only clinical use for physostigmine is for managing atropine/antimuscarinic poisoning. You won't encounter too many patients overdosed on atropine itself, but you'll see many poisoned with older antihistamines (e.g., diphenhydramine), older (tricyclic or tetracyclic) antidepressants (e.g., imipramine), some of the centrally acting antimuscarinics that are used for parkinsonism (e.g., benztropine and trihexyphenidyl), scopolamine (used for motion sickness), and most of the phenothiazine antipsychotics (e.g., chlorpromazine). Owing to the often strong antimuscarinic side effects of these drugs, treating overdoses of most of them probably will involve managing what amounts to "atropine poisoning"—and many other problems too.

500. The answer is e. (*Craig, pp 68–69, 126–130; Hardman, pp 180, 184–185; Katzung, pp 101–107, 989, 992.*) Most of the adverse responses to nerve gases (irreversible ACh esterase inhibitors such as soman and sarin) are due to a build-up of ACh at muscarinic receptors (i.e., ACh released from postganglionic parasympathetic nerves or sympathetic/cholinergic nerves innervating sweat glands). Those responses will be attenuated by atropine, because it is a highly specific competitive muscarinic antagonist. However, skeletal muscle stimulation (or eventual paralysis) involves nicotinic receptor activation. That will not be affected by atropine, and unless other supportive measures are provided, the patient is likely to die from ventilatory arrest/apnea.

501. The answer is b. (*Craig, pp 380–381, 383; Hardman, pp 452–455; Katzung, pp 394, 397–398, 985.*) Intravenously administered lorazepam is the drug of choice for treatment of status epilepticus, especially when the cause of this life-threatening seizure (and a specific antidote) are unknown. Lorazepam, like the benzodiazepines in general, increases the apparent affinity of the inhibitory neurotransmitter GABA for binding sites on brain cell membranes. The effects of lorazepam (or diazepam) are short-lasting. Immediately after giving the benzodiazepine either phenytoin or fosphenytoin should be given to provide longer seizure suppression and "coverage" because the effects of lorazepam wear off in a comparatively short time. Other drugs that can be used for status epilepticus include phenobarbital (not a drug of choice) and (paradoxically) lidocaine for refractory seizures (mainly a drug of last resort). None of the other drugs listed in the question are appropriate for status epilepticus, despite their widespread use for oral therapy of seizure disorders long term.

Bibliography

Craig CR, Stitzel RE (eds): *Modern Pharmacology with Clinical Applications,* 6th ed. Philadelphia, PA, Lippincott Williams & Wilkins, 2004.

Hardman JG, Limbird LE: *Goodman & Gilman's the Pharmacological Basis of Therapeutics,* 10th ed. New York, McGraw-Hill, 2001.

Katzung BG: *Basic and Clinical Pharmacology,* 9th ed. New York, McGraw-Hill, 2004.

Index